D1756484

Lymphoproliferative Diseases

IMMUNOLOGY AND MEDICINE SERIES

Immunology of Endocrine Diseases
Editor: A. M. McGregor

Clinical Transplantation: Current Practice and Future Prospects
Editor: G. R. D. Catto

Complement in Health and Disease
Editor: K. Whaley

Immunological Aspects of Oral Diseases
Editor: L. Ivanyi

Immunoglobulins in Health and Disease
Editor: M. A. H. French

Immunology of Malignant Diseases
Editors: V. S. Byers and R. W. Baldwin

Lymphoproliferative Diseases
Editors: D. B. Jones and D. H. Wright

Phagocytes and Disease
Editors: M. S. Klempner, B. Styrt and J. Ho

HLA and Disease
Authors: B. Bradley, P. T. Klouda, J. Bidwell and G. Laundy

Immunology of Sexually Transmitted Diseases
Editor: D. J. M. Wright

Lymphocytes in Health and Disease
Editors: G. Janossy and P. L. Amlot

Mast Cells, Mediators and Disease
Editor: S. T. Holgate

Immunodeficiency and Disease
Editor: A. D. B. Webster

Immunology of Pregnancy and its Disorders
Editor: C. M. M. Stern

Immunotherapy of Disease
Editor: T. J. Hamblin

Immunology of Prophylactic Immunization
Editor: A. J. Zuckerman

Immunology of Eye Diseases
Editor: S. Lightman

Immunology of Renal Diseases
Editor: C. D. Pusey

Biochemistry of Inflammation
Editors: J. T. Whicher and S. W. Evans

Immunology of ENT Disorders
Editor: G. Scadding

Immunology of Infection
Editors: J. G. P. Sissons, J. Cohen and L. K. Borysiewicz

IMMUNOLOGY
SERIES · SERIES · SERIES · SERIES AND SERIES · SERIES · SERIES · SERIES
MEDICINE

Volume 15

Lymphoproliferative Diseases

Edited by
D. B. Jones and D. H. Wright

University Department of Pathology
Southampton General Hospital

Series Editor: K. Whaley

KLUWER ACADEMIC PUBLISHERS

DORDRECHT/BOSTON/LONDON

1990

Distributors

---

for the United States and Canada: Kluwer Academic Publishers, PO Box 358, Accord Station, Hingham, MA 02018-0358, USA
for all other countries: Kluwer Academic Publishers Group, Distribution Center, PO Box 322, 3300 AH Dordrecht, The Netherlands

British Library Cataloguing in Publication Data

Lymphoproliferative diseases.
1. Man. Reticuloendothelial system. Malignant tumours.
Immunological aspects
I. Jones, D. B.   II. Wright, Dennis H. (Dennis Howard),
1931–   III. Series
616.99′442079

ISBN 0-85200-965-8

© 1990 by Kluwer Academic Publishers

Published in the United Kingdom by Kluwer Academic Publishers, PO Box 55, Lancaster, UK.

Kluwer Academic Publishers BV incorporates the publishing programmes of D. Reidel, Martinus Nijhoff, Dr W. Junk and MTP Press.

Typeset by Witwell Ltd, Southport.
Printed in the UK by Butler & Tanner Limited, Frome and London.

Contents

Series Editor's Note

The interface between Clinical Immunology and other branches of medical practice is frequently blurred and the general physician is frequently faced with clinical problems with an immunological basis and is often expected to diagnose and manage such patients. The rapid expansion of basic and clinical immunology over the past two decades has resulted in the appearance of increasing numbers of immunology journals and it is impossible for a non-specialist to keep apace with this information overload. The Immunology and Medicine series is designed to present individual topics of immunology in a condensed package of information which can be readily assimilated by the busy clinician or pathologist.

K. Whaley, Glasgow
March, 1990

List of Contributors

P. L. AMLOT
Department of Immunology
Royal Free Hospital, School of Medicine
Pond Street
London NW3 2QG
UK

K. J. M. BRITTEN
University Department of Pathology
Level E, S Block
Southampton General Hospital
Tremona Road
Southampton
Hants SO9 4XY
UK

J. C. CAWLEY
University Department of Haematology
Duncan Building
Royal Liverpool Hospital
Prescot Street
P.O. Box 147
Liverpool L69 3BX
UK

J. M. DAVIES
University Department of Haematology
Duncan Building
Royal Liverpool Hospital
Prescot Street
P.O. Box 147
Liverpool L69 3BX
UK

W. N. ERBER
Haematology Department
Royal North Shore Hospital
St Leonards
Sydney
New South Wales 2065
Australia

A. K. GHOSH
Immunology Department
Paterson Institute for Cancer Research
Christie Hospital and Holt Radium Institute
Wilmslow Road
Manchester M20 9BX
UK

J. GORDON
Department of Immunology
University of Birmingham Medical School
Vincents Drive
Birmingham B15 2TJ
UK

SU-MING HSU
Department of Pathology
P.O. Box 20708
University of Texas
Houston
Texas 77225
USA

P. G. ISAACSON
Department of Histopathology
University College and Middlesex School
of Medicine
University Street
London WC1E 6JJ
UK

D. B. JONES
University Pathology
Level E, South Block
Southampton General Hospital
Tremona Road
Southampton
Hant SO9 4XY
UK

B. L. MEPHAN
University Pathology
Level E, South Block
Southampton General Hospital
Tremona Road
Southampton
Hants SO9 4XY
UK

A. D. RAMSAY
Department of Histopathology
Southampton General Hospital
Tremona Road
Southampton
Hants SO9 4XY
UK

P. RICHARDSON
Department of Immunology
University of Birmingham Medical School
Vincents Drive
Edgbaston
Birmingham B15 2TJ
UK

J. L. SMITH
Regional Immunology Service
Tenovus Research Laboratory
Southampton General Hospital
Tremona Road
Southampton
Hants SO9 4XY
UK

W. J. SMITH
Department of Histopathology
University College and Middlesex School
of Medicine
University Street
London WC1E 6JJ
UK

J. SPENCER
Department of Histopathology
University College and Middlesex School
of Medicine
University Street
London WC1E 6JJ
UK

F. K. STEVENSON
Regional Immunology Service
Tenovus Research Laboratory
Southampton General Hospital
Tremona Road
Southampton
Hant SO9 4XY
UK

D. H. WRIGHT
University Department of Pathology
Southampton General Hospital
Tremona Road
Southampton
Hants SO9 4XY
UK

1
Introduction

Recent developments in the field of cellular pathology and molecular biology have had a major impact on our ability to diagnose lymphoreticular disease and on our understanding of many of the disease processes which contribute to lymphoreticular pathology. Twenty years ago, the immunological analysis of lymphoid proliferations was in its infancy. The techniques available, such as sheep red blood cell rosetting and immune adherence to frozen sections, now appear unbelievably crude when compared with our ability to accurately phenotype lymphocytes in suspension, in frozen section and, more recently, in formalin-fixed, paraffin-embedded tissue biopsies. Four international workshops have also standardized the nomenclature for the wide range of lineage-restricted and lineage-related monoclonal antibodies available, and have provided a basis for the sophisticated phenotypic analysis of lymphoid neoplasms in even the smallest routine laboratories. Our concepts relating to the pathogenesis of a number of human lymphomas have also changed substantially, and this has been aided by the development of systems for the classification of human lymphoma which are firmly based in our knowledge of the differentiation and biological behaviour of normal lymphoreticular cells.

In this monograph, we present contributions from many authors examining both leukaemia and lymphoma from an immunological perspective. It is our hope that some of these contributions will be of practical value in the laboratory investigation and diagnosis of lymphoreticular disease. Other contributions record our conceptual understanding of the histogenesis and pathogenesis of human lymphoma.

The categorization of B-cell neoplasia can be related, to some extent, to the differentiation stages of normal B-lymphocytes using synthesis of immunoglobulin as a marker. Even here, however, our understanding is not yet complete. Currently published studies of the molecules which regulate lymphocyte traffic and residence in different sites through the body show that there is a rational basis for the recognition of sub-groups of B-cell lymphoma (e.g. lymphomas of mucosa-associated lymphoid tissue) on the basis of their anatomical distribution, rather than on their morphology or phenotype alone. Our understanding of the normal maturation pathway of human T-cells has lagged behind that of the B-cell population. Presumably, this is due to the lack of a recognized and well-understood secreted product, such as immunoglobulin in the T-cell series. Our recently acquired ability to undertake a detailed phenotypic sub-division of the major T-cell lymphocyte sub-classes and the contribution of molecular biology in determining the sequential steps by which genes for T-cell receptor molecules are used by the maturing T-cell has gone some way to resolving the confusion which exists. Complications exist, however, in the direct comparison of T-cell neoplasms with their normal physiological counterparts. It is now well established that many phenotypic markers, present on maturing normal T-cells may be lost in T-cell lymphoma and this is particularly common in T-cell lymphoma of the peripheral T-cell type. It is also clear, from the failure of many groups to identify clonal T-cell receptor gene rearrangements in lymphoreticular lesions, which have the morphological, phenotypic and clinical characteristics of T-cell lymphoma, that a direct comparison between tumour cell and normal cell at the level of molecular biology may prove difficult. The way forward with this group of neoplasms would be to carefully analyse and document cases using all available immunological, molecular biological and karyotypic techniques and to correlate these findings with clinical features, response to treatment, progress and prognosis.

In many lymphomas the tumour cell population often represents a minority of the cells present in the biopsy. This is a feature which contributes to diagnostic confusion. Indeed, the use of such terms as, B-cell-rich, T-cell-lymphoma have evolved in response to the heterogeneity in cell types seen in certain specific cases. It would seem logical to assume that the non-neoplastic population has been attracted into the tumour by cytokines produced either by the tumour cells, themselves, or by other reactive cells. Little work has been undertaken in this area. Recent advances in the area of the basic biology of cytokines suggest that this will be an expanding area of investigation. In particular, our ability to investigate the synthesis and effects of biologically active molecules with specific gene probes and recombinant cytokines have moved this field of immunology beyond the use of biological assay systems, which often show great variability and where the data is often open to misinterpretation.

The lymphoma that most clearly demonstrates a marked disproportion between presumptive neoplastic cells and the reactive population is Hodgkin's disease. Efforts to identify the histogenesis of the Reed–Sternberg cells of Hodgkin's disease using the full battery of immunological and molecular biological techniques available to us have, so far, produced conflicting and inconclusive findings and have led many workers in this field to doubt the existence of Hodgkin's lymphoma as a single entity. In this volume we discuss the possibility that the cells recognized morphologically as Reed–Sternberg cells may, in fact, originate in more than one lineage. This may account for the problem, not infrequently encountered, of differentiating Hodgkin's disease from non-Hodgkin's lymphoma and suggests that pathologists may have to reconsider the established relationship between Hodgkin's disease and non-Hodgkin's lymphoma.

In conclusion, we hope that the immunopathological data presented in this volume will be of assistance, both at the level of diagnosis and also in provoking fresh discussion and investigation into the origin and pathogenesis of lymphoreticular disease.

2
Diagnosis of Leukaemia

J. M. DAVIES and J. C. CAWLEY

INTRODUCTION

Most malignancies of the blood and bone marrow are readily diagnosed and classified by traditional cytological and cytochemical methods. However, a number of additional techniques including ultrastructural, karyotypic and immunological marker analysis have been employed. All these additional methodologies, of which immunological analysis has been the most popular, have usually been performed for confirmatory rather than primary diagnostic reasons. However, genuine problems do occur sufficiently often for most haematological laboratories to have some interest in immunological marker techniques.

Major diagnostic difficulties arise in the form of the following questions:— Do the primitive cells represent an acute leukaemia, a lymphoma, some less acute haemic proliferation or, indeed, a non-haematological malignancy?— Is this acute leukaemia myeloid (AML) or lymphoid (ALL) and what is its subtype?— Is this chronic lymphocytosis a malignant proliferation and, if so, is it CLL or some other form of chronic lymphoproliferation?

Each of these diagnostic questions will be addressed from a morphological and immunological point of view, and the chapter will then conclude with a brief consideration of ultrastructural and cytogenetic studies.

ACUTE LEUKAEMIA VERSUS LESS ACUTE HAEMIC PROLIFERATION

Since myelodysplastic states (MDS) are common, one not infrequently encounters the question: Is this acute leukaemia or MDS? The FAB committee recommends that 30% of bone marrow cells must be 'blasts' to make a diagnosis of acute leukaemia[1]. Obviously this is an arbitary criterion, but it is nevertheless a useful one when it comes to instituting therapy. Immunological markers have little to contribute since the recognition of blasts is an essentially morphological one. Having said this, the recently introduced B1-3C5 monoclonal antibody (Mab) gives some guide to the number of primitive cells present[2].

ACUTE LEUKAEMIA VERSUS LYMPHOMA

The following question occasionally arises: Is this acute leukaemia or primitive non-Hodgkin's lymphoma (NHL) involving the blood or bone marrow? Morphology again often helps since primitive NHL cells lack myeloid features and have more abundant cytoplasm than ALL cells. Also, focal involvement of the marrow is suggestive of lymphoma. However, genuine difficulty sometimes remains and demonstration of surface immunoglulin then supports a diagnosis of NHL.

The presence of the CALL (CD10) antigen, while occasionally present in NHL, is suggestive of ALL. Conversely, the presence of CD21-CD23[3] B-cell antigens suggests NHL. The other well characterized B-cell antigens (CD19, 20, 22 and 24) are of no help since they are expressed by both ALL and NHL cells.

ACUTE LEUKAEMIA VERSUS NON-HAEMATOLOGICAL MALIGNANCY

Occasionally, one encounters a pancytopenic patient with a bone marrow which is heavily infiltrated by primitive cells whose origin is not clear, either because the patient is known to have a visceral cancer or because the cells seem morphologically atypical or are peculiarly clumped. In this context, demonstration of the leukocyte common antigen (LCA) is very helpful since its presence indicates that the infiltrating cells are of haemic origin. A variety of Mab to LCA are now available and some are reactive with paraffin-embedded material[4]. The latter antibodies are most useful for distinguishing between lymphomatous and carcinomatous lymph-node infiltrates.

Unfortunately, erythroid cells lack LCA and one cannot, therefore, definitively conclude that a proliferation is non-haematological because LCA is not expressed.

ACUTE MYELOID (AML) VERSUS ACUTE LYMPHATIC LEUKAEMIA (ALL)

Although the increasing use of anthracyclines in the treatment of ALL has reduced the therapeutic significance of this question, treatment strategies in the two diseases do still differ, so the question continues to be both therapeutically and biologically important. Furthermore, acute lymphoid, as opposed to myeloid, transformation of chronic granulocytic leukaemia (CGL) shows more response to chemotherapy.

Well established morphological and cytochemical criteria clearly distinguish AML and ALL in the great majority of instances, and fewer than 10% of cases remain unclassified after such conventional analysis[5].

6

The presence of the CALL antigen (CD10) and other lymphoid antigens (CD1–5, 7 and 8 (T-cell antigens[3]) and 19 and 20 (B-cell antigens)[3]) definitely identify the lymphoid origin of blasts. The presence of terminal deoxynucleotidyl transferase is now of less importance in identifying lymphoid cells since a significant proportion of AML blasts possess demonstrable enzyme activity[6].

The absence of lymphoid antigens is suggestive of AML, and this conclusion can be confirmed in up to 80% of cases by the demonstration of reactions with antimyeloid Mab such as My7 or 9[7]. In other instances, the non-lymphoid nature of the blasts can be demonstrated by the detection of glycophorin on primitive erythroid cells[8] and of platelet membrane glyco-proteins on megakaryoblasts[9]. In the very few cases where blasts lack lymphoid and myeloid (including erythroid and megakaryocytic) antigens, gene rearrangement studies may be helpful[10]. B- or T-gene rearrangement indicates a lymphoid origin, while the germ-line configuration is suggestive of AML[10].

The proportion of cases of acute leukaemia that remains truly unclassifiable after careful morphological, cytochemical and extensive immunological analysis is not yet clear, but is certainly small[10]. It is perhaps worth noting at this point that many cases of morphologically and cytochemically undifferentiated acute leukaemia are readily identified as ALL by immunological marker analysis[11].

Much work has been done concerning Ig, and T-cell-receptor gene rearrangement in the leukaemias; but the true diagnostic value of such techniques is probably confined to analysis of the clonality of chronic T-lymphocytosis (see later) and of the nature of certain lymphomas[12].

Subtypes of ALL

Mab allow nearly all cases of ALL to be identified as of thymic or B-cell origin. In this regard, CD7 Mab (e.g. WTI and 3AI) are the best indicators of T-lineage, while CD19 (e.g. leu 12 and B4) reagents are the most reliable B-lineage markers[9]. Although the recognition of thymic and B-precursor forms of ALL is of biological relevance in, for example, predicting the presence of a thymic mass, the therapeutic and prognostic importance of this sub-division of ALL is far from clear. Thy-ALL is frequently associated with a high peripheral blast count and such disease has an unfavourable prognosis. However, especially in adults, the presence of thymic antigens is of little independent prognostic or therapeutic significance (reviewed, for example, by Bloomfield[13]).

Among acute T-cell proliferations, the degree of maturation may have some bearing on the clinical behaviour of the tumour, in that proliferations possessing more mature T-cell antigens tend to behave in a lymphomatous fashion, having less tendency to become leukaemic[14]. However, the therapeutic importance of this observation is again minor since both highly and less immature proliferations are generally treated as high-risk ALL; furthermore, the correlation between phenotype and tissue distribution has recently been questioned[15].

Mab studies have now unequivocally shown that common ALL (CD10[+]) is

7

an early B-cell proliferation, a conclusion confirmed by Ig gene rearrangement studies[16]. It was established in the late 1970s that some 25% of cases of CALL show maturation in the form of synthesis of intracytoplasmic IgM, and Mab have confirmed the concept of maturation among morphologically similar cases of ALL[17]. However, as with Thy-ALL, these observations have little prognostic or therapeutic significance.

Subtypes of AML

It has long been recognized that AML can be subdivided according to the major lineage involved and to the degree of differentiation observed[5]. This type of classification is currently much used in the form set out in the FAB classifications[18], but its clinical and therapeutic value is limited. Acute promyelocytic (M3) and the monocytic leukaemias (M4/5) have distinctive clinical features in the form of coagulopathy and an increased tendency to extramedullary tissue involvement, respectively. However, the response to cytotoxic drugs is not sufficiently different in the various subtypes of AML as to alter the nature of chemotherapy employed.

My7 (CD13) and My9 (CD33) Mab react, to varying degrees, with 50–85% of cases of AML[19]; negativity raises the possibility of erythroid and megakaryoblastic proliferation (M6/7). Mab against HLA-DR or primitive antigens such as that detected by B1-3C5 help to distinguish M1 (primitive) AML from M2 (some differentiation) or M3 (promyelocytic) leukaemias, but the recognition of M2/3 really remains a morphological one.

A variety of anti-monocyte Mab may give some indication of the extent of any monocytic component present, but all are imperfect in this regard. For example, MO2 (CD14), perhaps the best such antibody, reacts with approximately 50% of M4/5 leukaemias, but also detects positivity in some 15% of M1/2 AML[19].

As mentioned earlier, anti-glycophorin and anti-platelet glycoproteins I, II and III are useful in identifying M6 and M7 variants, respectively.

Nature of a lymphocytosis

Not infrequently, the problem arises of the patient without marked organomegaly who has a persistent lymphocytosis involving cells of 'mature' appearance (i.e. relatively high nuclear–cytoplasmic ratio and condensed nuclear chromatin). The question then asked is whether or not this is a malignant lymphoid proliferation.

If the lymphoid cells prove to be B-cell in type, the demonstration of light-chain restriction conclusively indicates a clonal, and therefore neoplastic, origin. Heavy-chain isotypes are of no value in this regard since the B-cells may express any combination of M, D, G and A surface immunoglobulin.

When the lymphoid cells prove to be of T-cell origin, immunophenotyping cannot establish clonality, although aberrant antigen expression (e.g. $CD2^-$, $CD3^+$) or homogeneous subset markers (e.g. all CD8 positive) are suggestive of malignancy. The ability to demonstrate clonal rearrangements of the T-cell receptor gene has, therefore, been a significant diagnostic advance and has, for example, established the clonal nature of Tγ proliferations (often associated with neutropenia and macrocytosis)[20].

CHRONIC LYMPHOCYTIC LEUKAEMIA (CLL) VERSUS OTHER CHRONIC B-LYMPHOPROLIFERATIVE DISORDERS

The diagnosis of CLL is no longer completely straightforward[21]. Traditionally, the diagnosis is based on the presence in the blood and bone marrow of a persistent lymphocytosis without obvious precipitating cause. The lymphocytosis involves mainly small lymphocytes with scanty cytoplasm and condensed nuclear chromatin without conspicuous nucleoli, although it is recognized that a certain number of larger cells with more abundant cytoplasm, less condensed nuclear chromatin and nucleoli may be present. However, two difficulties immediately arise. Small lymphocytes with this morphological appearance are not homogeneous and comprise several different stages of lymphocyte development. Furthermore, no precise account is taken of the variability in the number and appearance of the larger cells that may be present.

Definitive diagnosis of CLL is, therefore, probably not possible at present, and the question: Is this CLL or a related disorder? is increasingly going to arise. Morphology can certainly help, and a number of distinct disorders can be identified. CLL can be distinguished from proliferations of centrocytic or lymphoplasmacytoid lymphocytes by the absence of nuclear clefting and of lymphoplasmacytoid differentiation. Furthermore, marrow involvement on trephine biopsy should not be paratrabecular (a feature of lymphoma as opposed to CLL) and larger cells should constitute less than 20% of all lymphocytes in the blood. When larger cells with a less condensed nuclear chromatin pattern and prominent nucleoli comprise more than 20% of all lymphocytes, the diagnosis is prolymphocytic transformation of CLL, prolymphocytic leukaemia or intermediate or high-grade lymphoma with peripheral blood involvement. The distinction between prolymphocytic transformations of CLL and the other possible diagnoses is that the former usually follows a phase of typical CLL and the larger 'prolymphocytes' bear the same surface markers as typical CLL cells.

Having said this, one is not infrequently left uncertain even after careful morphological examination. Unfortunately, immunological markers cannot yet give a definitive answer, although some pointers are now available. Possession of receptors for mouse erythrocytes (Mo) (no Mab is yet available to this receptor) is characteristic of CLL lymphocytes, but the receptor may be found on other cell types such as hairy cells[22] and centroblastic–centrocytic (CB–CC) cells[23]. The lymphocytes of all typical cases of CLL express the CD5 CB–CC (e.g. leu 1) antigen, but this structure is present on many other cell types including not only T-cells, but also the centrocytes of centrocytic cell leukaemia/lymphoma (but not those of CB–CC proliferations)[23]. The CD10 (CALLA) structure is also of some value in that typical CLL lymphocytes and the centrocytes of centrocytic cell leukaemia/lymphoma lack this antigen, while CB–CC (follicular lymphoma) cells are often positive, as are a proportion of centroblastic cells[24].

Lymphoplasmacytoid cells can be difficult to recognize morphologically, but can be readily identified by the presence of moderate to large amounts of intracytoplasmic immunoglobulin.

Hairy-cell leukaemia (HCL) is usually easily diagnosed morphologically, and genuine diagnostic difficulty only arises when hairy cells are very infrequent or when one is attempting to distinguish typical hairy-cell disease from the variants that have now been recognized[25]. These variants have acquired increased interest since at least some do not appear to respond to α-interferon. The diagnosis of HCL can be confirmed with CD25 and specific anti-HC reagents (e.g. anti HC-2[26]); hairy cells unlike most other B-cells, express moderate amounts of IL-2 receptor (CD25)[27].

A substantial number of other Mab, some with CD designations, are now available which result in limited staining among cells of B-lineage (e.g. CD6, 9 and 21–24). It is likely that in the immediate future these and new reagents will be used to classify the chronic lymphoproliferative disorders with increased precision. Meanwhile, typical CLL should have the following phenotype: Mo^+ $CD5^+$ $CD10^-$.

T-CLL

The morphological difficulties relating to the fact that small lymphocytes are not homogeneous in nature means that it is not surprising that some patients with obvious clinical lymphoma have circulating lymphocytes resembling those of typical B-CLL, but which in fact are of T-cell origin. Such cases may be associated with lymphoid infiltration of the skin (these T-cells are of helper $CD4^+$ phenotype), but this is not necessarily so. The presence of CD4 gives no indication of clonality, but such proliferations are often clearly malignant clinically and have been shown to have undergone clonal rearrangements of their T-cell receptor genes[28].

The Tγ ($CD8^+$) proliferations mentioned earlier are usually distinguishable on morphological grounds, since the cells are large, granular lymphocytes rather than the small, round cells of CLL.

ULTRASTRUCTURAL METHODS

Ultrastructural analysis of haematological malignancies has contributed little of genuine diagnostic importance. Possible exceptions include the demonstration of unexpected nuclear convolutions in chronic T-cell malignancy (Sezary Syndrome), the ribosome–lamella complexes typical, but not diagnostic, of HCL, and the platelet peroxidase of primitive megakaryocytic cells.

KARYOTYPING METHODS

The realization that chromosome breaks frequently occur at sites of cellular oncogenes has renewed interest in cytogenetic analysis. However, the strictly diagnostic value of such analysis is again limited.

Demonstration of the Philadelphia chromosomes (Ph) continues to be used in the confirmation of the diagnosis of CGL. Ph-negative CGL is often identifiable morphologically by the presence of marked dysplastic changes, and has a worse prognosis.

The presence of karyotype abnormalities in patients with peripheral cytopenias and modest dysplastic changes in the marrow favours a diagnosis of myelodysplasia. Recently, it has been appreciated that not only acute promyelocytic leukaemia, but also other morphological variants of AML, are associated with specific chromosomes abnormalities[29,30]. However, such abnormalities are once again of no primary diagnostic or therapeutic importance since their recognition has no effect on management.

CONCLUSIONS

(1) The diagnosis and the classification of the leukaemias is still primarily a morphological one, and immunological and other marker techniques are often used in a confirmatory way.

(2) Immunological markers have contributed substantially to the understanding of the biology of the leukaemias, but have had little true prognostic or therapeutic impact.

(3) Immunological markers are occasionally useful diagnostically in the following situations:
  (a) In distinguishing acute leukaemia from non-haematological malignancy;
  (b) In distinguishing AML from ALL;
  (c) In establishing the B-clonal nature of a lymphocytosis;
  (d) In distinguishing CLL from certain CLL-like disorders.

(4) Gene rearrangement studies are occasionally useful in establishing the clonality of certain T-lymphocytes and in typing malignancies with an equivocal immunological phenotype.

References

1. Bennett, J. M., Catovsky, D., Daniel, M. T., Flandrin, G., Galton, D. A. G., Gralnick, H. R. and Sultan, C. (1982). Proposals for the classification of the myelodysplastic syndromes. *Br. J. Haematol.*, **51**, 159–99

2. Tindle, R. W., Nichols, R. A. B., Chan, L., Campara, D., Catovsky, D. and Birnie, G. D. (1985). A novel monoclonal antibody BI-3C5 recognises myeoblasts and non-B non-T lymphoblasts in acute leukaemias and CGL blast crises, and reacts with immature cells in normal bone marrow. *Leuk. Res.*, **9**, 1–9

3. Reinherz, E. L., Haynes, B. F., Nadler, L. M. and Bernstein, I. D. (1986). *Leukocyte Typing II* (New York: Springer-Verlag).

4. Warnke, R. A., Gatter, K. C., Falini, B., Hildreth, P., Woolston, R-A., Pulford, K., Cordell, J. L., Cohen, B., DeWolf-Peeters, C. and Mason, D. Y., (1983). Diagnosis of human lymphoma with monoclonal antileukocyte antibodies. *N. Engl. J. Med.*, **309**, 1275–81

5. Hayhoe, F. G. J., Quaglino, D. and Doll, R. (1964). The Cytology and Cytochemistry of Acute Leukaemia: a study of 140 cases. (London: HMSO)

6. Erber, W. N., Mynheer, L. C. and Mason, D. Y. (1986). APAAP labelling of blood and bone marrow samples for phenotyping leukaemia. *Lancet*, **1**, 761–5

7. Foon, K. A. and Todd, R. F. (1986). Immunologic classification of leukemia and lymphoma. *Blood,* **68**, 1–31
8. Greaves, M. F., Sieff, C. and Edwards, P. A. W. (1983). Monoclonal antiglycophorin as a probe for erythroleukemia. *Blood,* **61**, 645–6
9. Vainchenker, W., Deschamps, J. F., Bastin, J. M., Guichard, J., Titeux, M., Breton-Gorins, J. and McMichael, A. J. (1982). Two monoclonal antiplatelet antibodies as markers of human megakaryocyte maturation: immunofluorescence staining and platelet peroxidase detection in megakaryocyte colonies and *in vivo* cells from normal and leukemic patients. *Blood,* **59**, 514–21
10. Chan, L.C., Pegram, S. M. and Greaves, M. F. (1985). Contribution of immunophenotype to the classification and differential diagnosis of acute leukaemia. *Lancet,* **1**, 475–9
11. Greaves, M. F., Bell, R., Amess, T. and Lister, T. A. (1983). ALL masquerading as AUL. *Leuk. Res.,* **7**, 735–46
12. Isaacson, P. G., O'Connor, N. T. J., Spencer, J., Bevan, D. H., Connolly, C. E., Kirkham, N., Polloch, D. J., Wainscoat, J. S., Stein, H. and Mason, D. Y. (1985). Malignant histiocytosis of the intestine: a T-cell lymphoma. *Lancet,* **11**, 688–91
13. Bloomfield, C. D. (1984). Acute Lymphoblastic Leukemia; clinical and histological features. In Goldman, J. M. and Priesler, H. D. (eds). *Leukaemias.* p. 163–189. (London: Butterworths)
14. Reinherz, E. L., Kung, P. C., Goldstein, G., Levey, R. H. and Schlossman, S. F. (1980). Discrete stages of human intrathymic differentiation. Analysis of normal thymocytes and leukemic lymphoblasts of T-cell lineage. *Proc. Natl. Acad. Sci.* USA, **77**, 1588–92
15. Roper, M. Crist, W. M., Metzgar, R., Ragab, A. H., Smith, S., Starling, K., Pullen, J., Levanthal, B., Bartolucci, A. A. and Cooper, M. D. (1983). Monoclonal antibody characterisation of surface antigens in childhood T-cell lymphoid malignancies. *Blood,* **61**, 830–7
16. Korsmeyer, S. J., Arnold, A., Bakhshi, A., Ravetch, J. V., Siebenlist, U., Heiter, P. A., Sharrow, S. O., Lebien, T. W. Kersey, J. H., Poplack, D. G., Leder, P. and Waldmann, T. A. (1983). Immunoglobulin gene rearrangement and cell surface antigen expression in acute lymphocytic leukemias of T cell and B cell precursor origins. *J. Clin. Invest.,* **71**, 301–13
17. Nadler, L. M., Korsmeyer, S. J., Anderson, K. C., Boyde, A. W., Slaughenhoupt, B., Park, E., Jensen, J., Corae, F., Mayer, R. J., Sallan, S. E., Ritz, J. and Schlossman, S. F. (1984). B cell origin of non-T cell acute lymphoblastic leukemia. A model for discrete stages of neoplastic and normal pre-B cell differentiations. *J. Clin. Invest.,* **74**, 332–40
18. Bennett, J. M., Catovsky, D., Daniel, M-T., Flandrin, G., Galton, D. A. G., Gralnick, H. R. and Sultan, C. (1976). Proposals for the classification of the acute leukaemias. *Br. J. Haematol.,* **33**, 451–8
19. Linch, D. C. and Griffin, J. D. (1986). Monoclonal antibodies reactive with myeloid associated antigens. In Beverley P. C. L. (ed). *Monoclonal antibodies.* p. 222–246. (Edinburgh: Churchill Livingstone)
20. Aisenberg, A. C., Krontiris, T. G., Mak, T. W. and Wilkes, B. M. (1985). Rearrangement of the gene for the beta chain of the T-cell receptor in T-cell chronic lymphocytic leukemia and related disorders. *N. Engl. J. Med.,* **373**, 530–3
21. Jansen, J., den Ottolander, G. J., Schuit, H. R. E., Waayer, J. L. M. and Hijamns W. (1984). Hairy cell leukaemia: its place among the chronic B cell leukaemias. *Sem. Oncol.,* **11**, 386–93
22. Burns, G. F. and Cawley, J. C. (1980). Spontaneous mouse erythrocyte-rosette formation: Correlation with surface immunoglobulin phenotype in hairy-cell leukaemia. *Clin. Exp. Immunol.,* **39**, 83–9
23. Stein, H., Gerdes, T. and Mason, D. Y. (1982). The normal and malignant germinal centre. *Clin. Haematol.,* **11**, 531–59
24. Ritz, J., Nadler, L. M., Bhan, A. K., Notis-McConarty, J., Pesando, J. and Schlossman, S. F. (1981). Expression of common acute lymphoblastic leukemia antigen (CALLA) by lymphomas of B-cell and T-cell lineage. *Blood,* **58**, 648–52
25. Cawley, J. C., Burns, G. F. and Hayhoe, F. G. J. (1980). A chronic lymphoproliferative disorder with distinctive features: a distinct variant of hairy-cell leukaemia. *Leuk. Res.,* **4**, 547–59
26. Posnett, D. N. and Marboe, C. C. (1984). Differentiation antigens associated with hairy cell leukemia. *Sem. Oncol.,* **11**, 413–15

27. Korsmeyer, S. J., Green, W. C. and Waldmann, T. A. (1984). Cellular origin of hairy cell leukemia malignant B cells that express receptors for T cell growth factor. *Sem. Oncol.*, **11**, 394–400

28. Waldmann, T. A., Davis, M. N., Bongiovanni, K. F. and Korsmeyer, S. J. (1985). Rearrangements of genes for the antigen receptor on T cells as marker of lineage and clonality in human lymphoid neoplasms. *N. Engl. J. Med.*, **313**, 776–83

29. Berger, R., Bernheim, A., Daniel, M-T., Valensi, F. and Flandrin, G. (1981). Cytologic characterisation and significance of normal karyotypes in t(8;21) acute myeloblastic leukemia. *Blood*, **59**, 171–8

30. Holmes, R., Keating, M. J., Cork, A., Broach, Y., Trujillo, J., Dalton, W. T., McCredie, K. B. and Freireich, E. J. (1985). A unique pattern of central nervous system leukemia in acute myelomonocytic leukemia associated with inv (16)(p13q22). *Blood*, **65**, 1071–8

3
The Diagnosis and Classification of Malignant Lymphomas

D. H. Wright

Before embarking on the controversies and complexities of the classification of lymphomas, it is worth stressing the need for accurate diagnosis and the means of achieving this. In terms of clinical management, the distinction between reactive processes and malignant lymphomas and between lymphomas and carcinomas is of greater importance than the detailed sub-classification of lymphomas. The histopathology of resected lymph nodes and other tissues remains the mainstay of lymphoma diagnosis, and the need for good fixation and high quality sections is paramount. The majority of pathologists rely on their standard haematoxylin and eosin (H&E) stain, but increasingly in Europe Giemsa is the stain of choice for the diagnosis of lymphoreticular disease. This technique certainly provides contrasts, and highlights features such as cytoplasmic basophilia that are not always apparent in H&E stained sections and it is worth using as an additional, if not as the primary, stain. In our laboratory the 'lymph node set' comprises H&E, Giemsa (methyl green pyronin may be substituted), reticulin (identifies basic architecture and reveals characteristic patterns of some lymphomas), periodic acid Schiff (reveals basement membranes, mucus in epithelial cells, IgM in some lymphomas).

The increasing use of Fine Needle Aspiration cytology (FNA) in diagnostic pathology has inevitably led to the question as to whether this technique should be used for the diagnosis of lymphoreticular disease. It might be thought that the difficulties of diagnosing malignant lymphomas on full lymph node biopsies would preclude the use of a method that yields relatively small cell samples. Nevertheless, aspiration cytology, because it is rapid and relatively non-invasive, has a role in diagnosis and management. It can be used to diagnose metastatic carcinoma with a high degree of reliability and is useful to screen for recurrence in patients already treated for malignant lymphomas. It can also be used to obtain samples for immunocytochemistry, cytogenetics, etc. As a means of making a reliable primary diagnosis of malignant lymphoma, it has limitations and should be followed up by lymph node biopsy whenever this is possible. The use of imprint cytology on lymph node biopsies will enable pathologists to become familiar with the cytomorphology of lymphoid cells, making them better equipped to tackle FNA cytology.

The greatly improved imaging techniques, developed in recent years, combined with aspiration biopsy presents pathologists with the problem of diagnosing lymphoreticular disease on relatively small samples. While often providing excellent cytomorphology, the assessment of architectural features, such as follicular growth patterns, is usually impossible on these small samples. Nevertheless, they have a very valuable role in patient management, particularly in detecting recurrent tumour and assessing cytological transformation. By avoiding the need for laparotomy, they save the patient from the morbidity associated with major surgery, and it behoves pathologists to maximize the information obtained from these biopsies.

Electron microscopy, until recently, had an important role in lymphoma diagnosis, particularly in differentiating between epithelial and lymphoreticular neoplasms. This role has since been taken over by immunohistochemistry (Chapter 7). The practice of immunohistochemistry is, itself, changing with the increasing availability of monoclonal antibodies reactive with epitopes that survive fixation and paraffin embedding. Until recently, the expense and technical difficulties of immunohistochemistry restricted its use to larger laboratories. At the present time, all laboratories should practise, or at least have easy access to, basic immunohistochemistry so that, for example, anaplastic carcinomas can be differentiated from large cell lymphomas with confidence. Too many patients still undergo unnecessarily radical surgery, or suffer inappropriate chemotherapy, because this distinction is not made correctly.

Cytogenetics have not achieved a role in the diagnosis of lymphomas, yet many non-random translocations are very characteristic of certain subtypes of lymphoma[1-3]. It is of considerable interest that these translocations frequently involve the immunoglobulin gene loci in B-cell lymphomas (e.g. 14:18 translocation in follicle centre cell lymphomas[4] and the 8:14, 8:2 or 8:22 translocations in Burkitt's lymphoma[5,6]) and the T-cell receptor loci in T-cell lymphomas. The other translocated fragment usually involves the site of a known or putative proto-oncogene. It is not always easy to obtain good chromosome spreads from malignant lymphomas for technical reasons. Translocations may, however, be detected by Southern blotting, digested DNA from the tumour and probing it with complementary DNA sequences to the site of the breakpoint (e.g. the BCL2 oncogene in follicle centre cell lymphomas)[7]. It has yet to be seen whether such techniques will be used for diagnostic purposes. The more familiar use of Southern blotting to detect immunoglobulin gene or T-cell receptor gene rearrangements certainly has a diagnostic role in a limited number of cases[8-11]. Clonal rearrangements identify clonal, presumed neoplastic proliferations, and some of the rearrangements are lineage specific.

One of the features of malignant lymphomas that confuses their recognition and diagnosis is the presence of large numbers of reactive, non-neoplastic cells that, in many lymphomas, out-number the neoplastic population. This mixture of cells is widely recognized in Hodgkin's disease and provides one of the criteria for the separation of the subtypes of this disease. Immunological and immunohistochemical analysis of non-Hodgkin's lymphomas has shown that many of these, particularly T-cell lymphomas, show similarly complex mixtures of reactive cells. Even B-cell lymphomas may be disguised by their reactive component and come to resemble T-cell lymphomas, the so-called T-cell-rich B-cell lymphomas[12]. In these complex lymphomas it may be difficult to identify the neoplastic population. In some instances, this recognition may be based on morphology, i.e. the atypical or blast cells are assumed to be the neoplastic population. Clonal populations may also be identified by immunoglobulin light chain restriction or by clonal rearrangements of the immunoglobulin or T-cell receptor genes.

CLASSIFICATION OF LYMPHOMAS

One of the reasons for the apparent dissatisfaction with lymphoma categorizations stems from the fact that different groups require different information from classifications. Clinicians need categorizations that will enable them to allocate patients to appropriate treatment groups. These treatment groups are usually based on experience of clinical trials acquired over long periods of time, hence the understandable reluctance of oncologists to overthrow established classifications. Essentially, clinicians require a classification that is reproduceable (between pathologists and by the same pathologist) that accurately identifies lymphomas in different treatment groups and that allows comparisons with other treatment centres. In practice, the clinical requirements for the categorization of non-Hodgkin's lymphomas are relatively simple. Apart from a few elaborations they need to know whether a lymphoma is follicular or diffuse and whether it is composed of small cells or large cells. Most patients can be assigned to appropriate treatment schedules on the basis of this information. It is not surprising, therefore, that the NCI sponsored study group, that established the Working Formulation (Table 1), found that all six classification systems studied (Kiel[13], (Table 2); Rappaport[14], (Table 3); Lukes and Collins[15], (Table 4); BNLI[16], (Table 5); Dorfmann[17], (Table 6); WHO[18], (Table 7)) were equally good in predicting prognosis[19].

While accepting the importance of this aspect of classification, it must be recognized that it reflects the relatively crude basis of most chemotherapeutic regimes. It is likely that, within the next few years, lymphokines produced by recombinant technology may be used in the treatment of lymphomas, together with refinements of chemotherapy. If this transpires more complex, biologically relevant classification of lymphomas will be required.

While specialists in lymphoreticular pathology have identified many new subtypes of non-Hodgkin's lymphomas, in recent years, general pathologists, who may see relatively few cases, often prefer to remain as 'lumpers', regretting the passing of the simpler classifications of previous times. However, the most important role of the pathologist, in the non-specialist centre, is to identify lymphomas as such and to distinguish them from other

Table 1 A working formulation of non-Hodgkin's lymphoma for clinical usage (equivalent or related terms in the Kiel classification are shown)

Working formulation	*Kiel equivalent or related terms*
Low grade	
(A) *Malignant lymphoma* Small lymphocytic consistent with CLL plasmacytoid	ML lymphocytic CLL ML lymphoplasmacytic/lympho- plasmacytoid
(B) *Malignant lymphoma, follicular* Predominantly small cleaved cell; diffuse areas; sclerosis	ML centroblastic-centrocytic (small), follicular ± diffuse
(C) *Malignant lymphoma, follicular* Mixed, small cleaved and large cell; diffuse areas; sclerosis	
Intermediate grade	
(D) *Malignant lymphoma, follicular* Predominantly large cell; diffuse areas; sclerosis	ML centroblastic–centrocytic (large), follicular ± diffuse
(E) *Malignant lymphoma, diffuse* Small cleaved cell; sclerosis	ML centrocytic (small)
(F) *Malignant lymphoma, diffuse* Mixed, small and large cell; sclerosis; epithelioid cell component	ML centroblastic–centrocytic (small), diffuse ML lymphoplasmacytic/–cytoid, polymorphic
(G) *Malignant lymphoma, diffuse* Large cell; cleaved cell; non-cleaved cell; sclerosis	ML centroblastic–centrocytic (large), diffuse ML centrocytic (large) ML centroblastic
High grade	
(H) *Malignant lymphoma* Large cell, immunoblastic; plasmacytoid; clear cell; polymorphous; epithelioid cell component	ML immunoblastic T-zone lymphoma lymphoepithelioid cell lymphoma
(I) *Malignant lymphoma* Lymphoblastic; convoluted cell; non-convoluted cell	ML lymphoblastic, convoluted cell type ML lymphoblastic, unclassified
(J) *Malignant lymphoma* Small non-cleaved cell; Burkitt's; follicular areas	ML lymphoblastic, Burkitt type and other B-lymphoblastic
Miscellaneous	
Composite	—
Mycosis fungoides	mycosis fungoides
Histiocytic	—
Extramedullary plasmacytoma	ML plasmacytic
Unclassifiable	—
Other	—

Table 2 Updated Kiel classification of non-Hodgkin's lymphomas

B	T
Low grade	**Low grade**
*Lymphocytic-chronic lymphocytic and prolymphocytic leukaemia; hairy cell leukaemia	Lymphocytic-chronic lymphocytic and prolymphocytic leukaemia
Lymphoplasmacytic/cytoid (LP immunocytoma)	Small, cerebriform cell – mycosis fungoides, Sezary's syndrome
Plasmacytic	Lymphoepithelial (Lennert's lymphoma)
*Centroblastic/centrocytic	Angioimmunoblastic (AILD, LgX)
– follicular ± diffuse	
– diffuse	T-zone
Centrocytic	Pleomorphic, small cell (HTLV–1±)
High grade	**High grade**
Centroblastic	Pleomorphic, medium and large cell (HTLV–1±)
*Immunoblastic	Immunoblastic (HTLV–1±)
*Large cell anaplastic (Ki–1+)	Large cell anaplastic (Ki–1±)
Burkitt lymphoma	
*Lymphoblastic	Lymphoblastic
Rare types	**Rare types**

*Indicates some degree of correspondence, either in morphology or in functional expression, between categories in two columns

Table 3 Rappaport classification

Nodular

    Lymphocytic, well differentiated
    Lymphocytic, poorly differentiated
    Mixed, lymphocytic and histiocytic
    Histiocytic

Diffuse

    Lymphocytic, well differentiated without
      plasmacytoid features
    Lymphocytic, well differentiated with
      plasmacytoid features
    Lymphocytic, poorly differentiated without
      plasmacytoid features
    Lymphocytic, poorly differentiated with
      plasmacytoid features
    Lymphoblastic convoluted
    Lymphoblastic, non-convoluted
    Mixed, lymphocytic and histiocytic
    Histiocytic without sclerosis
    Histiocytic with sclerosis
    Burkitt's tumour
    Undifferentiated

Malignant lymphoma, unclassified
Composite lymphoma

Table 4 Lukes and Collins classification

Undefined cell type
T-cell type, small lymphocytic
T-cell type, Sezary-mycosis fungoides (cerebriform)
T-cell type, convoluted lymphocytic
T-cell type, immunoblastic sarcoma (T-cell)
B-cell type, small lymphocytic
B-cell type, plasmacytoid lymphocytic
Follicular centre cell, small cleaved
Follicular centre cell, large cleaved
Follicular centre cell, small non-cleaved
Follicular centre cell, large non-cleaved
Immunoblastic sarcoma (B-cell)
Subtypes of follicular centre cell lymphomas
    1. follicular
    2. follicular and diffuse
    3. diffuse
    4. sclerotic with follicles
    5. sclerotic without follicles
Histiocytic
Malignant lymphoma, unclassified

Table 5 British National Lymphoma Investigation classification

Follicular lymphoma

    Follicle cells, predominantly small
    Follicle cells, mixed small and large
    Follicle cells, predominantly large

Diffuse lymphoma

    Lymphocytic, well differentiated
      (small round lymphocyte)
    Lymphocytic, intermediately differentiated
      (small, follicle lymphocyte)
    Lymphocytic, poorly differentiated (lymphoblast)
      (a) non-Burkitt
      (b) Burkitt's tumours
      (c) convoluted cell mediastinal lymphoma
    Lymphocytic/mixed small lymphoid and large cell
      (mixed follicle cells)
    Undifferentiated large cell (large lymphoid cell)
    Histiocytic cell (mononuclear phagocytic cell)
    Plasma cell (extramedullary plasma cells)
    Malignant lymphoma, unclassified
    Plasmacytoid differentiation
    Sclerosis, banded
    Sclerosis, fine

anaplastic tumours. To some extent, specific classification systems assist this process. When the term 'reticulum cell sarcoma' was in vogue it served as a 'waste paper basket' term, attracting a variety of anaplastic, large cell neoplasms. Specific classification categories require pathologists to be

Table 6 Dorfman classification

Follicular (or follicular and diffuse)

Small lymphoid
Mixed, small and large lymphoid
Large lymphoid

Diffuse

Small lymphocytic, without plasmacytoid differentiation
Small lymphocytic, with plasmacytoid differentiation
Atypical small lymphoid
Lymphoblastic, convoluted
Lymphoblastic, non-convoluted
Large lymphoid, without plasmacytoid differentiation
Large lymphoid, with plasmacytoid differentiation
Mixed small and large lymphoid
Histiocytic
Burkitt's lymphoma
Lymphoepithelioid cellular (Lennert's lymphoma)
Mycosis fungoides
Undifferentiated
Lymphoma associated with sclerosis
Malignant lymphoma, unclassified
Composite lymphoma

Table 7 WHO classification

Nodular lymphosarcoma, prolymphocytic
Nodular lymphosarcoma, prolymphocytic–lymphoblastic
Diffuse lymphosarcoma, lymphocytic
Diffuse lymphosarcoma, lymphoplasmacytic
Diffuse lymphosarcoma, prolymphocytic
Diffuse lymphosarcoma, prolymphocytic–lymphoblastic
Diffuse lymphosarcoma, lymphoblastic
Diffuse lymphosarcoma, immunoblastic
Diffuse lymphosarcoma, Burkitt's tumour
Mycosis fungoides
Plasmacytoma
Reticulosarcoma
Malignant lymphoma, unclassified
Composite lymphoma

---

accurate in identifying entities. The more precisely an entity is defined the less likely it is to act as a 'waste paper basket' term.

A major conceptual and practical problem in the classification of non-Hodgkin's lymphomas, 10 years ago, was the fact that, whereas the basis for lymphoma diagnosis is morphology, a major subdivision (between B- and T-cells) can only be reliably determined, in many instances by immunological means. This problem has been largely overcome by the development of lineage specific antibodies, reactive in routinely processed tissues[20,21]. A number of classification systems and the Working Formulation take no account of immunological phenotype. It is unlikely that this will provide a satisfactory basis for treatment in the near future.

Attempts have been made to subclassify B-cell non-Hodgkin's lymphomas (BNHL) according to their degree of immunological maturation, based on the hypothesis that the subtypes of BNHL represent B-cells arrested at different stages of maturation. Thus, lymphoblastic lymphomas, showing immuno-globulin heavy chain gene rearrangement and possibly expressing cyto-plasmic μ heavy chains represent the earliest stages of B-cell maturation and plasmacytic lymphomas the latest. Not all BNHL easily fit into this lineage related system and it is probable that there is more than one pathway to plasma cell maturation. Attempts to subclassify T-cell NHL, on their immunophenotype, have been less successful, since it appears that they do not express the phenotype of normal analogues[22,23]. Probably the most character-istic immunophenotypic feature of TNHL is the loss of antigens, indeed this may be a characteristic that permits the separation of neoplastic from reactive T-cell populations.

A major problem in the classification of NHL is not only knowing the histogenesis of the particular tumour, but having a suitable name for the cell of origin. This is well illustrated by the use of the term 'centrocyte' in the Kiel classification for the small cleaved cells of follicle centre cell lymphomas and for centrocytic lymphoma[24]. The cells of centrocytic lymphoma are not derived from follicle centre cells (hence are not centrocytes) and are immuno-logically distinct from the centrocytes of follicle centre cell lymphomas. Centrocytic lymphomas have also been designated as intermediate cell lymphomas because the cells were thought to be intermediate in size and shape between small lymphocytes and follicle centre centrocytes[25]. The term mantle zone lymphoma has also been used because centrocytic lymphomas frequently surround reactive germinal follicles forming a mantle before invading and destroying them[26]. Thus, a reasonably well defined clinicopatho-logical entity[27] is enveloped in semantic confusion because its cell of origin has no generally agreed name.

None of the classifications of NHL, currently in use, distinguish between nodal and extranodal lymphomas. Isaacson and Wright[28] propose that many extranodal lymphomas arise from the mucosa-associated lymphoid tissue. Subsequent work, by Spencer and Isaacson[29] (see Chapter 9), identified the origin of these tumours, not from follicle centre cells but from epitheliotropic centrocyte-like cells, yet extranodal lymphomas are usually categorized using the terminology of follicle centre cell lymphomas, e.g. blastic tumours of the stomach are usually categorized as centroblastic, whereas they presumably represent transformed centrocyte-like cells and, hence, have a different histo-genesis from nodal centroblastic lymphomas. It should be pointed out that nodal centroblastic lymphomas are morphologically indistinguishable from extranodal centroblastic lymphomas.

HODGKIN'S DISEASE

Thomas Hodgkin described six cases of lymphadenopathy in 1832[30]. Histolog-ical examination of tissue from these cases, 100 years later, showed that one was tuberculosis, one syphilis, one a non-Hodgkin's lymphoma and three Hodgkin's disease[31]. It is a reflection of our lack of understanding of Hodgkin's disease (HD), and our defective terminology, that the whole of our nomenclature of lymphoreticular neoplasms (Hodgkin's disease and non-Hodgkin's lymphomas) ultimately refers back to the clinical and gross anatomical description of six patients, 150 years ago, only three of whom had what is now accepted as Hodgkin's disease. Modern techniques of cell culture, immunohistochemistry and gene rearrangement studies have not clarified the histogenesis of Hodgkin's disease (see Chapter 8). In a small proportion of cases the distinction between Hodgkin's disease and non-Hodgkin's lymphoma (particularly of the T-cell phenotype) is difficult and ultimately decided on histopathological morphology. The diagnosis of Hodgkin's disease is based on the recognition of Reed–Sternberg cells, the nature of which is uncertain and the immunological phenotype and morphology of which may be closely mimicked by cells of non-Hodgkin's lymphomas. In this situation arguments become circular, and it should be borne in mind that at least some cases of Hodgkin's disease may be of the T-cell phenotype and, thus, arguably T-cell lymphomas.

The modern classification of Hodgkin's disease was introduced by Lukes, Butler and Hicks in 1966[32]. Their sub-categorization of the disease into six subtypes was condensed to four subtypes in the Rye classification[33]. This is now regarded as a mistake, since the original six subtypes reflect significant clinicopathological groupings. The earlier Jackson and Parker[34] classification of Hodgkin's disease provided very limited prognostic guidance, since the great majority of patients fell into the category of Hodgkin's granuloma. In a retrospective study Lukes, Butler and Hicks[32] found that their classification provided of significant prognostic information. However, in subsequent years, advances in treatment combined with an increasing proportion of cases falling into the nodular sclerosing category appear to have obliterated these differences. More recently, Haybittle et al.[35] have divided the NS category into Grade I (few RS and atypical cells) and Grade II (many RS and atypical cells) and shown significant prognostic differences between these groups.

Immunohistochemistry has shown that nodular lymphocyte/histiocyte predominant HD is a proliferation of B-cells and is distinct from other sub-types of HD[36]. Thus, it appears that HD is, in fact, at least two diseases. Two subtypes that are a source of diagnostic difficulty and confusion are diffuse L & H predominant HD and lymphocyte depleted (reticular) HD. Several review studies have shown that many cases diagnosed as reticular HD are, in fact, non-Hodgkin's lymphomas or anaplastic carcinomas[37,38].

B-CELL NON-HODGKIN'S LYMPHOMA (NHL)

The recognition that a large proportion of lymphomas arise from follicle centre cells provided a major conceptual advance in our understanding of NHL. In the Kiel classification these cells are known as centroblasts and centrocytes, whereas in the Lukes and Collins classification they are designated non-cleaved and cleaved cells, respectively. A disadvantage of the Kiel classification is that the terms imply a certain knowledge that a tumour is derived from follicle centre B-cells. While this is a reasonable assumption in a tumour with a nodular growth pattern, it is less certain with diffuse tumours. Thus, a diffuse blastic lymphoma might be of the T-cell phenotype or, if of B-cell origin, it might not be derived from the follicle centre.

Hui et al.[39] have recently suggested that centroblastic lymphomas should be divided into four morphological subtypes (monomorphic, polymorphic, multilobated, centrocytoid). At one time multilobated lymphomas were thought to be of the T-cell phenotype[40], whereas immunohistochemistry has shown that they are almost invariably B-cells. It is important to recognize the category, centroblastic/centrocytoid since these high-grade tumours are frequently misdiagnosed as centroblastic/centrocytic, diffuse, a low-grade lymphoma. This probably accounts for the widely varying reported incidence of diffuse centroblastic/centrocytic lymphoma. In centroblastic/centrocytoid lymphomas the tumour cells have irregular (cleaved) nuclei, but these have prominent nucleoli and the tumour cell cytoplasm is basophilic. The use of Giemsa stain aids the identification of this lymphoma.

The term 'immunoblastic lymphoma' is applied to a number of different entities and is not always precisely defined. Morphologically, immunoblasts are said to have a single, prominent, central nucleolus and basophilic cytoplasm. Variable numbers of such cells may be seen in centroblastic lymphomas[39]. It is probable that many pathologists designate such tumours as immunoblastic lymphoma, although they should be regarded as a subtype of centroblastic lymphoma. High-grade lymphomas, arising from the transformation of lymphocytic lymphoma (Richter's syndrome), or lympho-plasmacytic lymphomas, are usually designated as immunoblastic sarcomas, irrespective of their morphology.

The place of Burkitt's lymphoma (BL) in the classification of B-cell NHL is controversial. In the original Kiel classification it was included with the lymphoblastic lymphomas and the FAB classification of lymphoblastic leukaemia included 'Burkitt-like' tumours with bone marrow involvement (FAB3)[41]. Lymphoblastic neoplasms are derived from early stages of the T- or B-cell maturation pathways and are primarily bone marrow based. Burkitt's lymphoma cells have an immunophenotype of more mature B-cells and are primarily extramedullary. In recognition of these fundamental differences the updated Kiel classification[42] places BL in a category of its own.

Burkitt's lymphoma was described as a clinicopathological entity from Africa that characteristically involved extranodal sites, such as the jaws and abdominal viscera and rarely involved the peripheral lymph nodes. Tumours with a similar cytological and histological appearance were described from Europe and North America. Some of these cases have a similar anatomical distribution to the African cases, but a large number have nodal involvement or involvement of the nasopharynx and terminal ileum, sites that are rarely involved by African BL[43]. Mann et al.[44] noted an apparent transition between reactive germinal follicles and areas of BL in American patients with this tumour and, on this basis, they proposed that BL is a follicle centre cell lymphoma. Despite their morphologic similarities, it is my view that most cases of American BL are a different disease from African BL. While some of the American cases may be follicle centre cell derived, there are many features

24

of African BL that suggest that they are derived from cells of the mucosa associated lymphoid tissue[45].

T-CELL NON-HODGKIN'S LYMPHOMA (NHL)

The means of reliably identifying T-cell NHL have been available for a relatively short time and a clinicopathological database on which to construct a logical classification does not yet exist. The classification of T-cell lymphomas is essentially a compilation of entities, mainly recognized on the basis of their histology, with little knowledge of the relationship and transitions between these types. Presumably, this knowledge will accumulate in due course, provided that the tumours are accurately diagnosed and categorized. Three types of T-cell lymphoma are reasonably well characterized in terms of their clinical features and behaviour. These are T-lymphoblastic lymphoma, cutaneous T-cell lymphoma (Sézary's syndrome and mycosis fungoides) and HTLV1-associated adult T-cell leukaemia lymphoma. The latter shows a curious geographical localization to the southern islands of Japan and the Caribbean and also occurs in emigrants from these areas[46,47].

HISTIOCYTIC LYMPHOMA (SARCOMA)

In the Rappaport classification many large cell lymphomas are categorized as histiocytic lymphomas, although it is now recognized that the majority of these are of the B- or T-cell phenotype. The term 'histiocyte' was first used because it was thought that most large cell lymphomas were histiocyte-derived. In a little over a decade, first immunohistochemistry and then gene rearrangement studies have shown that true histiocyte lymphomas are extremely rare and that most earlier reports of histiocytic lymphomas are based on inadequate data and misconceptions[48]. The monocyte/macrophage system is composed of a large population of cells, and it is of interest that neoplasms of this sytem appear to be so rare in comparison with tumours of the lymphocyte lineage. This may be due to the end-cell nature of histiocytes with monocytic leukaemia reflecting the limited population able to undergo neoplastic transformation. It may be, however, that B- and T-cell lymphocytes are much more susceptible to neoplasia as a result of the rearrangement of the immunoglobulin or T-cell receptor genes during maturation. As stated above, many translocations present in lymphomas involve these genes and the sites of known or putative proto-oncogenes.

EXTRANODAL LYMPHOMAS

None of the existing classifications treat extranodal lymphomas as a separate group. It is assumed that classifications applied to nodal lymphomas can be applied to those at extranodal sites. As already discussed, many extranodal B-cell lymphomas arise from cells of the mucosa-associated lymphoid tissue

Table 8 Primary malignant lymphomas of the gastrointestinal tract

---

B-cell NHL
(1) Low-grade lymphoma of mucosa-associated lymphoid
     tissue
(2) High-grade lymphoma of mucosa-associated lymphoid
     tissue (with, or without, co-existing low-grade lymphoma)
(3) Immunoproliferative small intestinal disease
(4) Malignant lymphoma, centrocytic (with, or without,
     lymphomatous polyposis)
(5) Malignant lymphoma, centroblastic/centrocytic
(6) Plasmacytic lymphoma

T-cell NHL
(1) With, or without, enteropathy
(2) With, or without, eosinophilia

Classification of primary gastrointestinal lymphomas proposed at the meeting of the *European Association for Haematopathology* held in Geneva, April 1988

and have a different histogenesis and biological behaviour from nodal lymphomas (see Chapter 10). It is also apparent that a number of T-cell lymphomas have a specific predilection for extranodal sites. In the case of the cutaneous T-cell lymphomas (SS and MF), this has been known for some time. It also appears that the enteropathy-associated T-cell lymphomas (malignant histiocytosis of the intestine) is derived from a specific mucosal T-cell[49].

At a meeting of the *European Association for Haematopathology*, held in Geneva in April 1988, a classification or primary gastrointestinal lymphoma was proposed (Table 8). This scheme provides a reasonably simple working system within the limitations of our knowledge of intestinal lymphocyte populations. Immunoproliferative small intestinal disease has many similarities to tumours of mucosa-associated lymphoid tissue, as seen in Europe and North America[50]. The unique features of this condition are its frequent involvement of large segments of the small intestine, its geographical localization to the Middle-East and North Africa (with occasional cases elsewhere) and its association with the production of an abnormal IgA heavy chain. It is, as yet, unclear whether this condition has a genetic basis or is environmentally induced.

Lymphomatous polyposis of the gastrointestinal tract[51,52] is an uncommon neoplasm in which the neoplastic cells have the morphology and immuno-phenotype of the cells of centrocytic lymphoma. Presumably, however, the highly characteristic distribution of this tumour, forming multiple mucosal polyps throughout much of the intestinal tract with a predilection for the terminal ileum, indicates that it is derived from a different population of cells from that which gives rise to nodal centrocytic lymphoma and that the neoplastic cells must bear addressin molecules that direct them to mucosal sites.

Follicle centre cell lymphomas undoubtedly occur in the gastrointestinal tract, but are less common than reported since lymphomas of MALT have, in the past, been diagnosed as follicle centre cell lymphomas. Indeed, the propensity of the centrocyte-like cell of mucosa-associated lymphoid tumours (MALT) to invade and replace reactive follicles may give these neoplasms a follicular structure in some areas. Presumably, true follicle centre cell lymphomas arise from germinal centres in the gastrointestinal tract. It is, perhaps, surprising that these tumours are not more common, in view of the large amount of lymphoid tissue at this site. If non-endemic Burkitt's lymphoma (Burkitt-like) are follicle centre cell lymphomas, as suggested (Mann et al.[44]) they would be included in this group but, in view of the uncertainty of their histogenesis, it might be better that they should be allocated a separate category.

References

1. Rowley, J. D. (1982). Identification of the constant chromosome regions involved in human hematologic malignant disease. *Science*, **216**, 749–51
2. Yunis, J. J., Oken, M. M., Kaplan, M. E., Ensrud, K. M., Howe, R. R. and Theoligides, A. (1982). Distinctive chromosomal abnormalities in histologic subtypes of non-Hodgkin's lymphoma. *N. Engl. J. Med.*, **307**, 1231–6
3. Levine, E. G., Arthur, D. C., Frizzera, G., Peterson, B. A., Hurd, D. D. and Bloomfield, C. D. (1985). There are differences in cytogenetic abnormalities among histologic subtypes of the non-Hodgkin's lymphomas. *Blood*, **66**, 1414–22
4. Yunis, J. J., Frizzera, G., Oken, M. M., McKenna, J., Theologides, A. and Arnesen, M. (1987). Multiple recurrent genomic defects in follicular lymphoma. A possible model for cancer. *N. Engl. J. Med.*, **316**, 79–84
5. Manalova, Y., Manolov, G., Kieler, J., Levan, A. and Klein, G. (1979). Genesis of the 14q+ in Burkitt's lymphoma. *Hereditas*, **90**, 5–10
6. Lenoir, G. M., Preud, Homme, J. L., Bernheim, A. and Berger, R. (1982). Correlation between immunoglobulin light chain expression and variant translocation in Burkitt's lymphoma. *Nature*, **298**, 474–6.
7. Weis, L. M., Warnke, R. A., Sklar, J. and Cleary, M. L. (1987). Molecular analysis of the t(14;18) chromosomal translocation in malignant lymphomas. *N. Engl. J. Med.*, **317**, 1185–9
8. Arnold, A., Cossmann, J., Bakshi, A., Jaffe, E., Waldmann, T. A. and Korsmeyer, S. J. (1983). Immunoglobulin gene rearrangements as unique clonal markers in human lymphoid neoplasms. *N. Engl. J. Med.*, **309**, 1593–9
9. O'Connor, N. T. J., Wainscoat, J. S., Weatherall, D. J. *et al.* (1985). Rearrangement of the T-cell receptor beta-chain gene in the diagnosis of lymphoproliferative disorders. *Lancet*, **1**, 1295–7
10. Waldmann, T. A., Davis, M. M., Bongiovanni, K. F. and Korsmeyer, S. J. (1985). Rearrangement of genes for the antigen receptor on T-cells as markers of lineage and clonality in human lymphoid neoplasms. *N. Engl. J. Med.*, **313**, 776–83
11. Williams, M. E., Innes, D. J., Borowitz, M. J., Lovell, M. A., Swerdlow, S. H., Hurtubise, P. E., Brynes, R. K., Chan, W. C., Byrne, G. E., Whitcombe, C. C. and Thomas, C. Y. (1987). Immunoglobulin and T-cell receptor gene rearrangements in human lymphoma and leukemia. *Blood*, **69**, 79–86
12. Ramsay, A. D., Smith, W. J. and Isaacson, P. G. (1988). T-cell-rich B-cell lymphoma. *Am. J. Surg. Pathol.*, **12**, 433–43
13. Gerard-Marchant, R., Hamlin, I., Lennert, K., Rilke, F., Stansfeld, A. G. and van Unnik, J. A. M. (1974). Classification of non-Hodgkin's lymphomas. *Lancet*, **2**, 406–8
14. Rappaport, H. (1966). Tumors of the Hematopoietic System. *Atlas of Tumor Pathology*, Section 3, Fasc 8. (Washington DC: Armed Forces Institute of Pathology)
15. Lukes, R. J. and Collins, R. D. (1977). Lukes–Collins classification and its significance. *Cancer Treat. Rep.*, **61**, 971–9
16. Bennett, M. H., Farrer-Brown, G., Henry, K. and Jelliffe, A. M. (1974). Classification of non-Hodgkin's lymphomas. *Lancet*, **2**, 405–6

17. Dorfman, R. F. (1974). Classification of non-Hodgkin's lymphoma. *Lancet*, **1**, 1295
18. Mathé, G. Rappaport, H., O'Conor, G. T. *et al.* (1976). Histological and cytological typing of neoplastic diseases of haematopoietic and lymphoid tissues. In *WHO International Histological Classification of Tumours*, No 14. (Geneva: World Health Organisation)
19. Rosenberg, S. A., Bernard, C. W., Brown, B. W. *et al.* (1982). National Cancer Institute sponsored study of classification of non-Hodgkin's lymphomas. Summary and description of a working formulation for clinical usage. The non-Hodgkin's lymphoma pathologic classification project. *Cancer*, **49**, 2112–35
20. Norton, A. J. and Isaacson, P. G. (1987). Detailed phenotype analysis of B-cell lymphoma, using a panel of antibodies reactive in routinely fixed, wax-embedded tissue. *Am. J. Pathol.*, **128**, 225–40
21. Ng, C. S., Chan, J. K. C., Hui, P. K. and Lo, S. T. H. (1988). Monoclonal antibodies reactive with normal and neoplastic T-cells in paraffin sections. *Hum. Pathol.*, **19**, 295–303
22. Picker, L. J., Brenner, M. B., Weiss, L. M., Smith, S. D., Warnke, R. A. (1987). Discordant expression of CD3 and T-cell receptor beta-chain antigens in T-lineage lymphomas. *Am. J. Pathol.*, **129**, 434–40
23. Smith, J. L., Haegert, D. G., Hodges, E., Stacey, G. N., Howell, W. M., Wright, D. H., Jones, D. B. Phenotypic and genotypic heterogeneity of peripheral T-cell lymphoma. *Br. J. Cancer.* (In press)
24. Lennert, K. (1981). *Histopathology of Non-Hodgkin's Lymphomas (based on the Kiel Classification).* (Berlin: Springer-Verlag)
25. Weisenburger, D. D., Nathwani, B. N., Diamond, L. W., Winberg, C. D. and Rappaport, H. (1981). Malignant lymphoma intermediate lymphocytic type: A clinicopathologic study of 42 cases. *Cancer*, **48**, 1415–25
26. Weisenburger, D. D., Kim, H. and Rappaport, H. (1982). Mantle zone lymphoma: A follicular variant of intermediate lymphocytic lymphoma. *Cancer*, **49**, 1429–38
27. Swerdlow, S. H., Habeshaw, J. A., Murray, L. J., Dhaliwal, H. S., Lister, T. A. and Stansfeld, A. G. (1983). Centrocytic lymphoma: A distinct clinicopathologic and immunologic entity. A multiparameter study of 18 cases at diagnosis and relapse. *Am. J. Pathol.*, **113**, 181–7
28. Isaacson, P. and Wright, D. H. (1984). Extranodal malignant lymphoma arising from mucosa-associated lymphoid tissue. *Cancer*, **53**, 2515–24
29. Isaacson, P. G. and Spencer, J. (1987). Malignant lymphoma of mucosa-associated lymphoid tissue. *Histopathology*, **11**, 445–62
30. Hodgkin, T. (1832). On some morbid appearances of the absorbent glands and spleen. *Med. Chir. Trans.*, **17**, 68–114
31. Fox, H. (1926). Remarks on the presentation of microscopical preparations made from some of the original tissue described by Thomas Hodgkin, 1832. *Ann. Med. Hist.*, **8**, 370–4
32. Lukes, R. J., Butler, J. J. and Hicks, E. B. (1966). Natural history of Hodgkin's disease as related to its pathologic picture. *Cancer*, **19**, 317–44
33. Lukes, R. J., Craver, L. F., Hall, T. C., Rappaport, H. and Rubin, P. (1966). Report of the nomenclature committee. *Cancer Res.*, **26**, 1311
34. Jackson, H. Jr. and Parker, F. Jr. (1947). *Hodgkin's Disease and Allied Disorders.* (New York: Oxford University Press)
35. Haybittle, J. L., Hayhoe, F. G. J., Easterling, M. J., Jelliff, A. M., Bennett, M. H., Vaughan Hudson, G., Vaughan Hudson, B. and MacLennan, K. A. (1985). Review of British National Lymphoma Investigation studies of Hodgkin's disease and development of prognostic index. *Lancet*, **1**, 967–72
36. Pinkus, G. S. and Said, J. W. (1985). Hodgkin's disease, lymphocyte predominance type, nodular – A distinct entity. *Am. J. Pathol.*, **118**, 1–6
37. Greer, J. P., Kinney, M. C., Cousar, J. B., Flexner, J. M., Dupont, W. D., Graber, S. E., Greco, F. A., Collins, R. D. and Stein, R. S. (1986). Lymphocyte depleted Hodgkin's disease. Clinicopathologic review of 25 patients. *Am. J. Med.*, **81**, 208–14
38. Kant, J. A., Hubbard, S. M., Longo, D. L., Simon, R. M., DeVita, V. T., Jaffe, E. S. (1986). The pathologic and clinical heterogeneity of lymphocyte depleted Hodgkin's disease. *J. Clin. Oncol.*, **4**, 284–94
39. Hui, P. K., Feller, A. C. and Lennert, K. (1988). High-grade non-Hodgkin's lymphoma of B-cell type. I. Histopathology. *Histopathology*, **12**, 127–43

40. Weinberg, D. S. and Pinkus, G. (1981). Non-Hodgkin's lymphoma of large multilobated cell type. A clinicopathologic study of ten cases. *Am. J. Clin. Pathol.,* **76**, 190–6
41. Bennett, J. M., Catovsky, D., Daniel, M. T., Flandrin, G., Galton, D. A. G., Gralnick, H. R. and Sultan, C. (1976). Proposals for the classification of the acute leukaemias. *Br. J. Haematol.,* **33**, 451–8
42. Stansfeld, A. G., Diebold, J., Noel, H. *et al.* (1988). Updated Kiel classification for lymphomas. *Lancet,* **1**, 292–3
43. Levine, P. H., Kamaraju, L. S., Connelly, R. R., Berard, C. W., Dorfman, R. F., Magrath, I. and Easton, J. M. The American Burkitt's lymphoma Registry. Eight years experience. *Cancer,* **49**, 1016–22
44. Mann, R. B., Jaffe, E. S., Braylan, R. C., Nanba, K., Frank, M. M., Ziegler, J. L. and Berard, C. W. (1976). Non-endemic Burkitt's lymphoma, a B-cell tumor related to germinal centers. *N. Engl. J. Med.,* **295**, 685–91
45. Wright, D. H. (1985). Histogenesis of Burkitt's lymphoma: A B-cell tumour of mucosa-associated lymphoid tissue. In Lenoir, G., O'Conor, G. and Olweny, C. L. M. (eds): *Burkitt's Lymphoma: A Human Cancer Model,* IARC Scientific Publications No 60. (Lyon: International Agency for Research on Cancer)
46. Uchiyama, T., Yodoi, J., Sagawa, K., Tatsuki, K. and Uchino, H. (1977). Adult T-cell leukemia: Clinical and hematologic features of 17 cases. *Blood,* **50**, 481–92
47. Catovsky, D., Greaves, M. F., Rose, M. *et al.* (1982). Adult T-cell lymphoma-leukaemia in blacks from the West Indies. *Lancet,* **1**, 639–43
48. Weiss, L. M., Trela, M. J., Cleary, M. L., Turner, R. R., Warnke, R. A. and Sklar, J. (1985). Frequent immunoglobulin and T-cell receptor gene rearrangements in 'histiocytic' neoplasms. *Am. J. Pathol.,* **121**, 369–73
49. Isaacson, P. G., O'Connor, N. T. J., Spencer, J., Bevan, D. H., Connolly, C. E., Kirkham, N., Pollock, D. J., Wainscoat, J. S., Stein, H. and Mason, D. Y. (1986). Malignant histiocytosis of the intestine: A T-cell lymphoma. *Lancet,* **2**, 688–91
50. Isaacson, P. and Wright, D. H. (1983). Malignant lymphoma of mucosa-associated lymphoid tissue. A distinctive type of B-cell lymphoma. *Cancer,* **52**, 1410–16
51. Cornes, J. S. (1961). Multiple lymphomatosis polyposis of the gastrointestinal tract. *Cancer,* **14**, 249–57
52. Isaacson, P. G., MacLennan, K. A. and Subbuswamy, S. G. (1984). Multiple lymphomatous polyposis of the gastrointestinal tract. *Histopathology,* **8**, 641–56.

4
Analysis of Immunoglobulin Changes in Lymphoproliferative Diseases

J. L. SMITH and F. K. STEVENSON

IMMUNOGLOBULIN

Immunoglobulin (Ig) was the first and remains the most reliable marker of B-cells despite the increasing number of monoclonal antibodies directed at non-immunoglobulin determinants and used for the characterization of B-cells at various stages of differentiation. Essentially the Ig molecule is a four chain structure composed of two light chains and two heavy chains, with the carboxy terminal sequences of the heavy chains determining whether the molecule is destined for membrane insertion and surface expression or for export. Secreted Ig lacks the hydrophobic membrane insertion sequence and may exist in polymeric forms. The variable domains of the Ig heavy and light chains form the antigen combining site; the amino acid sequences and hence the tertiary structure of this site are unique and act as a marker for a single B-cell clone. Igs are also antigenic, and the variable regions are among the strongest immunogenic areas; antigenic sites in these regions are known as idiotypic determinants.

Ig is encoded by three unlinked families of genes found on chromosome 14 for the heavy chains, chromosome 2 for κ light chain and chromosome 22 for λ light chain. Within each family separate genes code for the variable (V), joining segment (J) and constant (C) regions of the Ig chain. The heavy chain germ line DNA also encodes for an additional diversity (D) segment between V and J regions[1]. The earliest event in the B-cell lineage is the rearrangement of the V, D, J and C region heavy chain genes in the stem cell. This usually occurs first for μ heavy chain resulting in the phenotypic expression of μ chain in the cytoplasm of pre B-cells without detectable light chain or surface Ig $(SIg)[2]$. These cells are also characterized by the presence of terminal deoxynucleotidyl transferase enzyme (TdT) common to all lymphoid stem cells[3]. Ig heavy chain gene rearrangement is followed by rearrangement of the κ light chain genes and if this is not productive rearrangement of the genes coding for λ light chain[4]. Phenotypically this event is followed by the disappearance of cytoplasmic μ chain and the expression of sparse SIgM.

The Ig found on the surface of lymphocytes giving rise to the majority of B-cell malignancies carries idiotypic determinants of such exquisite specificity that they can be regarded as tumour-specific. The potential for identifying and also treating established lymphoid tumours with anti-idiotypic antibody therefore exists, and was initially investigated in B-cell tumours with polyclonal antibody and then with monoclonal anti-idiotypic antibody[5,6].

Anti-idiotypic antibodies raised against a single tumour-derived Ig reveal a range of specificity, with some reacting with a significant proportion of normal polyclonal Ig whereas others appear specific for very private determinants not detectable in normal Ig. It is reasonable to assume that these determinants arise from amino acid sequences in the V region which are involved in recognition of antigen, i.e the complementarity-determining regions (CDRs). Determinants have been postulated to show a continuum of specificity, from more or less public to more or less private[7]. In this sense the terms refer to the frequency of a determinant on normal polyclonal Ig and not to the frequency of antibodies of the same specificity as the reference idiotypic Ig. For therapeutic purposes, most groups have opted for antibody to private determinants on the assumption that the idiotypic Ig (in the absence of secretory activity by the tumour) will not be present in serum to any significant extent, and that access of antibody to tumour cells, therefore, will not be blocked[8]. Further discussion on the use of anti-idiotypic antibodies for therapy and tumour monitoring will be found later in this chapter.

IMMUNOGLOBULIN EXPRESSION AND B-CELL DIFFERENTIATION: CORRELATION WITH TUMOUR HISTOLOGY

A schematic model of B-cell differentiation and Ig expression is given in Figure 1. This model encompasses two pathways of B-cell maturation, one dependent and the other independent of germinal centres. Thus the small resting B-cell on antigen activation may either migrate to the germinal centre where such cells are recognizable histologically as centrocytes and centroblasts[9] or directly give rise to immunoblasts. The generation of immunoblasts which commonly express both SIg and cytoplasmic Ig (CIg) is accompanied by the formation of memory cells capable of responding to secondary antigen challenge. These memory cells join the resting B-cell pool and while they are cytologically indistinguishable, many express different surface Ig heavy chain isotypes[10]. Further progress of immunoblasts to plasma cells takes place outside germinal centres with the loss of SIg and an increase in CIg levels. Resting and responding B-cells can express more than one heavy chain isotype but only one type of light chain. In contrast, plasma cells are usually committed to exporting a single Ig product. Allelic exclusion, a feature of B-cell Ig expression and production, appears to be complete at the pre-B cell stage of development[1].

In all cell types irrespective of the heavy chain isotype expressed, the type of light chain and the idiotypic determinants remain the same for each clone of developing B-cells. However, recent data on B-cell tumours suggests that subtle changes in idiotypic determinants can occur either spontaneously[11] or after treatment with anti-idiotype antibodies[12].

32

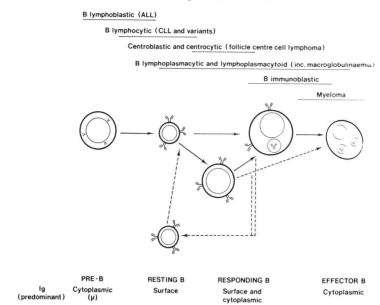

B lymphoblastic (ALL)

B lymphocytic (CLL and variants)

Centroblastic and centrocytic (follicle centre cell lymphoma)

B lymphoplasmacytic and lymphoplasmacytoid (inc. macroglobulinaemia)

B immunoblastic

Myeloma

	PRE-B	RESTING B	RESPONDING B	EFFECTOR B
Ig (predominant)	Cytoplasmic (μ)	Surface	Surface and cytoplasmic	Cytoplasmic

Figure 1 B cell differentiation and Ig expression: correlation with B cell tumour origin

Although there is some evidence that multiple heavy chain isotype expression occurs in neonatal life[13] the most common association is the dual expression of IgM and IgD on resting small B-lymphocytes. On encountering antigen resting B-lymphocytes exhibit a reduction in SIgD with maintenance of SIgM. However the sequence in which the various Ig heavy chain classes are expressed by SIgM-positive B-cells remains controversial[14]. Recent evidence suggests that direct switching from IgM to each of the other isotopes occurs[15] and that switching from IgG to IgA, or from one IgG subclass to another, do not represent major pathways[16].

Experimental evidence suggests that the dual expression of IgM and IgD derives from the splicing of a single primary ribonucleic acid (RNA) transcript of the rearranged heavy chain chromosome yielding two separate mRNAs for μ and δ[17]. However, the mechanism for expression of other multiple heavy chain isotype combinations is unclear as in this circumstance class switching is thought to result in deletion of intervening sequences by 'looping out' or unequal sister chromatid exchange[18]. Dual expression in these cases may result from the persistence of long lived mRNA in cells that have switched heavy chain expression. For further discussion of these mechanisms the reader is referred to a recent review by Vogler and Lawton[19].

CIg is usually found in responding cells at the immunoblastic and plasma cell stage. Mature plasma cells lose their capacity to express SIg and are fully committed to Ig export: the number of these cells in marrow producing IgG, A and M is linked to the relative levels of these Igs in serum. However, the amounts and type of Ig produced will vary with each tissue examined, the association of IgA with mucosal surfaces being a well known example[20]. The production of Ig especially polymeric Ig (IgM and IgA), for export is accompanied by the synthesis of J chain, a polypeptide of MW 16 000. J chain is involved with the control of polymerization and can be found in the cytoplasm of most normal and neoplastic cells involved in Ig production[21].

The majority of B-cell neoplasms appear as predominantly homogeneous populations thought to represent proliferations of cells 'frozen' at a particular stage of development. These neoplastic populations in common with proliferations of their normal B-cell counterparts express Ig of a single light chain class and individual idiotypic determinants[22], giving rise to the view that they derive from the neoplastic transformation and proliferation of a single cell. On the basis of Ig class, amount of cellular localization, the majority of lymphocytic tumours can be assigned a place within the framework of normal B-cell differentiation (Figure 1). This scheme does not allow for aberrant behaviour or for tumour pleomorphism other than that recognized in lymphomas of lymphoplasmacytic or lymphoplasmacytoid origin, where the tumour cells retain the capacity for continued maturation and differentiation comparable with normal cell development. Apparent tumour heterogeneity may also result from uncertainty surrounding normal cell development, for example, the opposing views of maturation within germinal centres. Some authors suggest the sequence from centroblasts to centrocytes and others the reverse[9,23].

Ig production and export can serve as useful parameters of B-cell maturity. In a study by Anderson and colleagues[24] the maturity of cell populations was reflected by the ratio of extracellular to intracellular Ig; immature cells synthesized relatively little Ig for export and had a ratio of < 1.0, in contrast plasma cells actively exporting Ig had a ratio of > 10.0. Some of these observations have been used by us for the analysis of tumour populations.

B-cell leukaemias and non-Hodgkin's lymphomas comprise a heterogeneous group of neoplasms displaying a wide variation in cell morphology, histology, immunological phenotype and prognosis. In this chapter tumours will be discussed as far as possible in relation to their putative cell of origin within the scheme of B-cell differentiation (Figure 1).

TUMOURS ARISING FROM B-CELLS

Leukaemia

B-cell leukaemias may be either lymphoblastic or lymphocytic. The former derive predominantly from pre-B-cells and can be distinguished from other lymphoblastic tumours by analysis of Ig gene rearrangement and presence of cytoplasmic μ chains. In contrast, the majority of B-lymphocytic leukaemias are thought to derive from resting B-cells expressing sparse SIg but lacking CIg.

Lymphoblastic leukaemia

These tumours present as acute lymphoblastic leukaemia (ALL) with the

34

phenotype of common ALL (cALL); this group forms 75% of childhood and 40% of adult ALL. The neoplastic cells are typically positive for TdT and the monoclonal antibody J5, which recognizes an antigen found on a population of lymphoid stem cells and mature B-cells[25]. In about 20% of cALL cases μ chain in the absence of light chain can be demonstrated in the cytoplasm of the neoplastic cells, identifying them as pre-B-cells[26]. Cytoplasmic γ and α chains have been found in subclones of cALL cells originally expressing cμ, suggesting that heavy chain switching can occur at the pre-B-cell stage[27].

Korsmeyer and colleagues[28] have demonstrated varying degrees of Ig gene rearrangement in cALL. In a study of 25 cases, 25 had undergone heavy chain rearrangement, 11 had further rearranged one light chain allele, but only 7 of 17 tested expressed a detectable Ig product. The failure to detect an Ig product may be explained by either aberrant rearrangement or by these cells being in a transient stage prior to active transcription or translation. Support for the latter explanation comes from evidence that neoplastic pre-B-cells are capable of further differentiation *in vitro* following exposure to a variety of differentiation factors, and that expression of both Ig heavy and light chains is found at a late stage of pre-B-cell differentiation (summarized in reference 29).

Pre-B ALL usually presents as either L_1 or L_2 in the French–American–British (FAB) classification. However, a small subgroup of ALL representing $<5\%$ of cases and belonging to the L_3 subgroup, have readily detectable SIg consistent with a mature B-cell origin. Tumour cells from the L_3 group are thought to represent a leukaemic phase of non-endemic Burkitt's lymphoma[30].

Lymphocytic leukaemia and variants

Tumours of resting B-cells such as chronic lymphocytic leukaemia (CLL) are a heterogeneous group when analysed for expression of Ig, with the majority expressing sparse SIgM or SIgM with IgD, some with no detectable Ig and a third group expressing SIgG or dense SIgM. This heterogeneity presumably reflects the cellular origin of these tumours, which can arise from either immature or mature B-(memory) cells. The large majority of CLL cells, however, express SIgM and IgD at a density of one-tenth of that expressed by normal blood lymphocytes, consistent with an immature cell origin[31]. Clinically these tumours present as an excess of round small lymphocytes in the peripheral blood. The lymphocytic lymphomas are thought to represent node based tumours of early B-cells and they share many phenotypic and cytological features with CLL; these tumours will be discussed with the non-Hodgkin's lymphomas in the next section.

Studies involving two different groups of CLL patients have been reported from this laboratory[32,33]. In both studies the patterns of Ig expression were similar and the most recent findings are summarized in Table 1. In this study of 200 cases the majority expressed either SIgM only (68 cases) or SIgM and IgD (85 cases); six were found to express SIgG alone and one case expressed IgA. A predominance of CLL cases with the phenotype SIgM κ compared to those with SIgM λ was also noted (Table 1). There is no clear explanation for this marked κ/λ imbalance in SIgM positive CLL, apart from the implication

Table 1 Surface Ig phenotype and Binet stage at presentation of 200 cases of CLL

SIg class		Number of patients		
Heavy chain isotype	κ/λ ratio	Total	Male/Female ratio	‡ Binet Stage A
μ	6.6	68	1.0	62
$\mu + \delta$	1.8	85	1.2	52
γ	ϕ	6	5.0	4
α	ϕ	1	†	†
*Undetectable	—	40	0.9	23

ϕ All κ
†   Female patient presenting at Stage A
*   Four patients had CIg crystalline inclusions
‡   Number of cases at Binet stage A at presentation

that this phenotype confers a survival advantage. A similar observation has been reported by Flanagan[34] for a group of CLL patients of similar age and sex distribution to those reported by ourselves.

A small number of cases in both studies co-expressed some SIgG with the other heavy chain isotypes, most commonly IgM and IgD. The true incidence and significance of SIgG on cells with SIgM and/or IgD is controversial. Studies from this laboratory suggest that in the cases studied with anti-idiotype this isotype was extrinsic[35,36]. However, multiple isotype expression on early normal B-cells has been reported[13] and the possibility that a small number of CLL cases co-express this isotype cannot be excluded[37].

CIg as detectable by routine techniques is uncommon in CLL. When found the CIg is likely to be in the form of crystalline inclusions or amorphous globules resembling Russell bodies. Clark and colleagues[38] reported a 10% incidence of crystalline Ig inclusions in a series of 30 cases of CLL. In our series the incidence was four cases in a total of 72 examined[39]. Crystalline Ig inclusions are of predominantly μ or occasionally α heavy chain isotype, but all have been associated with λ light chain[38,39]. Amorphous Ig Russell body inclusions are found less frequently, and isolated reports suggest these to be predominantly IgM κ[40], although IgM λ[41] and IgG κ[42] have been observed. Crystalline or amorphous inclusions occur in either all or a proportion of the neoplastic cells together with or in the absence of SIg. Normal cell counter-parts of this neoplastic cell type have not yet been defined and presumably this phenomenon represents a neoplastic cell secretary block.

Diffuse CIg and paraproteinaemia are easily detectable by conventional techniques in a small number of cases of CLL ($< 5\%$)[32,33,43]. We have reported a case where cells contained diffuse CIgD κ[44]. Weak diffuse CIgM has been reported by others in a varying number of cases depending on the sensitivity of the methods used for its detection[45]. However, we have shown that the majority of tumors of resting B-cells export whole Ig and/or free Ig light chains, when their presence is sought using biosynthetic techniques, radio-immunoassay or enzyme-linked immunosorbent assays (ELISA)[35,46]. Furthermore, CIg can be demonstrated in these cells at the ultrastructural level[47]. A full discussion of these findings will be found in a later section entitled Ig export. These tumours are also capable of responding to mitogens, growth factors and tumour promoting substances with acquisition of CIg and lymphoplasmacytoid features. Some aspects of this phenomenon will be discussed later in this chapter.

Conflicting results have come from attempts to correlate phenotypic expression of Ig in CLL with prognosis. In the series studied by Hamblin and colleagues[33] patients with neoplastic cells expressing SIgM κ present at Binet stage A[48] and have a longer acturial survival. These data suggest that SIgM κ is a characteristic associated with the more benign cases of CLL. While the syndrome of benign CLL is recognized by many authors, other reported series do not confirm this phenotypic association[49,50]. Differences between these reports will arise from the type of referral centre involved in the study, patients' age and the number of patients phenotyped. In the studies reported by Hamblin et al.[33] and Jayaswal et al.[32] a bias towards the more severe cases seen in series from tertiary referral centres, has been avoided. Both of these studies suggest that patients with undetectable SIg or with SIgM and IgD positive tumours have more aggressive disease then those cases expressing SIgM alone.

A varient of CLL, prolymphocytic leukaemia, often presents with spleno-megaly and is characterized by large cells with diffuse chromatin and a prominent nucleolus[51]. The neoplastic cells usually express dense SIgM. This leukaemia may present *de novo* or results from transformation of existing CLL and is refractory to treatment. The increase in SIg intensity associated with this cell type compared with CLL, is suggestive evidence for its more mature cell of origin and where it is preceded by CLL, an example of clonal differentiation[52].

Another variant, hairy cell leukaemia (HCL), is distinguished morpholog-ically by large cells with fine surface projections, often accompanied at presentation by splenomegaly and pancytopenia or monocytopenia: HCL is recognized as a distinct haematological and pathological entity[53]. The neoplastic cell shares morphological characteristics with lymphocytes and monocytes and in the past has caused considerable speculation over its origin. HCL can be shown to be of B-cell origin by Ig synthesis studies[54] and Ig gene rearrangement[55]. Many cases express SIgG and a high proportion express multiple heavy chain isotypes, but unlike CLL dual expression of SIgM and IgD occurs on a minority of cases. It is not uncommon to find surface expression of α and γ heavy chain isotypes together in this disease as well as the combinations $\alpha \gamma \delta$, $\alpha \mu \delta$ or $\alpha \gamma \mu \delta$[56]; however, it has not been clearly established whether all the isotypes expressed are of intrinsic origin, as the demonstration of monotypic SIg in this disease is notoriously difficult. The production of IgG by neoplastic cells in HCL can be unequivocally demonstrated in many cases expressing this isotype, suggesting an intrinsic origin[57]. Patients with neoplastic cells expressing heavy chain in combination with κ light chain have been reported to have a better prognosis than those expressing λ[56]. It is curious that this observation is similar to that reported for CLL.

LYMPHOPROLIFERATIVE DISEASES

Non-Hodgkin's lymphomas (NHL)

More than 80% of NHL are derived from B-cells and can be easily identified by their Ig phenotype (Figure 1). Current systems of classification relate morphology of neoplastic cells in NHL to normal patterns of differentiation and have been moderately successful in predicting T-, B- or histiocytic cell lineage. The classifications proposed by Lukes and Collins[23] and Lennert[9] are examples of this approach. In this chapter we have chosen to refer to the latter which is in common use in Southampton.

Routine histological and immunological assessment of 315 patients with proven NHL referred to the Southampton group of hospitals, revealed that 81% of these tumours were of B-cell origin, 12% of T-cell origin and the remaining 7% of histiocytic or uncertain origin. Histologically the B-cell tumours were represented by lymphocytic (19%) centroblastic/centrocytic (cb/cc) follicular (31%), cb/cc diffuse (12%), cb/cc follicular and diffuse (4%), cc diffuse (17%), cb diffuse (9%), immunoblastic (1%), lymphoblastic (3%) and immunocytoma (4%). For all tumours with cb, cc or cb/cc histology consistent with a B-cell origin[9] there was a 93% correlation between classification on morphology alone and B-cell immunophenotype.

Table 2 Histology and Ig phenotype of 202 cases of NHL

Histology	SIg Ig Heavy chain isotype									κ/λ ratio	Total	*CIg
	μ	$\mu+\delta$	$\mu+\gamma$	$\mu+\delta+\gamma$	δ	$\delta+\gamma$	γ	α	$\alpha+\delta+\gamma$			
Lymphocytic	16	20	2	1	1	0	5	0	0	2.1	46	2
φCentroblastic/ centrocytic (follicular)	22	11	8	2	2	1	7	1	2	1.9	56	4
Centroblastic/ centrocytic (diffuse)	16	4	2	0	0	0	4	0	0	1.2	26	4
Centroblastic/ centrocytic (follicular and diffuse)	3	1	0	0	0	0	1	0	0	0.7	5	0
Centrocytic	12	9	1	0	0	0	1	0	0	0.8	23	1
Centroblastic	21	4	2	0	0	0	2	0	0	1.9	29	2
Immunoblastic	3	1	0	1	0	0	1	0	0	1.0	6	3
Lymphoblastic	1	0	2	1	0	0	0	0	1	1.5	5	1
Immunocytoma	2	0	2	0	0	0	1	1	0	†	6	6

* Number of cases in which CIg was detected in 10–100% of the tumour cell population
φ Five cases of B-cell type not included in table, failed to express SIg or CIg
† All κ

Two hundred and two of the B-cell tumours were fully phenotyped for Ig heavy and light chain class and the data are given in Table 2. 82% of all tumours express IgM, 30% express SIgD, 23% express SIgG and 2% express SIgA. These percentages add up to more than 100% as many tumours expressed more than one SIg heavy chain isotype, however 47% of the tumours expressed SIgM alone, 25% expressed SIgM + IgD and 12% expressed SIgG alone. The SIg heavy chain phenotype of this tumour series is comparable with that reported recently by Kvaloy et al.[58] Similarly, the ratio of 1.39 for the SIg κ/λ light chain expression by the tumours in our study is comparable with the reported ratio of 1.58 by this group. We, like others[59], found SIg κ/λ ratio inversion for centrocytic but not for lymphocytic NHL[58].

Diffuse CIg positive neoplastic cells, detectable by conventional microscopy of labelled antibody stained preparation, were found in six out of six cases of immunocytoma and three out of six cases of immunoblastic NHL (Table 2). CIg positive cells occurred infrequently in FCC and lymphocytic NHL. In lymphocytic NHL, the presence of CIg was characterized by weak diffuse staining and absence of paraproteinaemia. In other lymphoma groups the presence of CIg did not always occur in the majority of cells and was occasionally associated with a paraproteinaemia. In this lymphoma study CIg was of either IgM or IgG class and corresponded to the SIg type of the tumour cell population; the variable occurrence of CIg positive cells reflects the heterogeneity within the tumour population as well as between tumours of the same histology.

Lymphocytic NHL

These tumours are thought to derive from either early immature resting B-cells or 'memory' B-cells following activation by antigen. They are analogous to CLL, and like CLL display similar expression of SIg heavy chain isotypes, dual expression of μ and δ being the most common and found on 44% of cases investigated; a small group (10%) express SIgG presumably reflecting the heterogeneity of the cell of origin in this disease (Table 2). These data are comparable with those reported for the CLL group (Table 1) and with other reported series[58,60]. Similar to the findings in CLL, the occurence of readily detectable CIg is rare (Table 2, reference 61) and the density of SIg on the majority of lymphocytic lymphoma cells is weak and of the order of 25% of that found on NHL cells of follicle centre cell type[61].

Follicle centre cell NHL

Cells of the follicle centre represent antigenically stimulated B-cells at an intermediate stage of differentiation and are histologically recognizable as a mixture of centroblasts and centrocytes in the *Kiel* classification[9]. Proliferations of this tumour type may occur with a diffuse or follicular growth pattern or occasionally as a mixture of both. These lymphomas express SIgM, IgD, IgA and IgG either alone or in combination, furthermore more than 70% of lymphomas expressing SIgG occur as proliferations of follicle centre cells (FCC) (Table 2). These data are consistent with the previously observed heterogeneity within this group of tumours[58,60] and provide further evidence that heavy chain class switching from μ to γ may be an important feature of this cell type[62].

Follicular proliferations of FCC lymphoma predominantly express SIgM (39% cases) and fewer cases (20%) express SIgM and IgD when compared with lymphocytic NHL (Table 2). SIgA was not commonly expressed in our series or in that reported by Kvaloy[58]. This isotype was expressed by one case of cb/cc follicular and together with δ and γ isotypes by a further two cases of this tumour type and by one case of lymphoblastic NHL (Table 2). These data are further examples of multiple isotype expression by neoplastic cells, a phenomenon shared by a small number of resting B-cell tumours.

We have recently reported five cases of cb/cc follicular NHL that failed to express detectable SIg or CIg; the B-cell nature of these tumours was demonstrated by Ig synthesis, Ig gene rearrangement and by monoclonal antibody staining[63]. In our series these Ig negative tumours represent 5% of all tumours of cb/cc follicular histology. A similar incidence has been reported by Tubbs and co-workers[64] who found one Ig negative cb/cc follicular NHL in a series of 53 cases examined. Several studies of reactive and neoplastic tissue have shown that follicle centre cells are either SIg or CIg positive[65]. It is, therefore, unexpected to find Ig negative tumours of this histology. While Ig negative B-cell CLL is thought to derive from an early B-cell we have no evidence that this is the case for Ig negative cb/cc follicular NHL. These tumours may represent a separate developmental lineage of B-lymphocytes within follicle centres or asynchrony between Ig expression and homing to sites of B-cell development. Alternatively, failure to express Ig by the majority of the neoplastic cells may arise as a consequence of an acquired defect in production by mechanisms similar to that observed in light chain myeloma, by aberrant Ig gene rearrangement or by factors unknown.

Diffuse FCC lymphomas represent a more aggressive phase of this tumour type, however, the histology of this group does not always correlate with a B-cell immunological phenotype. In our series of 315 patients, 7% of patients with this histology proved on immunological testing to have a T-cell NHL. The expression of heavy chain Ig isotypes by the B-cell cb/cc diffuse tumours was similar to that expressed by those with a follicular growth pattern (Table 2), an observation consistent with published data[58,60]. In cb and cb/cc diffuse and cb/cc follicular NHL the ratio of tumours bearing surface heavy chain in combination with κ light chain compared with those expressing λ was 1.9:1, 1.2:1 and 1.9:1, respectively (Table 2). The inverse ratio of 0.8:1 (Table 2) exhibited by cc NHL appears to be a well documented phenomenon[58,59].

Tumours of cc diffuse histology express predominantly surface μ and $\mu + \delta$ heavy chain isotypes. This pattern of expression is similar to that seen in tumours of cb/cc histology but the strength of staining is uniformly dense (Table 2, reference 65). In other series SIgD has not been found to be a major surface isotype[59]. Some authors regard cc diffuse NHL as a separate entity[59,65], which carries a more unfavourable prognosis than other FCC lymphomas; however, its Ig phenotype does not allow us to make this distinction[9].

In the Kiel classification centroblasts are thought to represent a transitional cell type between lymphocytes and centrocytes[9], however the SIg phenotype of cb NHL does not reflect this transition. These tumours predominantly express SIgM and fewer of these cases express both $\mu + \delta$ heavy chain isotypes compared with cc diffuse lymphomas (Table 2, references 58, 66).

In normal reactive tissue B-cells bearing SIgD with SIgM are found predominantly in the interfollicular area and mantle zone. These cells can also be found in primary follicles with subsequent loss of SIgD on the formation of secondary follicles[65,67]. While the neoplastic data suggest that SIgD appears on fewer tumours of FCC origin than lymphocytic NHL/CLL, the persistence of SIgD on neoplastic cells of NHL of FCC origin appears to contradict experimental evidence for expression of this isotype during a limited period of B-cell differentiation. In the study reported in Table 2, SIgD was often expressed at a lower density and on fewer cells than SIgM within each tumour population of FCC histology. This variability has been observed by others[61]. With the reservation that abnormal expression may arise from neoplastic transformation, the presence of cb/cc NHL clones that have maintained full or limited expression of IgD suggests that maturation pathways exist within follicle centres that are not commonly recognized. Alternatively variable expression of IgD within a tumour population may reflect tumour pleomorphism. Nevertheless, the presence of IgD on NHL of FCC origin suggests that this Ig class is not exclusively associated with immature or circulating cells, and, conversely, that the ability of cells to circulate is not solely dependent on expression of this Ig.

Immunoblastic NHL and immunocytoma

Tumours of this type may be associated with the entity of Waldenström's macroglobulinaemia and are thought to represent cells of mature or plasmacytoid cell origin, characterized by the presence of CIg and para-proteinaemia. Nevertheless, lymphomas with immunoblastic histology can be of T- or B-cell origin, and while the B-cell tumours predominantly express SIgM not all express CIg; furthermore, some of these B-cell tumours retain the capacity to express SIgD in association with IgM[58,66,68] (Table 2). The phenotypic heterogeneity of B-immunoblastic NHL has been compared with that within plasma cell tumours[69] and provides support for the suggestion that several different pathways of B-cell differentiation may give rise to plasma cells[70].

Lymphocytic lymphoma which has transformed to a high grade tumour of pleomorphic type is included within NHL of immunoblastic histology. This transformation, which is known as Richter's syndrome, is thought to be intraclonal[9], however a recent report indicates that this is not true of all cases[71]. The authors of this report describe a case where the transformed cells expressed a different Ig light chain from the co-existent lymphocytic tumour. Furthermore, DNA probes for Ig heavy chain revealed different rearrangement patterns in the two tumours. Further investigations of this type are required for clarification of this issue.

Neoplastic lymphoid cells in immunocytomas characteristically express SIg with readily detectable CIg. They represent a group of tumours exhibiting a

41

capacity for differentiation, many displaying an easily recognizable serum paraprotein. Within our series six tumours were fully phenotyped with respect to Ig (Table 2). All tumour populations included CIg positive lymphoplasmacytoid or plasma cells, but the phenotypes observed (Table 2) are not typical of those reported in the literature as many of these tumours also express SIgD and the κ/λ ratio does not appear to differ from that found for other NHL groups[9,58].

Lymphoblastic NHL

Lymphoblastic NHL comprised 5% of our lymphoma series. On immunological phenotyping the 17 cases were found to be of cALL (four cases), T-cell (six cases) or B-cell (seven cases) origin. While ALL and lymphoblastic NHL share many common features and are thought to represent different stages of a progressive disease, our data are consistent with the finding that T- and B-cell phenotypes of this disease are more commonly associated with tumour masses[72]. B-cell lymphoblastic NHL is characterized by the presence of SIg and absence of TdT and is derived from a more mature cell of origin than cALL. The five B-cell cases fully phenotyped for SIg expressed μ, γ, δ and α heavy chain isotypes (Table 2).

It is difficult to locate B-cell lymphoblastic NHL within the framework of B-cell differentiation (Figure 1). While these tumours have some features of Burkitt's lymphoma[30], Wright and Isaacson[73] believe they are histogenetically and clinically distinct and should be differentiated from this entity.

Plasma cell tumours: multiple myeloma

Plasmacytoma and myeloma represent tumours of effector B-cells characterized by the presence of malignant plasma cells, often associated with paraproteins in serum and/or Bence–Jones protein in urine. These plasma cell tumours have easily detectable CIg and do not usually express SIg. The nature of the clonogenic cell in myeloma is of considerable clinical importance since end-stage plasma cells might not be expected to proliferate rapidly, and there is some evidence that monoclonal B-lymphocytes expressing the same idiotype as the paraprotein are proliferating in the bone marrow of patients with myeloma[74]. Precursor B-cells have also been identified in the blood and marrow of some patients (reviewed in reference 74) and analysis of surface markers has suggested that such cells express the CALLA antigen[75]. Myeloma cells successfully established in culture can also expresss this antigen[76]. Thus an IgG secreting myeloma might be regarded as a differentiating B-cell tumour with cells expressing IgM, IgD and IgG of the same idiotype as the paraprotein[74]. Circulating B-cells may play a role in tumour spread and could be susceptible to regulatory signals.

BLOOD AND MARROW INVOLVEMENT IN NHL

It has been recognized for some time that immunological analysis of blood often reveals a subclinical leukaemia in many patients with NHL[77]. In a series of 95 cases of NHL we found that 44% had immunological detectable disease in the blood compared with haematological detection in 8% of these patients[78]. These findings are consistent with a recent report by Johnson[79]. Similarly, lymphoma detection in marrow aspirates can also be significantly improved by the application of immunological techniques. In our series 55% of patients with NHL had detectable marrow involvement compared with cytological and histological detection in 35% of these cases. These data reflect the wide dissemination of disease in the majority of patients with NHL. Blood involvement in the absence of immunologically involved marrow was an uncommon finding and was usually found in patients with mucosal associated lymphoma, reflecting the localized growth pattern associated with this tumour type[78,80].

The detection of peripheral circulating tumour cells with anti-idiotypic antibodies will be discussed later in this chapter, however an innovative approach has recently been described by Hu and colleagues[81]. These workers describe the use of gene rearrangement patterns for the detection of tumour involvement. This technique carried out on extracted DNA will not detect individual cell involvement, but will detect the presence of a proportion of neoplastic cells as low as 1%.

Ig GENE REARRANGEMENTS IN NHL

Ig gene rearrangements occur early in B-cell differentiation and are distinctive markers of B-cell lineage, clonality and differentiation status[4]. They have proved useful in the analysis of ALL, HCL and for NHL of indeterminate origin[4,28,82]. Nevertheless, investigation of both T- and B-cell NHL often reveals a dual genotypic pattern with tumours exhibiting both rearrangement of the T-cell receptor β chain gene and the J region of the heavy chain locus[83,84]. Approximately 10% of NHL exhibit this mixed rearrangement pattern which is more frequent among tumours of B- rather than T-cell origin. Despite this occurence tumours always display a B- or T-cell pheno-type, suggesting that this dual genotype may reflect a concomitant activation of common molecular mechanisms regulating the rearrangement of these loci[83].

IMMUNOGLOBULIN EXPORT

The export of Ig is usually associated with plasma or plasmacytoid cells and actively secreting cells can be identifed by the presence of CIg. The secretory process involves the packaging of Ig into vesicles in the Golgi apparatus and discharge of these vesicles by exocytosis. It is not generally recognized that the majority of resting and responding B-lymphocytes are also capable of exporting small but detectable amounts of Ig, and the presence of mRNA for both surface and secreted forms of Ig has been demonstrated in early B-cell lines[85].

In vitro studies of neoplastic cell Ig biosynthesis and secretion in this laboratory revealed that the majority (>90%) of B-cell tumours are capable

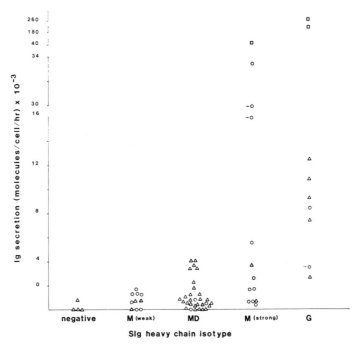

Figure 2 Correlation of tumour cell Ig export with SIg heavy chain isotype [Δ CLL, ○ NHL (→ ○ cb diffuse NHL), □ Immunocytoma]

of synthesizing and exporting free Ig light chains[46,86]. This finding was most pronounced in tumours of early B-cells including CLL and its variants[87]. This secretion of free monotypic light chains by cell populations from patients with CLL and NHL can lead to the presence of monoclonal light chains in urine, where they can serve as useful tumour markers and should be routinely looked for by sensitive methods such as isoelectric focusing where lymphocytic disease is included in the differential diagnosis[88].

Direct studies of the secretory capacity of cells from patients with CLL and NHL using ELISA revealed that the majority (13 out of 19 cases of CLL and 17 out of 24 cases of NHL) also secreted small amounts of pentameric IgM[86]. These low levels of secretion have been confirmed by others[89] and the presence of intracellular IgM in cells from such patients has been detected using immunoelectronmicroscopy[47,90]. A tendency of CLL cells to secrete more free light chain and less IgM than NHL was noted, but there was considerable heterogeneity in both groups. There was no clear trend relating secretory capacity to surface Ig expression until either the surface IgM was strong or the class expressed was IgG. For both these groups, which include neoplasms corresponding to more mature B-lymphocytes, the secretion of whole Ig was increased (Figure 2), and although the quantity of light chain synthesized remains similar, the ratio of free light chains to whole Ig in the extracellular fluid falls (Figure 3). In the group of tumours which express IgM and IgD at the cell surface (Figure 3) the ratio is very variable, consistent with the

44

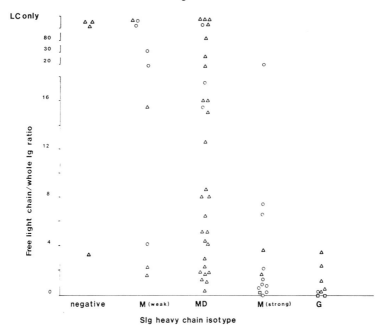

Figure 3 Correlation of tumour cell free light chain and whole Ig export (expressed as a molar ratio of light chain dimers to whole Ig monomers) with SIg heavy chain isotype. [Symbols as for Figure 2]

concept that tumours of this type represent an intermediate stage of B-cell differentiation[87,91]. In these studies, NHL of FCC origin also exhibited considerable heterogeneity with respect to total Ig production and to the ratio of free light chain to whole Ig. This heterogeneity supports the view that centrocytes may precede or follow centroblasts in B-cell maturation[92] rather than centroblasts always preceding centrocytes as suggested in the Kiel classification[9].

These findings are reflected by *in vitro* models of tumour maturation; exposure of normal or CLL cells to mitogens or phorbol ester results in the amplification of IgM production while the levels of free light chain export remain remarkably constant[45] so that the excess of light chain compared with whole Ig production is decreased[93].

Molecular analysis of the Ig produced by neoplastic B-cells from patients with CLL and NHL revealed the IgM to be in the pentameric form, and in several cases the tumour origin was confirmed by the use of anti-idiotypic antibodies[35]. Cells from a minority of patients also exported small amounts of IgD, and in most cases secretion was associated with the presence of λ chain[94], as found previously for IgD-secreting myeloma[95]. Whether secreted Ig arises from all cells within the clone or from a small number of more differentiated plasmacytoid cells has not been resolved[45], but minor populations of the latter were not found in the CLL and NHL patients investigated[35,94].

We have also observed the synthesis and export of free heavy chain by neoplastic and normal cells[96,97]. The neoplastic cells from a case of FCC-NHL were found to express free μ chains and could be demonstrated by biosynthetic studies to produce both μ and γ chains. In follow-up studies free γ, but not μ, chain could be found at the cell surface. These data suggest a heavy chain class switch in the absence of light chain expression and await more detailed studies on neoplastic and normal cells for the evaluation of their significance in normal B-cell differentiation[45,97]. Godal and colleagues have also reported a case of lymphoma expressing γ chains without light chains at the cell surface[98].

Heavy chain class switching in a lymphoma expressing SIgM has been observed by biosynthetic studies of an isolated case[99]. In this case there was evidence for dual synthesis of IgM and IgG by the neoplastic cell population.

IDIOTYPIC Ig AS A TUMOUR MARKER

Since most neoplastic B-cell populations secrete small amounts of idiotypic Ig, there is the potential for measuring levels of such soluble idiotypic Ig in the serum. This is effectively a tumour-specific marker and provides an objective measure of disease activity. Its use in a patient is illustrated in Figure 4: the patient presented with cb/cc follicular NHL which after initial chemotherapy relapsed with a marked leukaemic blood overspill. Following further treat-

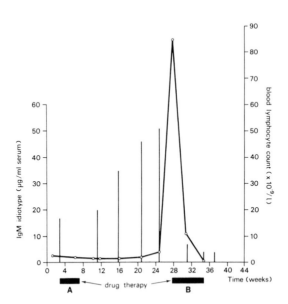

Figure 4 Levels of idiotypic IgM in the serum of patient Gol during two treatments with chemotherapy. (——O——) blood lymphocyte count ($\times 10^{-9}$ / l); vertical lines, idiotype IgM (μg/ml serum). Treatment consisted of **A**, adriamycin, 6-thioguanine and cytosine arabinoside; **B**, chlorambucil and prednisolone

ment the disease was characterized by long periods of apparent remission followed by relapse with increasing anaemia and a sudden increase in the blood white cell count presumably due to release of tumour cells from the bone marrow, since tumour cells could be shown to increase in this compartment prior to the blood. The graph shows such an episode following an ineffective and then an effective drug schedule and gives the levels of idiotypic IgM found in the serum over a period of 35 weeks (vertical bars). After the first drug combination (A) there seemed to be a good clinical remission, but we were surprised to find a continuing increase in idiotypic IgM in the serum. By week 20, anaemia was developing and tumour cells were found in large numbers in the blood at week 28. The patient was then given a different drug combination (B) and once again went into clinical remission. On this occasion, however, the idiotype levels fell and remission was maintained.

Methods for raising monoclonal anti-idiotypic antibodies have been described previously[78], but the approach has the disadvantage that a new antibody will be required for each patient. Recently we have examined antibodies which show specificity for the less private, cross-reacting idiotypes of Ig. These will recognize more than one lymphoma and by constructing a panel of such antibodies it should be possible to use them for monitoring disease in a range of patients. Another range of anti-idiotypic antibodies can be produced by using the urinary monoclonal light chains as immunogens. Preparation of these tumour-derived light chains from urine is relatively simple and antibodies raised against the idiotypic determinants have been found to recognize whole Ig on cell surfaces and in serum[100]. The use of anti-idiotypic antibodies as therapeutic agents for B-cell neoplasms has been reviewed recently[101] and will not be described here.

DIFFERENTIATION OF NEOPLASTIC CELL POPULATIONS

Neoplastic cells from ALL, CLL and NHL are able to undergo further differentiation in response to all or some of the following: B-cell growth factor, phorbol esters, T-cell factors, anti-Ig and interferon. For recent reviews on the subject the reader is referred to Zola[102] and Gordon[45].

CONCLUSIONS

In extensive studies of leukaemia and lymphoma Ig has proven to be a valuable marker of B-cell origin and clonality. Following Ig gene rearrangements, which are the earliest events in the commitment of cells to the B-cell lineage, Ig may be inserted into the membrane or exported. In most B-cells both processes are operative. In tumours of 'early' B-cells such as CLL, the neoplastic cells either express weak SIg or are SIg negative, fail to express significant CIg and export small amounts of Ig, which is often exclusively Ig light chain. Tumours of follicle centre cell origin express strong SIg with or without CIg while myeloma plasma cells are SIg negative and contain large amounts of CIg. In parallel with this observation maximum Ig export is

47

observed in myeloma. All Ig expressing tumours show Ig light chain restriction and the κ/λ ratio is consistent with the expected ratio of 2:1 with the exception of cc diffuse lymphoma in which the neoplastic cells predominantly express λ. The most commonly expressed Ig heavy chain isotype is μ. Ig heavy chain isotype expression does not relate to disease type and multiple expression of isotypes often occurs, in particular μ plus δ. Ig expressed by B-lymphocytic tumours carries clonal idiotypic determinants specific for that tumour. Anti-idiotypic antibodies raised to these determinants can be used for therapy or monitoring tumour load either by recognition of tumour cells bearing these determinants or by quantitation of secreted idiotypic Ig or fragments in serum or urine.

References

1. Honjo, T. (1983). Immunoglobulin genes. *Annu. Rev. Immunol.,* **1**, 499
2. Raff, M. C., Megson, M., Owen, J. J. T. and Cooper, M. D. (1976). Early production of intracellular IgM by B lymphocytic precursors in mouse. *Nature,* **259**, 224
3. Janossy, G., Bollum, F. J., Bradstock, K. F., McMichael, A., Rapson, N. and Greaves M. F. (1979). Terminal deoxynucleotidyl transferase positive cells in normal bone marrow have the antigenic phenotype of acute lymphoblastic leukaemia cells. *J. Immunol.,* **123**, 1525
4. Korsmeyer, S. J., Hieter, P. A., Sharrow, S. O., Goldman, S. K., Leden, P. and Waldman, T. A. (1982). Normal human B cells display ordered light chain gene rearrangements and deletions. *J. Exp. Med.,* **156**, 975
5. Hamblin, T. J., Abdul-Ahad, A. K., Gordon, J., Stevenson, F. K. and Stevenson, G. T. (1980). Preliminary experience in treating lymphocytic leukaemia with antibody to immunoglobulin idiotypes on the cell surfaces. *Br. J. Cancer,* **42**, 495
6. Miller, R. A., Maloney, D. G., Warnke, R. and Levy, R. (1982). Treatment of B-cell lymphoma with monoclonal anti-idiotype antibody. *N. Engl. J. Med.,* **306**, 517
7. Williamson, A. R. (1976). The biological origin of antibody diversity. *Annu. Rev. Biochem.,* **45**, 467
8. Gordon, J., Abdul-Ahad, A. K., Hamblin, T. J., Stevenson, F. K. and Stevenson, G. T. (1984). Mechanisms of tumor cell escape encountered in treating lymphocytic leukaemia with anti-idiotypic antibody. *Br. J. Cancer,* **49**, 547
9. Lennert, K., Mohri, N., Stein, H., Kaiserling, E. and Muller-Hermelink, H. K. (1978). *Malignant Lymphomas other than Hodgkin's Disease,* (Berlin: Springer-Verlag)
10. Gearhart, P. J. and Cebra, J. J. (1981). Most B cells that have switched surface immunoglobulin isotypes generate clones of cells that do not secrete IgM. *J. Immunol.,* **127**, 1030
11. Raffeld, M., Neckers, L., Longo, D. L. and Cossman, J. (1985). Spontaneous alteration of idiotype in a monoclonal B cell lymphoma. *N. Engl. J. Med.,* **312**, 1653
12. Meeker, T. C., Lowder, J., Cleary, M., Stewart, S., Warnke, R., Sklar, J. and Levy, R. (1985). Emergence of idiotype variants during treatment of B-cell lymphoma with anti-idiotype antibodies. *N. Engl. J. Med.,* **312**, 1658
13. Gathings, W. E., Lawton, A. R. and Cooper, M. D. (1977). Immunofluorescent studies of the development of pre-B cells, B lymphocytes and immunoglobulin isotype diversity in humans. *Eur. J. Immunol.,* **7**, 804
14. Gearhart, P. J., Hurwitz, J. L. and Cebra, J. J. (1980). Successive switching of antibody isotypes expressed within the lines of a B cell clone. *Proc. Natl. Acad. Sci. USA,* **77**, 5424
15. Kuritani, T. and Cooper, M. D. (1982). Human B cell differentiation. *J. Exp. Med.,* **155**, 839
16. Mayurri, M., Kuritani, T., Kubagawa, H. and Cooper, M. D. (1983). IgG subclass expression by human B lymphocytes and plasma cells: B lymphocytes precommited to IgG subclass can be preferentially induced by polyclonal mitogens with T cell help. *J. Immunol.,* **130**, 671
17. Liu, C. P., Tucker, P. W., Muchinsi, J. F. and Blattner, F. R. (1980). Mapping of heavy chain genes for mouse immunoglobulins M and D. *Science,* **209**, 1348

18. Obata, M., Kataoka, T., Nakai, S., Yamagishi, H., Takahashi, N., Yamawaki-Kataoka, Y., Nikaido, T., Shimizu, A. and Honjo, T. (1981). Structure of a rearranged γ_1 chain gene and its implication to immunoglobulin class switch mechanism. *Proc. Natl. Acad. Sci. USA*, **78**, 2437

19. Vogler, L. B. and Lawton, A. R. (1985). Ontogeny of B cells and humoral immune functions. *Clin. Immunol. Allergy*, **5**, 235

20. Korsnid, F. R. and Brandtzaeg, P. (1980). Immune systems of human nasopharyngeal and palatine tonsils: histomorphometry of lymphoid components and quantification of immunoglobulin producing cells in health and disease. *Clin. Exp. Immunol.*, **39**, 361

21. Brandzaeg, P. and Berdal, P. (1975). J chain in malignant human IgG immunocytes. *Scand J. Immunol.*, **4**, 403

22. Salsano, F., Froland, S. S., Natvig, J. B. and Michaelsen, T. E. (1974). Same idiotype of B lymphocyte membrane IgD and IgM. Formal evidence for monoclonality of chronic lymphocytic leukaemia cells. *Scand. J. Immunol.*, **3**, 841

23. Lukes, R. J. and Collins, R. D. (1974). Immunologic characterization of human malignant lymphomas. *Cancer*, **34**, 1488

24. Anderson, J., Buxbaum, J., Citronbaum, R., Douglas, S., Forni, L., Melchers, F., Pernis, B. and Stoff, D. (1974). IgM producing tumours in the BALBc mouse. A model for B cell maturation. *J. Exp. Med.*, **140**, 742

25. Greaves, M. F., Delia, D., Robinson, J., Sutherland, R. and Newman, R. (1981). Exploration of monoclonal antibodies: A 'who's who' of haematopoetic malignancy. *Blood Cells*, **7**, 757

26. Vogler, L. B., Crist, W. M., Bockman, D. E., Pearl, E. R., Lawton, A. R. and Cooper M. D. (1978). Pre B cell leukaemia. *N. Engl. J. Med.*, **298**, 872

27. Kubagawa, H., Mayumi, M., Crist, W. M. and Cooper, M. D. (1983). Immunoglobulin heavy chain switching in pre-B leukaemias. *Nature*, **301**, 340

28. Korsmeyer, S. J., Arnold, A., Bakhashi, A., Ravetch, J. V., Sibenlist, U., Hieter, P. A., Sharrow, S. O., Le Bien, T. W., Kersey, J. H., Poplack, D. G., Leder, P. and Waldmann, T. A. (1983). Immunoglobulin gene rearrangement and cell surface antigen expression in acute lymphocytic leukaemias of T cell and B cell precursor origins. *J. Clin. Invest.*, **71**, 301

29. Bernard, A., Boumsell, L., Dausset, J., Milstein, C. and Schlossman, S. F. (eds). (1984). *Leukocyte Typing* (Berlin: Springer-Verlag)

30. Gralnick, H. R., Galton, D. A. G., Catovsky, D., Sultan, C. and Bennett, J. M. (1977). Classification of acute leukaemia. *Ann. Intern. Med.*, **87**, 740

31. Chen, Y. H. and Heller, P. (1978). Lymphocyte surface immunoglobulin density and immunoglobulin secretion *in vitro* in chronic lymphocytic leukaemia (CLL). *Blood*, **52**, 601

32. Jayaswal, U., Roath, S., Hyde, R. D., Chisholm, D. M. and Smith, J. L. (1977). Blood lymphocyte surface markers and clinical findings in chronic lymphoproliferative disorders. *Br. J Haematol.*, **37**, 207

33. Hamblin, T. J., Oscier, D. G., Gregg, E. O. and Smith, J. L. (1986). Cell markers in a large single centre series of CLL. *Br. J. Haematol.* (in press)

34. Flanegan, N. G., Ridway, J. C., Kozlowski, C. L. and Copsey, P. C. (1982). Clinical and immunological feature in patients with chronic lymphocytic leukaemia presenting in an area of high incidence. *Clin. Lab. Haematol.*, **4**, 343

35. Stevenson, F. K., Hamblin, T. J., Stevenson, G. T. and Tutt, A. L. (1980). Extracellular idiotypic immunoglobulin arising from human leukaemic B lymphocytes. *J. Exp. Med.*, **152**, 1484

36. Stevenson, F. K., Hamblin, T. J. and Stevenson, F. T. (1981). The nature of immunoglobulin G on the surface of B lymphocytes in chronic lymphocytic leukaemia. *J. Exp. Med.*, **154**, 1965

37. Ling, N. R. (1983). Immunoglobulin as a differentiation and clonal marker. *J. Immunol. Meth.*, **65**, 1.

38. Clarke, C., Rydell, R. R. and Kaplan, M. E. (1973). Frequent association of IgM with crystalline inclusions in chronic lymphocytic leukaemia. *N. Engl. J. Med.*, **289**, 113

39. Cawley, J. C., Smith, J. L., Goldstone, A. H., Emmines, J., Hamblin, T. and Hough, D. (1976). IgA and IgM cytoplasmic inclusions in a series of cases of chronic lymphocytic leukaemia. *Clin. Exp. Immunol.*, **23**, 78

40. Smith, J. L., Gordon, J., Newell, D. G. and Whisson, M. (1977). The biosynthesis and

characterization of unreleased IgM in a case of CLL. *Br. J. Haematol.*, **37**, 217
41. Berrebi, A., Talmor, M., Vorst, E., Rasnitzky, P. and Shtalnid, M. (1983). IgM lambda globular cytoplasmic inclusions in chronic lymphocytic leukaemia resembling immunocytoma. *Scand. J. Haemtol.*, **30**, 43
42. Nies, K. M., Marshall, J., Oberlin, M. A., Halpern, M. S. and Brown, J. C. (1976). Chronic lymphocytic leukaemia with gamma chain cytoplasmic inclusions. *Am. J. Clin. Pathol.*, **65**, 948
43. Bartolini, C., Flanini, G., Gentiloni, N., Barone, C., Gambassi, G. and Terranova, T. (1980). Non Hodgkin's lymphoma associated with double monoclonal immunoglobulin. *Acta Haematol.*, **63**, 49
44. Gordon, J., Smith, J. L., Newell, D., Chisholm, M., Corte, G., Warley, A. and Richardson, N. (1977). Biosynthesis and characterization of intracellular IgDκ in a case of CLL. *Clin. Exp. Immunol.*, **30**, 70
45. Gordon, J. (1984). Molecular aspects of immunoglobulin expression by human B cell leukaemias and lymphomas. *Adv. Cancer Res.*, **41**, 71
46. Gordon, J., Howlett, A. R. and Smith, J. L. (1978). Free light chain synthesis by neoplastic cells in chronic lymphocytic leukaemia and non Hodgkin's lymphoma. *Immunology*, **34**, 397
47. Newell, D. G., Hannam-Harris, A. C. and Smith, J. L. (1983). The ultrastructural location of immunoglobulin in chronic lymphocytic leukaemia cells: changes in light and heavy chain distribution induced by mitogen stimulation. *Blood*, **61**, 511
48. Binet, J. L., Catovsky, D., Chandra, P., Dighiero, G., Montserrat, E., Rai, K. K. and Sawitsky, A. (1981). Chronic lymphocytic leukaemia: Proposals for a revised prognostic staging system. Report from the International Workship on CLL. *Br. J. Haematol.*, **48**, 365
49. Caligaris-Cappio, F., Gobbi, M., Bergni, L., Campana, D., Lauria, F., Fierro, M. T. and Foa, R. (1984). B-chronic lymphocytic leukaemia patients with stable benign disease show distinctive membrane phenotype. *Br. J. Haematol.*, **50**, 655
50. Han, T., Ozer, H., Gavigan, M., Gajera, R., Minowada, J., Bloom, M. L., Sadomoni, N., Sandberg, A. A., Gomez, G. A. and Henderson, E. S. (1984). Benign monoclonal B cell lymphocytosis – a benign variant of CLL: clinical, immunoglobulin phenotypic and cytogenic studies in 20 patients. *Blood*, **64**, 244
51. Galton, D. A. G., Goldman, J. M., Wiltshaw, E., Catovsky, D., Henry, K. and Goldenberg, G. J. (1974). Prolymphocytic leukaemia. *Br. J. Haematol.*, **27**, 7
52. Ghani, A. M., Krause, J. R. and Brody, J. P. (1986). Prolymphocytic transformation of chronic lymphocytic leukaemia. A report of three cases and a review of the literature. *Cancer*, **57**, 75
53. Bouroncle, B. A., Wiseman, B. K. and Doan, C. A. (1958). Leukaemic reticuloendotheliosis. *Blood*, **13**, 609.
54. Gordon, J. and Smith, J. L. (1978). Free immunoglobulin light chain synthesis by neoplastic cells in leukaemic reticuloendotheliosis. *Clin. Exp. Immunol.*, **31**, 244
55. Korsmeyer, S. J., Greene, W. C., Cossman, J., Hsu Su-Ming, Neckers, L., Depper, J. M., Leonard, W. J., Jaffe, E. S. and Waldmann, J. A. (1983). Rearrangement and expression of immunoglobulin genes and expression of TAC antigen in hairy cell leukaemia. *Proc. Natl. Acad. Sci., USA*, **80**, 4522
56. Jansen, J., Schuit, H. R. E., Hermans, J. and Higmans, W. (1984). Prognostic significance of immunologic phenotype in hairy cell leukaemia. *Blood*, **63**, 1241
57. Cawley, J. C., Burns, G. F., Bevan, A., Worman, C. P., Smith, J. L., Gray, L., Barker, C. R. and Hayhoe, F. G. J. (1979). Typical hairy cell leukaemia with IgG κ paraproteinaemia. *Br. J. Haematol.*, **43**, 415
58. Kvaloy, S., Langholm, R., Kaalhus, O., Marton, P. F., Host, H. and Godal, T. (1985). Immunologic subsets in B cell lymphomas defined by surface immunoglobulin isotype and complement receptor – their relationship to survival. *Scand. J. Haematol.*, **35**, 137
59. Svedlow, S. H., Habeshaw, J. A., Murray, L. J., Dhaliwal, H. S., Lister, T. A. and Stanfeld, A. G. (1983). Centrocytic lymphoma: A distinct clinicopathologic and immunologic entity. A multiparameter study of 18 cases at diagnosis and relapse. *Am. J. Pathol.*, **113**, 181
60. Payne, S. V., Smith, J. L., Jones, D. B. and Wright, D. H. (1977). Lymphocyte markers in non-Hodgkin's lymphomas. *Br. J. Cancer*, **36**, 57

61. Godal, T., Lindmo, T., Marton, P. F., Landaas, T. O., Langholm, R., Hoie, J. and Abrahamsen, A. F. (1981). Immunological subsets in human B cell lymphomas. *Scand. J. Haematol.*, **14**, 481

62. Kraal, G., Weissman, I. L. and Butcher, E. C. (1981). Germinal centre B cells: antigen specificity and changes in heavy chain class expression. *Nature*, **298**, 377

63. Gregg, E. O., Al-Saffar, N., Jones, D. B., Wright, D. H., Stevenson, F. K. and Smith, J. L. (1984). Immonoglobulin negative follicle centre cell lymphoma. *Br. J. Cancer*, **50**, 735

64. Tubbs, R. R., Fishleder, A., Weiss, R. A., Savage, R. A., Sebek, B. A. and Weick, J. K. (1983). Immunohistologic cellular phenotypes of lymphoproliferative disorders. *Am. J. Pathol.*, **113**, 207

65. Stein, H., Gerdes, J. and Mason, D. Y. (1982). The normal and malignant germinal centre. *Clin. Haematol.*, **11**, 531

66. Porwit-Ksiazek, A., Christensson, B., Lindenmalm, C., Mellstedt, H., Tribukait, B., Biberfield, G. and Biberfield, P. (1983). Characterization of malignant and non neoplastic cell phenotypes in highly malignant non Hodgkin's lymphomas. *Int. J. Cancer*, **32**, 667

67. Sitia, R., Abbott and Hammerling, K. (1979). The ontogeny of B lymphocytes v. lipopolysaccharide induced changes of IgD expression on murine B lymphocytes. *Eur. J. Immunol.*, **9**, 859

68. Habershaw, J. A., Bailey, D., Stansfeld, A. G. and Greaves, M. F. (1983). The cellular content of non Hodgkin's lymphomas: A comprehensive analysis using monoclonal antibodies and other surface marker techniques. *Br. J. Cancer*, **47**, 327

69. Burns, G. F., Worman, C. P., Roberts, B. E., Raper, C. G. L., Barker, C. R. and Cawley, J. C. (1979). Terminal B cell development as seen in different human myelomas and related disorders. *Clin. Exp. Immunol.*, **35**, 180

70. Beiske, K., Rudd, E., Drack, A., Marton, P. F. and Godal, T. (1984). Induction of maturation of human B cell lymphomas *in vitro*. Morphologic changes in relation to immunoglobulin and DNA synthesis. *Am. J. Pathol.*, **115**, 362

71. van Dougen, J. J. M., Hovijkaas, H., Michiels, J. J., Grosveld, G., de Klein, A., van der Kwart Th. H., Prins, M. E. F., Abels, J. and Hagemayer, A. (1984). Richter's syndrome with different immunoglobulin light chains and different heavy chain gene rearrangements. *Blood*, **64**, 571

72. Crist, W. M., Kelly, D. R., Ragab, A. H., Roper, M., Dearth, J. C., Castleberry, R. P. and Flint, A. (1981). Predictive ability of Lukes Collins classification for immunological phenotypes of childhood non-Hodgkin's lymphoma. An institutional series and literature review. *Cancer*, **48**, 2070

73. Wright, D. H. and Isaacson, P. G. (1984). Biopsy pathology of the lymphoreticular system. (London: Chapman and Hall)

74. Mellstedt, H., Holm, G., Pettersson, D. and Peest, D. (1982). Idiotype-bearing lymphoid cells in plasma cell neoplasia. *Clin. Haematol.*, **11**, 65

75. Caligaris-Cappio, F., Tesio, L., Bergui, L., Malavasi, F., Campana, D. and Janossy, G. (1985). Characterization of CALLA and malignant plasma cell precursors. In Radl. J., Hymans, W., van Camp, B. (eds) *Topics in Ageing Research in Europe*, vol. 5, p. 119. (Rijswijk: Eurage)

76. Durie, B. G. M. and Grogan, R. M. (1985). CALLA-positive myeloma: an aggressive subtype with poor survival. *Blood*, **66**, 229

77. Garre, H. J. V., Scarffe, J. H. and Newton, R. K. (1979). Abnormal peripheral blood lymphocytes and bone marrow infiltration in non Hodgkin's lymphoma. *Br. J. Haematol.*, **42**, 4

78. Stevenson, G. T., Smith, J. L. and Hamblin, T. J. (1983). *Immunological investigation of lymphoid neoplasms*. (Edinburgh: Churchill Livingstone)

79. Johnson, A., Cavallin-Stahl, E. and Akerman, M. (1985). Flow cytometric light chain analysis of peripheral blood lymphocytes in patients with non Hodgkin's lymphoma. *Br. J. Cancer*, **52**, 159

80. Herbert, A., Wright, D. H., Isaacson, P. G. and Smith, J. L. (1984). Primary malignant lymphoma of the lung. Histopathology and Immunology of 9 cases. *Hum. Pathol.*, **15**, 415

81. Hu, E. Thompson, J., Horning, S., Trela, M., Lowder, J., Levy, R. and Sklar, J. (1985). Detection of B cell lymphoma in peripheral blood by DNA hybridization. *Lancet*, **2**, 1092

82. Cleary, M. I., Chao, J., Warnke, R. and Sklar, J. (1984). Immunoglobulin gene rearrange-

ment as a diagnostic criterion of B cell lymphoma. *Proc. Natl. Acad. Sci., USA,* **81**, 593
83. Pellicci, P., Knowles, D. M. and Favera, R. D. (1985). Lymphoid tumours displaying gene rearrangements of both immunoglobulin and T cell receptor genes. *J. Exp. Med.,* **162**, 1015
84. O'Connor, N. J., Weatherall, D. J., Feller, A. C., Jones, D., Pallesen, G., Stein, H., Wainscoat, J. S., Gatter, K. C., Isaacson, P., Lennert, K., Ramsey, A. and Wright, D. H. (1985). Analysis of gene rearrangement in the diagnosis of T cell lymphoma. *Lancet,* **1**, 1295
85. Perry, R. P. and Kelley, D. E. (1979). Immunoglobulin messenger RNAs in murine cell lines that have characteristics of immature B cells. *Cell,* **18**, 1333
86. Stevenson, F. K., Gregg, E. O., Smith, J. L. and Stevenson, G. T. (1984). Secretion of immunoglobulin by neoplastic B lymphocytes from lymph nodes of patients with lymphoma. *Br. J. Cancer,* **50**, 579
87. Hannam-Harris, A. C., Gordon, J. and Smith, J. L. (1980). Immunoglobulin synthesis by neoplastic B lymphocytes: Free light chain synthesis as a marker of B cell differentiation. *J. Immunol.,* **125**, 2177
88. Stevenson, F. K., Spellerberg, M. and Smith, J. L. (1983). Monoclonal immunoglobulin light chain in urine of patients with B lymphocytic disease: its source and use as a diagnostic aid. *Br. J. Cancer,* **47**, 607
89. Johnstone, A. P., Jensenius, J. C., Millard, R. E. and Hudson, L. (1982). Mitogen-stimulated immunoglobulin production by chronic lymphocytic leukaemic lymphocytes. *Clin. Exp. Immunol.,* **47**, 697
90. Yasuda, N., Kanoh, T., Shirakawa, S. and Uchin, H. (1982). Intracellular immunoglobulin in lymphocytes from patients with chronic lymphocytic leukaemia: an immunoelectron microscopic study. *Leuk. Res.,* **6**, 659
91. Gregg, E. O. (1984). Immunoglobulin production by neoplastic human B lymphocytes. *PhD Thesis,* University of Southampton
92. Hannam-Harris, A. C., Gordon, J., Wright, D. H. and Smith, J. L. (1982). Correlation between Ig synthesis patterns and lymphoma classification. *Br. J. Cancer,* **46**, 167
93. Hannam-Harris, A. C. and Smith, J. L. (1981). Induction of balanced immunoglobulin chain synthesis in free light chain producing lymphocytes by mitogen stimulation. *J. Immunol.,* **126**, 1848
94. Stevenson, F. K., Stevenson, G. T. and Tutt, A. L. (1982). The export of immunoglobulin D by neoplastic B lymphocytes. *J. Exp. Med.,* **156**, 337
95. Pernis, B., Governa, D. and Rowe, D. S. (1969). Light chain types in plasma cells that produce IgD. *Immunology,* **16**, 685
96. Hannan-Harris, A. C. and Smith, J. L. (1981). Free immunoglobulin light chain synthesis by foetal liver and cord blood lymphocytes. *Immunology,* **43**, 417
97. Gordon, J., Hamblin, T. J., Smith, J. L., Stevenson, F. K. and Stevenson, G. T. (1981). A human B cell lymphoma synthesizing and expressing surface μ chain in the absence of detectable light chain. *Blood,* **58**, 552
98. Godal, T., Lindmo, T., Marton, P. F., Landaas, T. O., Langholm, R., Hoie, J. and Abrahamsen, A. F. (1981). Immunological subsets in human B cell lymphomas. *Scand. J. Immunol.,* **14**, 481
99. Gordon, J. and Smith, J. L. (1980). Immunoglobulin synthesis by neoplastic cells: models of a clonal transformation from IgM to IgG synthesis. *J. Clin. Pathol.,* **331**, 539
100. Tutt, A. L., Stevenson, F. K., Smith, J. L. and Stevenson, G. T. (1983). Antibodies against urinary light chain idiotypes as agents for detection and destruction of human neoplastic B lymphocytes. *J. Immunol.,* **131**, 3058
101. Stevenson, F. K. and Stevenson, G. T. (1986). Therapeutic strategies for B cell malignancies involving idiotype–anti-idiotype interactions. *Intern. Rev. Immunol.,* **1**, 303
102. Zola, H. (1985). Differentiation and maturation of human B lymphocytes. A review. *Pathology,* **17**, 365

52

5
Immunoenzymatic Analysis of Haematological and Cytological Preparations

A. K. GHOSH and W. N. ERBER

INTRODUCTION

The cytological evaluation of peripheral blood and bone marrow smears contributes a major part in the diagnosis and management of patients with haematological disorders. Lymphomas and leukaemias may also be complicated by pleural and peritoneal effusions. A cytological examination of serous fluid often clarifies a diagnosis which would otherwise be obscure. However, in many cases it is difficult even for the experienced haematologist or cytologist to make a differential diagnosis on morphological criteria alone. The introduction in the early 1970s of immunocytochemical techniques for studying cellular antigens has proved of great value in the diagnosis and classification of haematological neoplasms. More recently, the appearance of monoclonal antibodies (Mab) which could precisely define lymphoid antigens and be used to generate immunoenzyme labelling techniques have extended the scope of immunocytochemical methods.

Initially these investigations were based on the use of immunofluorescent procedures applied to cells in suspension. This approach precludes the simultaneous visualization of most morphological detail. The full potential of immunocytochemical techniques in the assessment of haematological disorders can only be realized if there is simultaneous evaluation of the morphological appearance of positive and negative cell populations. This is also of importance in studying bone marrow trephine samples where it is necessary to visualize marrow architecture[1].

In this chapter we describe our experience with immunoenzymatic techniques in the analysis of lymphoid neoplasms in haematological and cytological preparations. We have used techniques that combine optimal visualization of morphological detail with labelling of cellular antigens by monoclonal antibodies and applied these to peripheral blood samples, bone marrow smears, trephine biopsies and serous effusions. These techniques can be readily applied in routine haematological and cytological laboratories. As the methods used are not yet widely applied, the technical aspects of immuno-cytochemistry will be considered first. The technical problems facing the haematologist and cytologist are similar and will be discussed together.

TECHNICAL ASPECTS OF IMMUNOENZYMATIC STAINING

Monoclonal antibodies

Table 1 lists some of the monoclonal and polyclonal antibodies that can be used for the immunocytochemical analysis of haematological disorders. Monoclonal antibodies are preferred because of the greater specificity of their reactivity and consequent cleaner labelling pattern. In addition, hybridoma tissue culture supernatant is used in preference to ascitic fluid which contains contaminating polyclonal immunoglobulin and gives non-specific reactivity if used at high concentrations.

Immunocytochemical labelling techniques

Immunofluorescence, immunoperoxidase and immunoalkaline phosphatase techniques have all been widely used in the analysis of haematological samples and to a lesser extent cytological samples. The immunoenzymatic procedures, utilizing horseradish peroxidase and alkaline phosphatase, offer two major advantages for the analysis of haematological samples:

(1) The reaction product of the enzyme can be examined with a light microscope and enables simultaneous visualization of cellular detail and the antigen label;
(2) The immunoenzymatic reaction product is stable on storage enabling slides to be re-examined after a period of time.

Immunoperoxidase techniques have been used extensively in diagnostic pathology samples, but their limited use in haematology is primarily due to the presence of endogenous peroxidase in erythroid cells, granulocytes and monocytes. This endogenous enzyme activity gives rise to unwanted background staining that interferes with the interpretation of results and is difficult to block (by treatment with peroxidase inhibitors, e.g. methanol) without denaturing some antigens or distorting cellular morphology.

Recently, alkaline phosphatase labelling techniques have been found to overcome this problem. In contrast to endogeneous peroxidase, endogenous alkaline phosphatase survives poorly in fixed cell smears and tissue sections, and residual activity can be inhibited by levamisole without destroying either antigenicity or cellular morphology. In addition, the vivid red immuno-alkaline phosphatase reaction product is more easily seen than the immunoperox-idase reaction product, making the technique particularly suitable for labelling antigens in cell smears.

The majority of labelling procedures performed in the authors' laboratory on haematological and cytological samples have been by the alkaline phospha-

Table 1 Monoclonal and polyclonal antibodies used for labelling haematological and cytological samples

Antibody	CD no.	Specificity	Source
B Cell Markers			
DAKO-Pan B	CD22	B-cells	Dakopatts
Tu1	CD23	follicle mantle zone B cells	Dr A. Ziegler
DAKO-CALLA	CD10	CALLA	Dakopatts
DAKO-IgM		IgM	Dakopatts
DAKO-kappa		kappa light chains	Dakopatts
DAKO-lambda		lambda light chains	Dakopatts
T Cell Markers			
DAKO-T6	CD1	cortical thymocytes	Dakopatts
DAKO-T11	CD2	SRBC receptor (Pan T)	Dakopatts
UCHT1	CD3	Pan T	Dr P. Beverley
DAKO-T4	CD4	T-Helper/inducer	Dakopatts
DAKO-T1	CD5	Pan T	Dakopatts
DAKO-T2	CD7	Pan T	Dakopatts
DAKO-T8	CD8	T-suppressor/cytotoxic	Dakopatts
OKT10		T10	Ortho Diagnostics
Myelomonocytic Markers			
DAKO-macrophage		monocytes	Dakopatts
DAKO-p150, 95	CD11c	monocytes, neutrophils	Dakopatts
Myeloperoxidase[a]		myeloperoxidase	Dr I. Olsson
Platelet Markers			
DAKO-Gp1b		glycoprotein 1b	Dakopatts
C17		glycoprotein 111a	Dr P. Tetteroo
Miscellaneous			
CR3/43		HLA/DR	Dr D. Y. Mason
TdT[a]		terminal transferase	Supertechs
DAKO-EMA		epithelial membrane antigen (EMA)	Dakopatts
DAKO-LC	CD45	leukocyte common antigen	Dakopatts
HC2		hairy cells	Dr D. Posnett
B3/25	CD9	transferrin receptor	Dr I. Trowbridge
RER		rough endoplasmic reticulum	Dr G. Janossy
DAKO-ACT1	CD25	IL-2 receptor	Dakopatts
LICR.LON.R10		glycophorin A	Dr P. Edwards
AP-7/6/7		alkaline phosphatase	Dr D. Y. Mason
APAAP		alkaline phosphatase: anti-alkaline phosphatase	Dakopatts
Rabbit anti-mouse Ig[a]		rabbit anti-mouse Ig	Dakopatts
MR12/53		mouse anti-rabbit	Dr D. Y. Mason

[a] = polyclonal antisera

tase: anti-alkaline phosphatase technique (APAAP) (Figure 1). This method is very sensitive and enables small amounts of antigen to be detected. In addition, the sensitivity can be enhanced by repeating the second and third incubation stages (anti-mouse Ig and APAAP complexes) enabling the detection of antigens which are present at levels too low to be demonstrated by other methods.

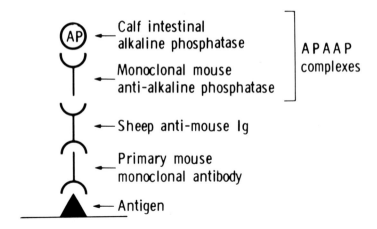

Figure 1 Schematic representation of the APAAP alkaline phosphatase; anti-alkaline phosphatase labelling procedure

Staining of cell smears

Most previous work on the detection of cellular antigens in haematological samples was primarily performed by immunofluorescent labelling procedures on living cells in suspension. These techniques suffer several drawbacks for their routine use in diagnostic haematology or cytology laboratories. These disadvantages include the necessity to label samples shortly after collection, the inability to visualize morphological detail of labelled and unlabelled cells and the impermanence of fluorescence preparations.

Immunocytochemical labelling techniques have been developed that enable cell smears, rather than cells in suspension to be labelled. Labelling of air-dried cell smears prepared from haematological or cytological samples offers considerable advantages over conventional immunofluorescent labelling in terms of practical convenience and with regard to the morphological detail that can be recognized.

Preparation of samples (see technical appendix)

Haematological samples

Immunocytochemical labelling can be performed on conventionally prepared blood and bone marrow smears, cytocentrifuged preparations of mononuclear cells, white-cell enriched preparations and cryostat sections of bone marrow trephines.

Cytological samples

Equally good results can be obtained with cytocentrifuge preparations or conventionally prepared cerebrospinal fluid (CSF) and cell aspirate smears. The

Table 2 Applications of immuno-enzymatic labelling in haematology

---

(1) *Lymphocyte enumeration*
  – analysis of normal white cell populations
  – assessment of abnormal T-cell subsets, e.g. AIDS
  – investigating lymphocytosis of unknown aetiology
  – diagnosis of congenital abnormalities of the immune system,
    e.g. Di George Syndrome

(2) *Diagnosis and classification of haematological neoplasms*
  – acute leukaemias
  – chronic leukaemias
  – myelomas

(3) *Detection of neoplastic cells in bone marrow aspirates*
  – e.g. carcinoma, rhabdomyosarcoma, neuroblastoma

(4) *Analysis of bone marrow trephines*

---

smears remain stable at room temperature for one week and for long periods (greater than one year) if stored unfixed at $-20°C$. The stability of the antigens in frozen cell smears enables positive control samples to be stored.

Interpretation of labelling

The interpretation of immunoenzymatic labelling is straightforward, but it is important to assess the staining reactions in conjunction with positive and negative controls. Positive controls are cell smears known to express a particular antigen, e.g. a known case of common ALL; and negative controls consist of slides from which the primary antibody has been omitted or replaced by buffer or an irrelevant Mab, (non-reactive). In fixed cell smears both surface membrane and intra-cellular antigens can be visualized (e.g. μ chains in pre-B cells). In many cases it is not possible to distinguish between these two types of labelling, but occasionally intracytoplasmic collections of antigen can be visualized that appear to be localized to one area, often the Golgi region. The detection of intracytoplasmic antigen may lead to a reassessment of the antigen profile of some haematological neoplasms as specific cellular antigens may be detected in the cytoplasm prior to their insertion into the plasma membrane (e.g. T-cell antigens in T-cell ALL).

APPLICATIONS OF IMMUNO-ENZYMATIC LABELLING IN DIAGNOSTIC HAEMATOLOGY

This section describes some of the practical applications of immunoenzymatic techniques that have been performed on haematological samples in the authors' laboratory using the APAAP immunoalkaline phosphatase[2] labelling technique (Table 2).

Lymphocyte enumeration

The major lymphoid cell populations (T-cells and their subsets and B-cells)

Table 3 Cellular origin of lymphocytes in cases of 'lymphocytosis of unknown aetiology'

| | Antigens detected | | | | | |
	T3 CD3	T1 CD5	T4 CD4	T8 CD8	HLA-DR	Pan B CD22
Reactive T-cells	+	+	+/−	+/−	+	−
B-CLL	−	+	−	−	+	+
T-CLL	+	+	+ or	+	−	−

can be readily identified in routinely prepared blood smears without preliminary white cell separation. This provides a convenient method for analysing the relative proportions of lymphoid cells in normal peripheral blood and in different disease states[3].

In *normal* blood samples a mean T-helper/suppressor ratio of 1.95 is obtained which agrees with previously published values obtained by immunofluorescence labelling of peripheral blood mononuclear cells in suspension[4,5]. In contrast, in patients with *infectious mononucleosis* a reversal of the T-helper/suppressor ratio can be detected, with a relative excess of HLA-DR positive T-suppressor cells[6-10]. This reversed T-helper/suppressor ratio can also be detected in patients with the *acquired immune deficiency syndrome*[3,11,12].

Enumeration of lymphoid populations in blood smears is a useful method for the assessment of patients with *lymphocytosis of unknown aetiology*. In

Table 4 Expression of cellular antigen in acute leukaemias

	CALL	B-ALL	T-ALL	AML	AMML	AMKL	AUL	ERYTHRO
No. of cases	57	1	12	24	28	12	7	1
ANTIGENS								
CD10	+	−	−/+	−	−	−	−	−
μ chain	−/+[1]	+	−	−	−	−	−	−
HLA-DR	+	+	−	+	+	+/−	+	+
CD22 (Pan B)	+	+	−	−	−	−	−	−
*TdT	+	−	+	−/(+)	−	−	+/−	−
CD7 (Pan T)	−	−	+	−/(+)	−	−	−	+
Myeloperoxidase	−	−	−	+	+	−	−	−
CD11c	−	−	−	+/−	+	−/+	−	−
Monocyte antigen	−	−	−	−	+	−	−	−
Platelet Gp IIIa	−	−	−	−	−	+	−	−
Glycophorin A	−	−	−	−	−	−	−	−

*	= Polyclonal antisera
1	= Intracytoplasmic μ chain in some cases of pre-B-ALL
Gp	= Glycoprotein
+	= All cases positive
+/−	= Majority of cases positive (>80%)
−/+	= Majority of cases negative (>80%)
−/(+)	= Very occasional cases positive (0–10%)
−	= All cases negative

these cases the cellular origin of the lymphoid cells can be established using a panel of anti-T-cell and anti-B-cell antibodies (Table 3), and whether the patient has a reactive lymphocytosis or an early stage of chronic lymphocyte leukaemia (CLL) can be determined.

Since the technique of labelling routinely prepared blood smears requires only a very small volume of blood (i.e. enough to make a smear), this method can be used in the diagnosis of congenital abnormalities of the immune system, such as *Di George syndrome*, where there is an absence of T-cells. In these cases a heel-prick blood sample is sufficient for the diagnosis to be established.

Classification of haematological neoplasms in cell smears

The majority of acute and chronic haematological neoplasms can be immuno-phenotyped by immunoalkaline phosphatase labelling peripheral blood and bone marrow smear preparations[13,14]. The details of the results obtained in immunophenotyping more than 250 cases of haematological neoplasm using the APAAP technique are detailed below and listed in Tables 4 and 5.

Acute leukaemias

Common acute lymphoblastic leukaemia (CALL)

All cases of CALL express the CALL antigen (CD10, CALLA) on the majority of blast cells, but the percentage of positive cells and the intensity of the label is very variable. HLA-DR is expressed in all cases and the CD19 and CD22 B-cell

Table 5 Classification of chronic haematological neoplasms by immunoenzymatic labelling

No. of cases	B-CLL 39	B-PLL 6	HCL 14	T-CLL 4	T-PLL 2	MYELOMA 25
ANTIGENS						
HLA-DR	+	+	+	–	–	–
CD22 (Pan B)	+	+	+	–	–	–
CD23	+/–	–	–	–	–	–
μ chain	+	+	+/–	–	–	–
δ chain	+	+/–	–	–	–	–
CD5 (T1)	+/–	+/–	–	+	+	–
CD3 (T3)	–	–	–	+	+	–
CD7 (Pan T)	–	–	–	–/+	+	–
CD11c	–/+	–	+	–	–	–
RER	–	–	–	–	–	+
EMA	–	–	–	–	–	+/–

RER = Rough endoplasmic reticulum
EMA = Epithelial membrane antigen
+ = All cases positive
+/– = Majority of cases positive
–/+ = Majority of cases negative
– = All cases negative

antigens in 60% and 95% of cases, respectively. The majority of CALL cases show nuclear expression of TdT and 20% have intracytoplasmic μ chain. No cases of CALL express T-cell or myeloid antigens.

T-cell acute lymphoblastic leukaemia (T-ALL)

All cases of T-ALL studied by the APAAP immunoalkaline phosphatase technique have been shown to express the CD7 pan-T antigen on a high percentage of blast cells (Figure 2). In addition, the majority (75%) of cases react with anti-CD2, CD3 and CD5 T-cell antibodies, and a smaller number of cases (33%) express the CD1 cortical thymocyte marker. The large number of cases expressing the 'mature' T-cell antigens (CD3 and CD5) is probably due to the detection of intracytoplasmic antigen that would not be visualized by immunofluorescent labelling of cells in suspension. Nuclear TdT is present in all cases of T-ALL, and B-cell and myeloid antigens are absent.

B-cell acute lymphoblastic leukaemia (B-ALL)

One case of B-ALL, with the typical FAB L3 morphological appearance, has been studied by immunoalkaline phosphatase labelling. The blast cells in this

---

Figure 2 Immunoalkaline phosphatase labelling of a peripheral blood smear from a case of T-cell acute lymphoblastic leukaemia with antibody DAKO-T2 (CD7). All the leukaemic cells are positively labelled. (Note one negative nucleated late normoblast – arrowed)

Figure 3 Peripheral blood smear from a case of megakaryoblastic blast crisis of chronic myeloid leukaemia labelled with monoclonal anti-platelet glycoprotein IIIa (antibody C17). Three strongly labelled blast cells and many abnormal platelets are seen

Figure 4 Peripheral blood smear from a case of erythroleukaemia labelled with anti-glycophorin A. Note the positively labelled blast cell (arrowed), nucleated red cell precursors (asterisks) and red blood cells

Figure 5 Peripheral blood smears from a case of hairy cell leukaemia. **(a)** Strong labelling of the hairy cells for the CD11c antigen (antibody KB90). Note one negative normal lymphocyte (arrowed). **(b)** The Pan B (CD22) antigen is strongly expressed by the hairy cells

Figure 6 APAAP labelling of bone marrow trephine cryostat sections from a case of T-cell lymphoma. **(a)** Strong staining of all the lymphoma cells with DAKO-T8 (CD8). **(b)** Labelling with DAKO-Macrophage shows positive marrow macrophages but the lymphoma cells (arrowed areas) to be negative

Figure 7 Bone marrow smear from a case of metastatic neuroblastoma. **(a)** A single clump of cells is seen in the Romanowsky stained film. **(b)** Staining with anti-leukocyte common antibody shows positively labelled lymphoid cells but the clump of malignant cells to be negative. **(c)** Labelling with the anti-neuroblastoma antibody UJ13A shows a positive cell clump and negative normal haemopoietic marrow cells

Figure 8 Immunoalkaline phosphatase labelling of a pleural effusion smear from a patient with centroblastic/centrocytic lymphoma. **(a)** Strong staining of lymphoma cells for HLA-DR (antibody CR3/43). **(b)** Reactive T-lymphocytes (antibody UCHTI) amongst neoplastic cells

Figure 9 Strongly labelled malignant cells in a pleural effusion from a patient with carcinoma of the lung detected with antibody DAKO-EMA

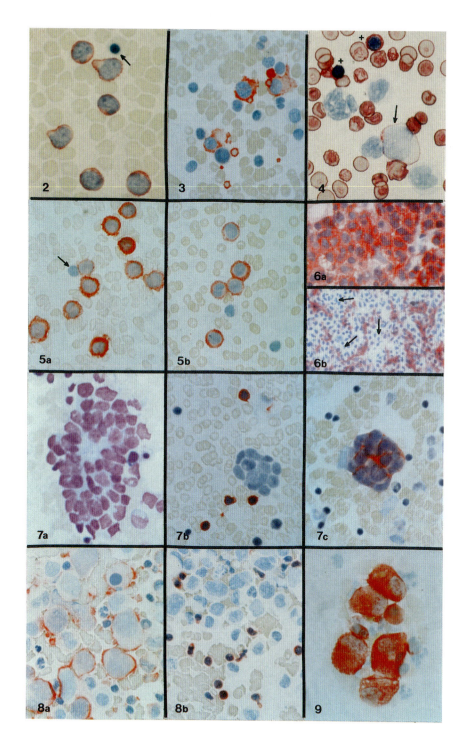

case expressed HLA-DR, the CD19 and CD22 B-cell antigens and surface IgM, but lacked TdT, CD10 and T-cell markers.

Acute myeloblastic leukaemia (AML)

Twenty-four cases of AML were identified by their typical myeloid morphological features, cytochemical expression of myeloperoxidase and lack of non-specific esterase (NSE) activity. All these cases were shown to react with the polyclonal anti-myeloperoxidase antibody (using the APAAP technique), but the number of positive cells (10–100%) and the cellular distribution of the enzyme was very variable. Antibody KB90 (recognizing the CD11c p150, 95 MW molecule present on neutrophils, monocytes and hairy cells[15]) reacted with the myeloblasts in 42% of the cases tested, but DAKO-Macrophage, an anti-monocyte antibody[16], was negative in all cases. HLA-DR was strongly expressed by the blast cells in the majority (95%) of cases and TdT reacted with smaller number of cases (30%). Two anti-T-cell antibodies, anti-CD2 and anti-CD7, reacted with myeloblasts in a small number of cases (25% and 20%, respectively). None of the cases expressed CD10, B-cell or IgM antigens.

Acute myelomonocytic (AMML) and monocytic leukaemia (AMOL)

Twenty-eight cases of acute leukaemia were diagnosed as containing a monocytic component on the morphologic appearance of the blast cells and the NSE activity of more than 10% of the blasts. All cases reacted with the anti-monocyte antibody DAKO-Macrophage (in contrast to the absence of expression of this antigen in cases of AML). The number of positive cells was variable, but all cases gave a granular intracellular labelling pattern. In all cases myloperoxidase, HLA-DR and the CD11c reagent (KB90) were positive on blast cells. None of the cases expressed TdT, CD10, CD7 or other T-cell antigens.

Eight of the cases tested with the anti-platelet glycoproteins Ib and IIIa antibodies showed a small number of positive lymphoid-like cells in the peripheral blood. The strong immunocytochemical labelling of these atypical 'lymphocytes' (small cells with an open nuclear chromatin pattern and ragged cytoplasm[17] with anti-platelet antibodies suggested that they were the megakaryocytic lineage (promegakaryoblasts) and represented dual lineage differentiation of the leukaemic clone.

Acute megakaryoblastic leukaemia (AMKL)

Twelve cases of AMKL were detected by immunocytochemical labelling with anti-platelet glycoprotein antibodies[17]. Antibody C17 (glycoprotein IIIa) labelled blast cells (10–50%) in all cases tested (Figure 3), and AN51 (glycoprotein Ib) detected megakaryoblasts in a smaller number (83%) of cases. In addition, all cases expressed HLA-DR on varying numbers of blast cells (10–80%), and the CD11c and CD2 antigens were present on megakaryoblasts in occasional cases. None of the cases expressed CD10 antigen, myeloperoxidase, B-cell antigens or TdT.

Erythroleukaemia

One case of acute leukaemia fulfilled the FAB morphological criteria for erythroleukaemia[18]. The majority of blast cells expressed the CD7 antigen and smaller numbers expressed glycophorin A (Figure 4), HLA-DR and transferrin receptor. The malignant cells were unreactive with myeloperoxidase, anti CD10, TdT, anti-B cell, anti-CD3 and anti-platelet glycoprotein antibodies.

Acute undifferentiated leukaemia (AUL)

Seven cases of AUL have been identified in the present study. All expressed HLA-DR and six (86%) had nuclear, or a combination of nuclear and cytoplasmic, expression of TdT. None expressed any specific cell markers, e.g. B- and T-cell antigens, myeloperoxidase, platelet glycoproteins and glycophorin A.

Mixed leukaemias

The majority of cases of acute leukaemia can be classified into one of the major phenotypic subgroups described above. However, small numbers have a mixed phenotype. These cases have been studied by double labelling, utilizing immunoperoxidase and immunoalkaline phosphatase techniques sequentially and shown to be either biclonal (characterized by a heterogeneous mixture of myeloid and lymphoid blast cells) or biphenotypic (a homogeneous) population of blast cells expressing features of lymphoid and myeloid cells).

Chronic haematological neoplasms

B-cell chronic lymphocytic leukaemia (B-CLL)

The leukaemic cells in B-CLL strongly express HLA-DR and show weaker reactivity for the B-cell antigen CD22. The majority of cases (89%) have positive labelling with anti-CD5 antibodies, the intensity varying from case to case, from strong to very weak. In 80% of cases the leukaemic cells react with the anti-CD23 antibody Tu2 confirming the follicular mantle zone origin of the B-CLL cell. IgM is strongly expressed in all cases and IgD more weakly. Monoclonality of the malignant lymphoid cells can be shown in each case by expression of either kappa or lambda light chains. The anti CD11c antibody, KB90, is weakly expressed in approximately 20% of the cases and the CD3 antigen absent from the leukaemic cells.

B-cell prolymphocytic leukaemia (B-PLL)

Cases of B-PLL, identified on clinical and morphological criteria, all show strong positivity for HLA-DR and have weaker expression of the CD22 B-cell antigen. The malignant cells show variable intensity of expression of the CD5 antigen, but all cases are positive. IgM is strongly expressed by the prolymphocytes in all cases and IgD positive in some cases (67%). None of the cases express the CD23 antigen, commonly seen on B-CLL cells, nor the CD11c molecules, and the cells show no reactivity with anti-CD3 and CD7 anti-T-cell antibodies.

Hairy cell leukaemia (HCL)

Fourteen cases of HCL have been immunophenotyped by the APAAP technique on blood or bone marrow smears[19]. All show strong expression of pan-B (CD22) antigen, HLA-DR and the CD11c antigen (Figure 5a,b) and, in addition, 86% show weak labelling with CD25 anti-IL-2 receptor (Tac) antibodies and a granular intracytoplasmic labelling pattern with the anti-monocyte antibody DAKO-Macrophage. The anti-hairy cell antibodies HC1 and HC2[20,21] label hairy cells in a smaller number of cases (36% and 82% respectively). CALLA is expressed on 50% of the cases, IgM on 70% and the CD2 antigen on small numbers of hairy cells (10–30%) in 40%. In all cases the hairy cells lack the CD5 and CD23 antigens (seen in B-CLL) and TdT.

T-cell chronic lymphocytic leukaemia (T-CLL)

Cases of CLL can be identified as being of T-cell origin by the expression of a number of mature T-cell markers. All cases strongly express the CD2, CD3 and CD5 anti-T-cell antigens and the antigen recognized by antibody Tu33[22]. In the present study two cases (of four tested) were of suppressor phenotype and expressed the CD7 antigen; the other two cases were malignant T-helper cells and lacked the CD7 antigen. None of the cases expressed HLA-DR, CD22 or CD23 (seen on B-CLL cells), or the cortical thymocyte marker (CD1, T6) or TdT expressed by immature T-cells and in cases of T-ALL.

T-cell prolymphocytic leukaemia (T-PLL)

Two cases of PLL, identified on clinical and morphological criteria, showed immunocytochemical features characteristic of mature T-cells. The leukaemic cells in these cases were CD2, CD3, CD7 and CD4 positive T-helper cells. None of the leukaemic cells expressed HLA-DR, B-cell markers, the CD1 antigen or TdT.

Sézary syndrome

The two cases of Sézary syndrome in the present study had immunocytochemical characteristics similar to those T-helper CLL. These cells were CD2, CD3, CD7 and CD4 positive and lacked the CD7 antigen and HLA-DR.

Chronic myeloid leukaemia (CML)

Blast cells from patients with CML in blast crisis can be immunologically pheno-typed using the APAAP technique and be shown to have lymphoid, myeloid or mixed phenotypes. In five cases studied the blast cells resembled CALL, expressing CD10 antigen, HLA-DR, CD22 antigen and TdT, and in one case the cells resembled T-ALL (CD7 and TdT positive, but lacking myeloperoxidase and HLA-DR). In nine cases blast cells had a myeloid phenotype (HLA-DR and myeloperoxidase positive) and, in addition, five of these cases expressed mono-cytic (DAKO-Macrophage) and megakaryoblastic features (platelet glycoprotein IIIa) on small numbers (5–10%) of blast cells. Two cases had a pure megakary-oblastic blast crisis (platelet glycoprotein IIIa positive and myeloperoxidase, DAKO-Macrophage, CD10 and TdT negative) and one case was undifferentia-ted, expressing only HLA-DR and TdT. None of the cases showed any reactivity with the anti-glycophorin A antibody. These findings confirmed that the blast cells in CML can express either lymphoid or myeloid features[23-26].

Multiple myeloma

Immunophenotyping bone marrow samples from cases of multiple myeloma shows that the majority of cases share a common antigenic profile. All cases of myeloma lack expression of the leukocyte common antigen, HLA-DR, CD22 and CD5 antigens (seen on other chronic lymphoproliferative disorders of B-cell origin), but express rough endoplasmic reticulum and the T10 antigen. In addition, epithelial membrane antigen (EMA)[27] and the plasma cell associated antigen PC-1 are expressed by myeloma cells in approximately 80% of cases.

Detection of metastatic cells in bone marrow aspirates

The detection of metastatic cells in bone marrow aspirates is not a problem for haematologists when numerous malignant cells are present, and especially if they form prominent clusters[28]. However, when infiltrating metastatic cells are only present in small numbers and do not form clusters, or when the bone marrow aspirate is hypocellular, it is very difficult, if not impossible, for the haematologist to confidently make a diagnosis.

Immunoalkaline phosphatase labelling of bone marrow smears can reveal small numbers of matastatic cells with great clarity, and enables a diagnosis of metastatic infiltration to be made in cases which are not readily diagnosable on conventional examination. This method of analysis of bone marrow allows single cells and clumps of metastatic cells of both epithelial (e.g. carcinoma) and non-epithelial origin (e.g. neuroblastoma, Ewings sarcoma and rhabdomyosarcoma) to be identified. In addition, this method is of value for identifying the true nature of poorly differentiated neoplasms in the

Table 6 Monoclonal antibodies useful in the diagnosis of metastatic infiltration of the bone marrow

Specificity	Antibody	Source	Diagnostic value
Epithelium	Le61	Dr E. Lane	carcinoma
	DAKO-CK1	Dakopatts	carcinoma
Desmin	DAKO-Desmin	Dakopatts	rhabdomyosarcoma
Neural filaments	DAKO-NF	Dakopatts	neural tumours
Neuroblastoma	UJ13A	Dr J. Kemshead	neuroblastoma

marrow. Monoclonal antibodies useful in the diagnosis of metastatic infiltration of the marrow, therefore, include anti-epithelial, anti-neuroblastoma and anti-desmin antibodies (Table 6 and Figure 7a–c).

Analysis of bone marrow trephines

The introduction of methods for the immunocytochemical analysis of frozen sections of bone marrow trephines[1] has enabled phenotypic studies to be performed in haematological disorders in which a conventional marrow aspiration yields a 'dry tap'. Immunocytochemical studies of bone marrow trephines have proved to be of value in the diagnosis of acute and chronic lymphoproliferative disorders, myelofibrosis, metastatic infiltration of the marrow and in phenotyping neoplastic lymphoid proliferations (Figure 6a,b). In addition, these methods enable information to be obtained on the architecture of the bone marrow, the phenotype of marrow cells that do not readily enter suspension (e.g. dendritic reticulum cells) and the antigenic characteristics of marrow cells that are only present in small numbers (e.g. megakaryocytes).

APPLICATIONS OF IMMUNOENZYMATIC LABELLING IN CYTOLOGICAL PREPARATIONS

This section describes some practical applications of immunoenzyme techniques in the diagnosis of lymphoproliferative disorders in cytological preparations (Table 7).

Cerebrospinal fluid (CSF)

Samples of CSF containing only small numbers of cells may be analysed by immunoenzymatic techniques. It is often not feasible to test such samples in suspension by standard immunofluorescent techniques because of the paucity of cells. Immunostaining CSF samples is of practical value in the diagnosis of cases of acute leukaemia, neuroblastoma and in distinguishing carcinoma from lymphoma[13,29,30]. In one case of acute lymphoblastic leukaemia in which central nervous system relapse had occurred, only a small sample of CSF was obtained. Although only two cytospin preparations were made from this sample this was sufficient to allow staining for CD10 antigen, revealing

Table 7 Applications of immunoenzymatic labelling in cytology

---

(1) Analysis of cerebrospinal fluid

(2) Analysis of serous effusions
       — distinction between reactive and neoplastic lymphoproliferative states
       — classification of lymphoid neoplasms
       — identification of tumour cell type

(3) Analysis of fine needle aspirates

---

numerous leukaemic cells, and for CD3 antigen, showing the presence of only a minor population of T-lymphocytes[13]. In a study of 17 patients with suspected neoplastic meningitis, a study of the CSF with a panel of Mabs including antibodies to lymphoid, epithelial and neuroectodermal antigens, a positive diagnosis could be made in 16 cases. The immunoenzymatic labelling enabled the neoplastic cells to be correctly identified in cases where the morphological appearance alone made a definite diagnosis difficult. Additional Mabs can also be used to provide further diagnostic information, e.g. for the phenotyping of lymphomas[30].

Serous effusions

Distinction between reactive and neoplastic lymphoproliferative states

Effusions containing numerous lymphocytes may be due to inflammatory processes (including tuberculosis), non-specific reactions complicating other diseases (including carcinoma) or chronic lymphocytic leukaemia or lymphoma. Analysis of the relative proportions of T- and B-lymphocytes may aid in distinguishing between reactive and neoplastic lymphoid infiltrates.

In a study from the authors' laboratory, immunoalkaline phosphatase staining of T- and B-cells in lymphocytic effusion samples from a control group of 19 patients with non-lymphoid malignancy or with benign conditions (such as cardiac failure) reported a mean of 85.26% T-cells and 11% B-cells[31]. These results are comparable to those previously reported for serous effusion samples using separated cells and immunofluorescence. Domagala et al.[32], reported a mean of 80.2% rosette forming lymphocytes (T-cells) and 7.4% immunoglobulin bearing cells (B-cells) in a control group of patients with non-malignant effusions, and Krajewski et al.[33] detected 84% T-cells and 4.5% B-cells in a similar group of patients. In contrast, enumeration of T- and B-cells from fluid samples from patients with chronic lymphocytic leukaemia or lymphoma revealed a different pattern to that seen in 'reactive' effusions (Table 8).

Classification of lymphoid neoplasms

The cytology of serous fluids alone cannot reliably diagnose subtypes of lymphoma (according to the Kiel classification), but in some cases it is possible to give an indication of the cell-type involved[34]. Immunoenzymatic labelling with Mabs may be used to provide additional or confirmatory information. Using these techniques it is possible to distinguish between T-cell and B-cell lymphoid neoplasms (Figure 8a,b) with specific Mabs, and the latter can be further analysed for the presence of surface immunoglobulin and type of light chain present.

An effusion containing high-grade lymphoma cells may occasionally develop in a case being treated as a low-grade lymphoma on the grounds of a previous histological report, and in such cases the cytological diagnosis provides essential supplementary information. In one example, a patient presented with a pleural effusion in which lymphoma cells were identified on cytological examination. A previous histological report had diagnosed mixed cellularity type Hodgkin's

Table 8 Immunocytochemical labelling patterns of serous effusions with monoclonal antibodies to T- and B-cells

Diagnosis	T-cells (pan T) %	B-cells (pan B) %	Interpretation
Non-lymphoid disease	85	11	reactive T-cells
B-CLL	1	99	neoplastic B-cells
T-CLL	95	1	neoplastic T-cells
Centroblastic lymphoma	Neg*	Pos*	neoplastic B-cells
Burkitt type lymphoma	1	99	neoplastic B-cells
Histiocytic lymphoma[+]	Neg*	Neg*	probably neoplastic histiocytes

Values represent percentages of positive lymphoid cells
*In these cases it was not possible to make accurate counts of the percentage of positive cells – for example, because of cell clumping or thick smears. Pos and Neg refer to the reactivity of unequivocal neoplastic cells
[+]Neoplastic cells from this patient were positive with DAKO-Macrophage Mab

disease. Immunostaining the pleural fluid with monoclonal antibodies to T- and B-cell antigens and the CD30 antibody Ki-1 to Hodgkin and Reed–Sternberg cells showed that the lymphoma cells were IgM and kappa positive, CD30 negative; supporting the cytologist's report of a non-Hodgkins lymphoma.

Identification of tumour cell types

Occasionally serous effusions are found to contain morphologically identifiable tumour cells but of unknown origin. The differential diagnosis between lymphoma and carcinoma in the majority of these cases can be made using immunoenzymatic labelling with a suitable panel of Mabs. Antibodies of practical value in this context are anti-leukocyte common antigen and anti-epithelial membrane (milk fat globule membrane) antigen (Figure 9), the former reacting with malignant lymphoma cells and the latter with carcinoma cells[35].

Fine needle aspirates

Fine needle aspirates do not usually present a diagnostic problem to the cytologist when numerous neoplastic cells are present. However, in some cases a diagnosis may be difficult to make on cytology alone, e.g. anaplastic tumours and some of the small round cell tumours. Although our experience with immunostaining of fine needle aspirates is limited the techniques mentioned in this chapter are suitable for labelling air-dried smears or cytospin preparations of washed cells. One example where immunoenzymatic staining of a fine needle aspirate was of value in establishing the diagnosis was a thyroid aspirate from a patient with a rapidly enlarging thyroid, who also had breast carcinoma. In this case immunoenzymatic staining was able to confirm that the malignant cells were of lymphoid origin (CD45 +ve, lambda +ve, kappa –ve) and not a metastasis from the breast carcinoma. The epithelial antibodies tested gave negative staining reactions.

CONCLUSION

Immunocytochemical methods using monoclonal antibodies are now widely used by haematologists, cytologists and pathologists for the diagnosis of haematological disorders. The methods described in this Chapter should prove to be of great value in the assessment of haematological and cytological samples. These techniques have a number of advantages over conventional immunofluorescent procedures including the ability to routinely label prepared blood smears, bone marrow smears and cytological preparations; samples can be stored for unlimited periods prior to labelling; cellular morphology is optimally preserved and can be visualized simultaneously with the antigen label; and the labelled preparations are permanent. These features, together with the general availability of monoclonal antibodies, should make these immunoenzymatic techniques accessible to routine diagnostic haematology and cytology laboratories. In future these methods will play an increasingly important role in the diagnosis of haematological disorders.

TECHNICAL APPENDIX

Immunoenzymatic techniques for staining blood, bone marrow and cytological samples.

Cell smear preparation

Whole blood, bone marrow, serous fluid (CSF) and fine needle aspirate smears

(1) Smears are prepared as for routine haematological or cytological examination and air-dried.

White cell-enriched smears

(1) Whole blood is mixed with an approximately equal volume of dextran solution and red cells are allowed to sediment.
(2) The supernatant white cell-rich plasma is aspirated, centrifuged and smears are then prepared from the white cell pellet.

Mononuclear cell smears

(1) Mononuclear cells are isolated from peripheral blood or bone marrow samples by centrifugation on Triosil Ficoll.
(2) The mononuclear cell preparation is washed twice in isotonic buffer or in tissue culture medium. The cells are resuspended in the washing medium which should contain 1% bovine serum albumin (or other protein) to prevent cell clumping, and cytocentrifuged or smeared onto clean glass slides.

Marrow trephines

(1) Unfixed bone marrow trephine samples are carefully snap-frozen by immersion in liquid nitrogen.
(2) Frozen marrow samples should be stored at $-70°C$ until sectioning.
(3) Cryostat sections (approximately 5–8 μm) are cut from snap frozen bone marrow trephine samples.
(4) Air dry slides at room temperature for between 2 and 24 hours.

Storage

(1) If slides are not to be stained immediately, they can be stored at $-20°C$ for prolonged periods without loss of antigenic reactivity.
(2) Shortly before staining, slides are removed from the freezer, and warmed to room temperature and then unwrapped.
(3) Slides are fixed in methanol:acetone (1:1) or methanol:acetone: formalin (19:19:2) for 90 seconds and then transferred to Tris buffered saline to avoid drying of the smears. Bone marrow trephine sections may be fixed in acetone at room temperature for 10 minutes and then allowed to air dry.

Immunoenzymatic staining techniques

Many preparations can be stained by both immunoperoxidase and immuno-alkaline phosphatase labelling methods, but in some instances (e.g. blood and bone marrow smears) immunoalkaline phosphatase labelling is preferable.

Immunoalkaline phosphatase staining technique

APAAP method (Figure 1)

(1) Apply the primary monoclonal antibody to the slide and incubate for 30 minutes.
(2) Wash in Tris buffered saline (TBS).
(3) Add anti-mouse Ig antiserum. It may be necessary to add normal human serum (1:5 to 1:20) to block cross-reactivity against human immuno-globulin. Incubation is carried out for 30 minutes.
(4) Wash in TBS.
(5) Add APAAP complexes (Dakopatts a/s) and incubate for 30 minutes.
(6) Wash in TBS.
(7) Add alkaline phosphatase substrate and incubate for 15 minutes.
(8) Wash in tap water and counterstain with haematoxylin.
(9) Wash in tap water, transfer to distilled water and mount in an aqueous mounting medium. NB Do not dehydrate and mount in non-aqueous mountant as the reaction product will be dissolved.

'Enhanced' APAAP method

This technique may be of value if labelling by the standard APAAP technique is relatively weak.

(1) Perform the incubation steps 1–6 as detailed above for the APAAP method.
(2) Repeat steps 3–6, but shorten the incubation period for steps 3 and 5 to 10 minutes each.
(3) Perform steps 7–9 as detailed above under APAAP method.

Alkaline phosphatase substrate

Dissolve 2 mg naphthol–AS–MX phosphate in 0.2 ml dimethyl formamide in a glass tube. Add 9.8 ml 0.1 mol/l Tris buffer pH 8.2. This solution is made fresh each time. Immediately before staining, dissolve Fast Red TR salt at a concentration of 1 mg/ml and filter directly onto the slide. If it is necessary to block endogenous alkaline phosphatase activity levamisole should be added to the substrate solution at a concentration of 1 mmol/l.

References

1. Falini, B., Martelli, M. F., Tarallo, F., Moir, D. J., Cordell, J. L., Gatter, K. C., Loreti, G., Stein, H. and Mason, D. Y. (1984). Immunohistological analysis of human bone marrow trephine biopsies using monoclonal antibodies. *Br. J. Haematol.*, **56**, 365–86
2. Cordell, J. L., Falini, B., Erber, W. N., Ghosh, A. K., Abdulaziz, Z., MacDonald, S., Pulford, K. A. F., Stein, H. and Mason, D. Y. (1984). Immunoenzymatic labelling of monoclonal antibodies using immune complexes of alkaline phosphatase and monoclonal anti-alkaline phosphatase (APAAP complexes). *J. Histochem. Cytochem.*, **32**, 219–29
3. Erber, W. N., Pinching, A. J. and Mason, D. Y. (1984). Immunocytochemical detection of T and B cell populations in routine blood smears. *Lancet*, **1**, 1042–6
4. Hoffman, R. A., Kung, P. C., Hansen, W. P. and Goldstein, G. (1980). Simple rapid measurement of human T lymphocytes and their subclasses in peripheral blood. *Proc. Natl. Acad. Sci. USA*, **77**, 4914–17
5. Reinherz, E. L. and Schlossman, S. F. (1980). Regulation of the immune response. Inducer and suppressor T-lymphocyte subsets in human beings. *N. Engl. J. Med.*, **303**, 370–3
6. Johnsen, H. E., Madsen, M., Kristensen, T. and Kissmeyer-Nielson, F. (1978). Lymphocyte sub-populations in man. Expression of HLA-DR determinants on human T cells in infectious mononucleosis. *Acta Pathol. Microbiol. Scand. (C)*, **86**, 307–14
7. Reinherz, E. L., O'Brien, C., Rosenthal, P. and Schlossman, S. F. (1980). The cellular basis for viral-induced immunodeficiency: analysis by monoclonal antibodies. *J. Immunol.*, **125**, 1269–74
8. Crawford, D. H., Brickell, P., Tidman, N., McConnel, I., Hoffbrand, A. V. and Janossy, G. (1981). Increased numbers of cells with suppressor T cell phenotype in the peripheral blood of patients with infectious mononucleosis. *Clin. Exp. Immunol.*, **43**, 291–7
9. DeWaele, M., Thielmans, C. and Van Camp, B. K. (1981). Characterisation of immunoregulatory T cells in EBV-induced infectious mononucleosis by monoclonal antibodies. *N. Engl. J. Med.*, **304**, 460–2
10. Hirt, A., Imbach, H., Morell, A. and Wagner, H. P. (1981). Infectious mononucleosis: Sequential immunologic, cytochemical and cytokinetic studies on single lymphoid cells in peripheral blood. *Blood*, **58**, 602–6
11. Pinching, A. J., McManus, T. J., Jeffries, D. J., Moshtael, O., Donaghy, M., Parkin, J. M., Munday, P. E. and Harris, J. R. (1983). Studies of cellular immunity in male homosexuals in London. *Lancet*, **2**, 126–30
12. Pinching, A. J. (1983). T cell ratios in AIDS. *Br. Med. J.*, **287**, 1716–17
13. Moir, D. J., Ghosh, A. K., Abdulaziz, Z., Knight, P. K. and Mason, D. Y. (1983). Immunoenzymatic staining of haematological samples with monoclonal antibodies. *Br. J. Haematol.*, **55**, 395–410

14. Erber, W. N., Mynheer, L. C. and Mason, D. Y. (1986). APAAP labelling of blood and bone-marrow samples for phenotyping leukaemia. *Lancet*, **1**, 761–5
15. Falini, B., Pulford, K., Erber, W. N., Posnett, D. N., Pallesen, G., Schwarting, R., Annino, L., Cafolla, A., Canino, S., Mori, A., Minelli, O., Ciani, C., Voxes, E. E., Golomb, H. M., Delsol, G., Stein, H., Martelli, M. F., Grignani, F. and Mason, D. Y. (1986). Use of a panel of monoclonal antibodies for the diagnosis of hairy cell leukaemia. An immunocytochemical study of 36 cases. *Histopathology*, **10**, 671–87
16. Franklin, W. A., Falini, B., Pulford, K. A. F., Clarke, L. C., Stein, H., McGee, J. O'D., Bliss, E. A., Gatter, K. C. and Mason, D. Y. (1985). Heterogeneity of the mononuclear phagocytes. In Grignani, F., Martelli, M. F. and Mason, D. Y. (eds). *Monoclonal Antibodies in Haematopathology*. Serono Symposium No. 26. pp. 191–199. (New York: Raven Press)
17. Erber, W. N., Breton-Gorius, J., Villeval, J. L., Oscier, D. G. and Mason, D. Y. (1986). Detection of cells of megakaryocyte lineage in haematologic malignancies by immuno-alkaline phosphatase labelling cell smears with a panel of monoclonal antibodies. *Br. J. Haematol.*, **65**, 87–94
18. Bennett, J. M., Catovsky, D., Daniel, M. T., Flandrin, G., Galton, D. A. G., Gralnick, H. R. and Sultan, C. (1985). Proposed revised criteria for the classification of acute myeloid leukemia. *Ann. Intern. Med.*, **103**, 626–9
19. Falini, B., Schwarting, R., Erber, W., Posnett, D. N., Martelli, M. F., Grignani, F., Zuccaccia, M., Gatter, K. C., Cernetti, C., Stein, H. and Mason, D. Y. (1985). The differential diagnosis of hairy cell leukaemia with a panel of monoclonal antibodies. *Am. J. Clin. Pathol.*, **83**, 289–300
20. Posnett, D. N., Chiorazzi, N. and Kunkel, H. G. (1982). Monoclonal antibodies with specificity for hairy cell leukaemia cells. *J. Cell Invest.*, **70**, 254–61
21. Posnett, D. N., Wang, C. Y., Chiorazzi, N., Crow, M. K. and Kunkel, H. G. (1984). An antigen characteristic of hairy cell leukaemia cells is expressed on certain activated B cells. *J. Immunol.*, **133**, 1635–40
22. Stein, H., Gerdes, J. and Mason, D. Y. (1982). The normal and malignant germinal centre. In Janossy, G. (ed.) *Clinics in Haematology*. Vol. II, pp. 531–559. (Philadelphia: W. B. Saunders)
23. Greaves, M. F., Verbi, W., Reeves, B. R., Hoffbrand, A. V., Drysdale, H. C., Jones, L., Sacker, L. S., and Samaratunga, I. (1979). 'Pre-B' phenotypes in blast crisis of Ph[1] positive CML: Evidence for a pluripotent stem cell 'target'. *Leuk. Res.*, **3**, 181–91
24. Griffin, J. D., Todd III, R. F., Ritz, J., Nadler, L. M., Canellos, G. P., Rosenthal, D., Gallivan, M., Beveridge, R. P., Weinstein, H., Karp, D. and Schlossman, S. F. (1983a). Differentiation patterns in the blastic phase of chronic myeloid leukaemia. *Blood*, **61**, 85–91
25. Griffin, J. D., Tantravahi, R., Canellos, G. P., Wisch, J. S., Reinherz, E. L., Sherwood, G., Beveridge, R. P., Daley, J. F., Lane, H. and Schlossman, S. F. (1983b). T-cell surface antigens in a patient with blast crisis of chronic myeloid leukemia. *Blood*, **61**, 640–4
26. Bettelheim, P., Lutz, D., Majdic, O., Paietta, E., Linkesch, W., Neumann, E., Lechner, K. and Knapp, W. (1985). Cell lineage heterogeneity in blast cell crisis of chronic myeloid leukaemia. *Br. J. Haematol.*, **59**, 395–409
27. Delsol, G., Gatter, K. C., Stein, H., Erber, W. N., Pulford, K. A. F., Zinne, K. and Mason, D. Y. (1984). Human lymphoid cells express epithelial membrane antigen. *Lancet*, **2**, 1124–8
28. Ghosh, A. K., Erber, W. N., Hatton, C. S. R., O'Connor, N. T. J., Falini, B., Osborn, M. and Mason, D. Y. (1985). Detection of metastatic tumour cells in routine bone marrow smears by immunoalkaline phosphatase labelling with monoclonal antibodies. *Br. J. Haematol.*, **61**, 21–30
29. Hancock, W. W. and Medley, G. (1983). Monoclonal antibodies to identify tumour cells in CSF. *Lancet*, **2**, 739–40
30. Coakham, H. B., Garson, J. A., Brownell, B., Allan, P. M., Harper, E. I., Lane, E. B. and Kemshead, J. T. (1984). Use of monoclonal antibody panel to identify malignant cells in cerebrospinal fluid. *Lancet*, **1**, 1095–8
31. Ghosh, A. K., Spriggs, A. I. and Mason, D. Y. (1985). Immunocytochemical staining of T and B lymphocytes in serous effusions. *J. Clin. Pathol.*, **38**, 608–12
32. Domagala, W., Emeson, E. E. and Koss, L. G. (1981). T and B lymphocyte enumeration in the diagnosis of lymphocyte-rich pleural fluids. *Acta Cytol.*, **25**, 108–10

33. Krajewski, A. S., Dewar, A. E. and Ramage, E. F. (1982). T and B lymphocyte markers in effusions of patients with non-Hodgkin's lymphoma. *J. Clin. Pathol.,* **35**, 1216–19
34. Spriggs, A. I. and Vanhegan, R. I. (1981). Cytological diagnosis of lymphoma in serous effusions. *J. Clin. Pathol.,* **34**, 1311–25
35. Ghosh, A. K., Spriggs, A. I., Taylor-Papadimitriou, J. and Mason, D. Y. (1983). Immunocytochemical staining of cells in pleural and peritoneal effusions with a panel of monoclonal antibodies. *J. Clin. Pathol.,* **36**, 1154–64

6
Cell-mediated Immunity in Lymphomas

P. L. AMLOT

INTRODUCTION

In 1902 Dorothy Reed noted that several patients with Hodgkin's disease were unresponsive to tuberculin when tested by intradermal injection for delayed cutaneous hypersensitivity (DCH). Subsequently, Parker (1932) confirmed this lack of a tuberculin reaction in most patients with Hodgkin's disease, and suggested that their susceptibility to tuberculosis may be due to an immunological deficit. In those days Hodgkin's disease was so commonly associated with tuberculosis (TB) that it was regarded by some as an atypical form of TB. However, it was not untill 1956 that Schier et al. demonstrated that this unresponsiveness to tuberculin was part of a more general anergy involving any antigen which normally elicited DCH responses[1]. This finding implied a general deficiency of cell-mediated immunity in Hodgkin's disease. Since then a rapidly growing literature has analysed and examined the possible causes of this immunodeficiency, and at the same time has shown that this phenomenon occurs in other forms of lymphoma. It is now known that the severity of the immunodeficiency was compounded by extensive radiotherapy as well as by treatment with steroids and cytotoxic drugs which many of these patients had received. This review will give an individual interpretation of the vast literature on this subject and it will be biased towards Hodgkin's disease, partly reflecting the greater number of reported studies on Hodgkin's disease and partly because the immunodeficiency has been more clearly defined in this disease than in other lymphomas.

CLINICAL ASPECTS

Opportunistic infections occur in Hodgkin's disease (HD) and non-Hodgkin's lymphomas (NHL) caused by organisms such as *Pneumocystis carinii, Cryptococcus neoformans,* Nocardia, *Candida albicans,* Cytomegalovirus and Aspergillus. Unlike tuberculosis, such infections are rarely seen in normal immunocompetent individuals and they are also unusual in untreated patients with HD or NHL unless the patients have become severely debilitated as a result of widespread disease. The deficiency of cell-mediated immunity (CMI) frequently seen in lymphoma patients underlies this susceptibility to opportunistic infections. The combination of persistent and unresponsive lymphomatous disease together with extensive cytotoxic or radiotherapy leads to the highest incidence of superinfection. Common pathogenic bacteria are the cause of most infections in lymphoma patients, and the more unusual 'opportunistic' infections, although widely reported in the literature, account for only a minority of infections[2]. Shingles caused by *Herpes zoster* is another disease attributable to a deficiency of immunity. This occurs in about 10–15% of untreated patients and rises to 40% of those treated patients who have also undergone splenectomy as part of the assessment of their disease. The deficiency in CMI can be so severe that fatal cases of Graft-versus-Host disease have followed transfusions of fresh blood into patients undergoing treatment for HD[3]. All these examples indicate a significant deficiency in cellular immunity which is compounded by therapy. Such clinical manifestations of immunodefiency are not normally seen in the many benign and malignant diseases in which abnormal *in vitro* lymphocyte responses have been described.

ASSESSMENT OF IMMUNITY *IN VIVO*

Impaired CMI in patients with lymphomas has been demonstrated dramatically by allogeneic skin grafting[4]. Delayed rejection was seen in most cases and some patients accepted their grafts indefinitely. However, immunity has usually been measured by DCH responses towards a panel of delayed hypersensitivity recall antigens, contact sensitizers or by immunization with previously unencountered antigens. (The term 'recall' antigens means those antigens to which a normal person is likely to have been exposed and become sensitized.) The earliest reported studies were performed on patients who had already received therapy for their lymphomas and they revealed a very high incidence of anergy. However, the therapy these patients had received was potently immunosuppressive and the direct influence of the disease upon immunity (or of immunodeficiency as part of lymphomagenesis) could not be assessed until untreated patients were examined. ('Untreated' in this context means patients whose immunological investigations were carried out before therapy was started.) Two large studies, involving over 100 untreated patients each, were performed in the early 1970s and addressed the questions as to whether (a) immunodeficiency affected the expression or outcome of HD, and (b) immunodeficiency occurs early in HD or may even precede it.

The first study performed at the National Cancer Institute[5] found that anergy to a panel of five delayed recall antigens (Mumps, *Candida albicans*, Histoplasmin, PPD and Coccidiodin) only occurred in 12% of patients with HD, a figure much lower than previously expected from studies on treated patients. In the earliest stage (Stage I) of HD there was no anergy and the incidence of anergy increased with spread of disease, but even in the most advanced stage (Stage IV) was only found in 27% of patients. Furthermore, using a contact skin sensitizer (dinitrochlorobenzene) 67% of patients were able to develop cell-mediated immunity compared with 95% of normal controls. This study found no relationship between skin test reactivity at diagnosis and the patient's subsequent survival, frequency of relapse or duration of remission. The absence of anergy in the earliest stages of disease also suggested that immunodeficiency was acquired as a result of disease spread and was not a premorbid, predisposing factor.

The second study carried out at the Stanford Medical Center[6] also used sensitization with dinitrochlorobenzene, but at a lower sensitizing dose than had previously been used so that only 83% of the normal controls developed a positive skin test response. Using this more sensitive technique only 40% of patients with early stages of HD (Stages I and II) reacted, compared to approximately 20–30% of patients with more advanced disease (Stages III or IV) or those having 'B' symptoms (fever, night sweats or weight loss). This study only showed a modest, though significant, impairment of CMI as a result of disease spread, but in disagreement with the first study suggested that an impairment of CMI existed in the earliest stages and may even predate the onset of HD.

There is no doubt that sensitization with antigens to which the recipient has not previously been exposed is a much more discriminating method of assessing immunocompetence than testing with recall antigens. It requires the induction as well as the expression of the immune response and, therefore, tests both afferent and efferent arms of immunity. In relation to the aforementioned studies we have tested the DCH response to Keyhole Limpet haemocyanin (KLH) induced by immunization of 66 controls, 55 untreated patients with HD and 48 untreated patients with NHL[7] and the results are shown in Table 1. Both patients with HD as well as NHL show a much lower incidence of sensitization than controls, but HD differs from both the other groups in that patients who do develop DCH do so more slowly and more feebly. Another interesting feature seen only in patients with HD was the appearance of *delayed* DCH. This occurred in about 10% of patients and

Table 1 Induction and strength of the DCH response in lymphomas

DCH Response	% with a positive DCH response		
	Controls	Hodgkin's	NHL
Onset day 6–8[A]	47	4	25
Onset day 9–14[A]	21	16	4
Response to challenge[B]	88	20	40
Of responders:			
DCH elicited by 1 μg[C]	24	0	21

[A]DCH developing at the site of immunization with 0.2 mg Keyhole Limpet haemocyanin (KLH) i.d. without further challenge. [B]Challenged with 1 or 10 μg KLH i.d. on day 14 after primary immunization and read 2 days later. [C]Highly sensitized subjects responded to 1 μg and the remainder to 10 μg KLH

consisted of DCH responses occurring 4–7 days (instead of the usual 2 days) after challenge with recall antigens or KLH.

The immune defect in HD selectively affects CMI leaving humoral immunity relatively intact (at least until widespread disease and debilitation occur). Antibody responses that are largely T-cell independent (to natural antigens such as pneumococcal polysaccharides or synthetic antigens such as DNP-Ficoll) are normal in HD unless they have undergone splenectomy or treatment[8,9] although they may be decreased in some types of NHL without either splenectomy or treatment. The effect of HD upon T-cell dependent antibody responses is more controversial. Most investigators agree that secondary antibody responses in HD are normal, but there is disagreement over the effect upon primary antibody responses[10]. When we examined primary DCH and antibody responses to KLH in parallel, the proportion of antibody responders was less in both HD and NHL and the IgG responses were more severely affected than IgM (Table 2). These results imply that the early antibody response (which is relatively T-cell independent) was unaffected while the subsequent T-cell sensitization, which normally provides help to boost and switch the antibody response from IgM to IgG, was deficient in patients with lymphomas. Therefore, T-cell sensitization, both for DCH and for providing help in antibody production, was abnormal and of the two, T-cells involved in DCH were more severely affected and could occur early in the disease in otherwise fit young adults, whereas defects in antibody responses tended to occur in debilitated patients with advanced disease. Furthermore, unresponsiveness to KLH was found more often in patients with advanced disease (stages III and IV or with 'B' symptoms). Using KLH we had a similar sensitization rate to the Stanford study (summarized above), yet in agreement with the NCI study we found no relationship between DCH responses to either recall antigens or KLH and the patient's response to treatment, relapse rate or survival.

Biological response modifiers such as thymic hormones, levamisole, transfer factor, BCG or prostaglandin synthetase inhibitors have been given to patients with active lymphomatous disease but have made no significant difference to CMI *in vivo* although these agents can alter *in vitro* tests.

Table 2 Antibody responses to Keyhole Limpet haemocyanin in lymphomas

| Antibody | Day | % of antibody responders | | |
		Controls	Hodgkin's	NHL
IgM	7	21	18	9
	14	35	33	22
	21	47	22*	24*
IgG	7	18	14	14
	14	74	46*	43*
	21	81	48*	49*

*Significantly fewer antibody responders compared with controls

76

CHANGES OF LYMPHOCYTE POPULATIONS IN LYMPHOMAS

Lymphocytes have been identified which are responsible for cell mediated immunity (T-cells) as distinct from those involved in humoral immunity (B-cells). Subsequently T-cells have been further subdivided into T-helper/inducer (CD4), T-suppressor (CD8), natural killer (NK) and other subpopulations. The 'markers' used for identification of lymphocytes are described elsewhere in this book. The studies described here will deal solely with information relevant to cell-mediated immunity. Obviously, in the non-Hodgkin's lymphomas (e.g. chronic lymphocytic leukaemia, centroblastic-centrocytic lymphoma or the Sezary syndrome) there may be gross replacement of normal blood, bone marrow, lymph node or splenic lymphocytes by neoplastic B- or T-cells.

Lymphocytopenia occurs in HD and NHL. In the former it is associated with a poor prognosis and occurs more frequently in advanced stage (stage IV) disease and with 'B' symptoms[11]. The deficiency of CMI seen in HD and NHL would lead one to expect that there might be a selective depletion of T-cells in this disease. There is, however, only a modest relative reduction in T-cells, while in lymphocytopenic patients there is an absolute fall in all types of lymphocytes. The lymphocytopenia is not accompanied by a fall in blood monocytes and this may be responsible for some of the abnormalities of *in vitro* function described later. The absolute numbers of lymphocytes and their subsets can vary in the blood of normal healthy individuals, but there is usually little variation in the ratio of T-helper to suppressor cells (CD4/CD8). However, in HD there is often an absolute and relative decrease of T-helper cells (CD4)[12-14] with normal numbers of T-cytotoxic/suppressor cells (CD8) causing a decrease in the ratio of CD4/CD8 below the normal range (1.7–2.4). This imbalance of blood lymphoctyes persists and is accentuated by treatment for HD[15]. A monoclonal expansion of B- or T-cells is found in the blood of about half the patients with NHL.

On the other hand, when tissues from patients with HD have been examined, the reverse of the situation in the blood has been found. In the spleen and lymph nodes there is an overall increase in the proportion of T-cells mostly of T-helper phenotype (CD4) which predominates over T-cytotoxic/suppressor cells[12,13,16]. T-cells in the tissues often show evidence of activation by the expression of the transferrin receptor, OKT10 or HLA-DR antigens[16,17]. Activated T-helper cells are commonly found in clusters around Reed–Sternberg or Hodgkin cells. Some of these activated cells have the phenotype of immature, cortical thymocytes, for in addition to the T10 antigen, a proportion form stable E-rosettes at 37°C[18]. Clustering of T-helper cells is not restricted to RS and HD cells but may occur around the normal antigen presenting accessory cells or around the Langerhans cells in the skin of patients with mycosis fungoides. In both these cases the cells around which T-cells cluster express HLA Class II antigens strongly. The alteration in T-cell distribution in HD occurs in both involved and uninvolved spleens and lymph nodes[19]. In the lymph nodes from patients with B-cell NHL the T-cytotoxic/suppressor cells (CD8) may predominate and these T-cells are often HLA-DR positive, indicating activation[20]. Remember that these results exclude those cases where a monoclonal expansion of a malignant lymphocyte population is found.

This alteration in the balance of T-cells found in blood compared with the other lymphoid compartments (lymph nodes or spleen) has been termed 'ecotaxopathy'[21]. The concept of ecotaxopathy develops the idea that in disease states there may be an altered migration pattern of lymphocytes induced by chemotactic factors or by adherence to specific receptors within lymphoid organs, leading to an abnormal distribution of lymphocytes within the body. This appears to be the case in HD and probably in some NHL. Turnover studies *in vivo*, using radioactively labelled lymphocytes, have revealed a higher turnover rate and shorter life for lymphocytes in lympho-cytopenic patients with HD[22].

It should be noted that children with HD differ from adults in that there is no progressive lymphopenia, T-cell numbers are normal or increased and conversely the B-cell number may be decreased[23].

LYMPHOCYTE FUNCTIONAL STUDIES *IN VITRO*

In order to better understand the defective cell-mediated immunity of lymphoma patients, the purified peripheral blood mononuclear cells (composed mostly of lymphocytes) have been examined *in vitro* under which conditions the environment can be more carefully controlled. The numerous studies performed have all found that lymphocyte proliferation stimulated by mitogens, phytohaemagglutinin (PHA) or concanavalin A (Con A), was impaired and the impairment was augmented in patients who had received treatment. Most investigators were unable to discern any relationship between the impaired *in vitro* responses and clinical parameters such as the stage of disease spread, response to treatment, DCH responses or prognosis. In children with HD the PHA response recovers with successful treatment and this recovery implies a good prognosis[23]. In adults it has generally been found that *in vitro* responses do not predict the clinical stage or outcome of the disease, but there have been two exceptions to this general finding. Firstly, it was reported from Stanford that, by using suboptimal stimulating concentrations of PHA and measuring protein synthesis, the lymphocytes from patients with early stages (I, II) of HD responded better than those with advanced stages (III, IV) although there was no correlation with 'B' symptoms, lymphocyte count or DCH[24]. Secondly, a Swedish study reported that those patients whose lymphocyte proliferative response to Con A was below an arbitrarily set level had a poorer 5 year survival than those above the set level[25].

In all these studies mitogens were used because they can induce lymphocyte proliferation or protein synthesis without the patient having to be sensitized by previous exposure (as would be the case with antigens). In this sense such a system is an artificial examination of CMI except that the mitogens used are specific T-cell activators, and in turn T-cells are responsible for CMI.

When the proliferative ability of lymphocytes from patients with HD or NHL were tested by a variety of stimuli they were found to be hyporesponsive towards mitogens, soluble antigens and in the autologous mixed lymphocyte reaction (AMLR) but responded *normally* in the allogeneic mixed lymphocyte reaction (MLR)[26,27]. The AMLR and MLR measure T-cell proliferation of the T-helper cell subset (CD4) induced by non-T-cells expressing MHC Class II antigens on their membranes (HLA-DR, DP, DQ). In the AMLR, autologous or self-Class II antigens are the stimulus whilst in the MLR allogeneic or foreign-Class II antigens are stimulatory. T-helper cells (CD4) are stimulated by soluble antigens and probably even mitogens in association with self-Class II antigens. It seems reasonable to deduce that T-helper cells responsive to self-Class II antigens (directly in the AMLR or indirectly in association with soluble antigens or mitogens) are either absent, reduced or defective in the blood of patients with HD or NHL, while those responsive to foreign Class II antigens are normally present.

On the other hand when lymphocytes from lymph nodes or spleens of patients with HD were examined for mitogen-induced proliferation their responses were found to be normal or increased[28,29]. This agrees with the increased proportions of phenotypically determined T-cells and T-helper cells found in these lymphoid compartments, and suggests that T-helper cells reactive with autologous Class II antigens are enriched in lymphoid organs such as spleens or lymph nodes of patients with lymphomas, especially in HD.

EFFECT OF MONONUCLEAR ADHERENT CELLS ON LYMPHOCYTE PROLIFERATION *IN VITRO*

The impaired response to PHA or Con A by peripheral blood mononuclear cells from lymphoma patients implies an intrinsic defect or maldistribution of T-lymphocytes since these mitogens are T-cell specific. However, such purified cell preparations normally contain between 5–20% of monocytes, and there is abundant evidence that cells capable of adhering to glass or plastic surfaces *in vitro* and derived mostly from monocytes are able to suppress lymphocyte proliferation. Could the impaired lymphocyte response in lymphomas be caused by suppression induced by monocytes/adherent cells? Further purification of the peripheral blood mononuclear cells by removal of adherent cells on glass wool markedly enhanced the proliferative response to PHA, and further analysis suggested that the adherent cells induced suppression by producing prostaglandins[30]. Two complementary pieces of evidence have shown that prostaglandins interfere with an early step in lymphocyte activation: (1) the addition of prostaglandin synthetase inhibitors (e.g. indomethacin) to lymphocyte cultures from patients with HD enhanced proliferative responses to PHA despite the presence of the suppressive adherent cells, and (2) by the addition of exogenous prostaglandin (especially PGE$_2$) which could mimic the defect in HD by suppressing normal lymphocyte responses. However, none of these manipulations completely corrected the hyporesponsiveness found in HD[31,32].

One of the reasons why defective *in vitro* responses in lymphomas cannot be attributed entirely to inhibition induced by adherent cells is that these cells have two completely opposite effects depending upon their relative proportion

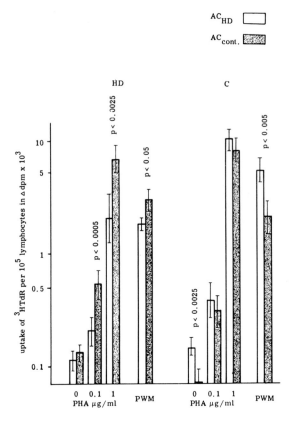

Figure 1 Interaction between adherent cells and lymphocytes in mitogenesis.
AC: Adherent cells after incubating peripheral blood mononuclear cells on plastic for 1 h at 37°C; **HD:** Hodgkin's disease; **C:** Healthy controls; **PHA:** Phytohaemagglutinin; **PWM:** Pokeweed mitogen; ^{3}**HTdR:** Tritiated thymidine. Significance values were obtained by Student's paired t-test using $\log_{10}$ transformed values of triplicate ^{3}HTdR uptakes by lymphocytes with AC_{HD} or AC_{cont}

compared to lymphocytes. At low proportions (approximately 1–10%) these cells are essential to most mitogen- and all antigen-induced proliferation. Complete removal of all adherent cells suppresses or abolishes mitogenesis[33]. At higher proportions (greater than 20%) they suppress mitogenesis, the MLR and antigen-induced proliferation. Apart from any altered function shown by monocytes/adherent cells in HD, it should be remembered that the lymphocytopenia often present in HD leads to a high proportion of monocytes relative to lymphocytes when the blood mononuclear cells are separated for studies *in vitro*. We have carried out experiments to test the effect of adherent cells upon mitogenesis, in which lymphocytes from healthy volunteers and patients with HD were cultured in the presence of their own adherent cells or those from a paired adherent cell preparation obtained from the opposite group. The results can be seen in Figure 1. In the presence of

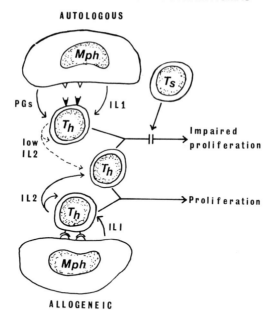

Figure 2 Proposed mechanism of impaired antigen, mitogen or AMLR proliferation of blood lymphocytes compared with the normal MLR. T_h: T-helper cells (CD4); T_s: T-suppressor cells (CD8); Mph: Macrophages derived from monocytes *in vitro*; PGs: Prostaglandins; IL1: Interleukin 1; IL2: Interleukin 2; △: Autologous Class II antigens; ◠: Allogeneic Class II antigens: ⋎: Blocked receptors on T-helper cells or decreased numbers of T_h cells with receptors for autologous Class II antigens

allogeneic adherent cells, mitogen responses by HD lymphocytes became normal, while they were remarkably decreased in the presence of their auto- logous adherent cells. However, lymphocytes from healthy volunteers were not suppressed at all by adherent cells from patients with HD, indeed in pokeweed mitogen stimulated cultures the response was increased (Amlot and Chivers, unpublished observations). This suggests that there is an abnormal interac- tion, in at least some patients with HD or NHL, between T-cells and their own adherent cells. Although monocyte/adherent cell depletion has been shown to augment mitogenesis it has no effect upon the deficient AMLR in HD[34]. These observations taken together would fit with the hypothesis that in the peripheral blood of patients with HD there exists a deficiency of T-helper cells capable of recognizing or blocked from recognizing autologous Class II antigens (Figure 2).

It may be that the interaction of an imbalanced lymphocyte population reacting with monocytes in the presence of mitogens induces prostaglandin synthesis[35] and this may lead to part of the diminished mitogen responsiveness seen in lymphoma patients. Preincubation of peripheral blood mononuclear cells for at least 24 hours augments mitogenesis[36], and this may work by abrogating any prostaglandin mediated effect because increased levels of prostaglandins need to be present within the first 6 hours of culture to cause significant suppression. There appears to be no defect in the production of interleukin 1 (IL-1) by mononuclear cells from patients with lymphomas, but interleukin 2 (IL-2) production by their T-cells is decreased[37]. Since T-cell proliferation by lymphocytes from lymphoma patients becomes normal in the presence of exogenous IL-2, the deficiency in IL-2 production is evidently critical.

Monocyte function, when examined separately from T-cell proliferation assays, revealed that in patients with lymphomas there is: (a) a normal or increased antibody-dependent cytotoxicity, (b) abnormal chemotaxis in some patients, and (c) decreased intracellular killing of pathogens such as *Staphylococcus aureus*[38]. In HD the abnormal chemotaxis is compounded by increased serum levels of chemotactic factor inactivator[39]. The deranged chemotaxis may be relevant to the *delayed* DCH which occurs in HD and was described earlier in this chapter.

In lymphomas *in vitro* suppressive influences have been detected other than those caused by adherent cells. Non-adherent suppressor cells occurring spontaneously or induced by concanavalin A or by the MLR are increased in about half the patients with depressed mitogenic responses and this suppression is mediated by T-suppressor cells (CD8)[40-42]. It is this form of suppression that persists for many years after treatment of HD and NHL and correlates with an increase of T-suppressor cells in the blood. Adherent cell suppression disappears after successful treatment of lymphomas so that addition of prostaglandin synthetase inhibitors has no effect on the lymphocyte hyporesponsiveness found in patients during remission following treatment.

SPONTANEOUSLY PROLIFERATING CELLS IN THE BLOOD

Uptake of thymidine (a precursor in DNA synthesis) is often increased in lymphocyte cultures from patients with HD or NHL. This increase in spontaneous DNA synthesis in blood mononuclear cells is similar to that seen in subjects undergoing intensive antigenic stimulation[43]. Increased spontaneous DNA synthesis is often associated with lymphopenia and decreased mitogen responses[25], the combination of which carries a poor prognostic outlook. DNA synthesizing cells are removed by the spleen[44] which is the primary site of migration for T-cells emerging from the thymus. Although it is attractive to conjecture that these cells are responding to tumour related antigens, their frequent presence in lymphopenic patients suggests that these may be immature cells whose production is stimulated in order to compensate for the deficit in lymphocyte number. The gradual depletion of normal lymphoid tissues and lymphocytes which occurs as HD progresses could be caused by a deficient production or a shorter lymphocyte lifespan. The increased turnover of lymphocytes found by an *in vivo* study suggests that the shorter lymphocyte lifespan accounts for lymphopenia in HD[22]. What mechanism accounts for the consumption of lymphocytes in the tissues of HD is unknown, but there is a parallel in the lymphocyte lysis which occurs in the acquired immunodeficiency disease syndrome (AIDS) induced by the Human Immunodeficiency

Virus (HIV). The histological appearances of HD and AIDS are very different, but it has been claimed that monoclonal antibodies reacting with the p18 antigen of HIV also reacts with Reed–Sternberg (RS) or Hodgkin's cells in HD tissues [44a]. Further work will tell what relation this has to the AIDS virus, and whether the p18 antigen detected in RS or HD cells represents a framework structure of a retrovirus similar to HIV (affecting human T-cells and causing a milder immunodeficiency than AIDS) or whether it is just one of the many red herrings that litter the history of research into HD.

CELL-MEDIATED CYTOTOXICITY

Mononuclear leukocytes which are able to kill other nucleated cells are called cytotoxic cells and *in vitro* assays have shown that this function is accomplished by a number of phenotypically distinct cells. Among these cytotoxic cells are: cytotoxic T-lymphocytes (CTL); monocytes and lymphocytes able to mediate antibody-dependent cellular cytotoxicity (ADCC); and natural killer cells (NK). Studies performed using peripheral blood mononuclear cells from lymphoma patients have shown that:

(1) CTL can be generated normally during the mixed lymphocyte reaction although there may be a decrease in lectin-induced cytotoxicity;
(2) Monocyte-mediated ADCC is increased compared with normal individuals while lymphocyte-mediated ADCC is normal[45];
(3) Natural killer cell (NK) activity is decreased in lymphomas[46,47].

The decrease in NK activity in the blood of lymphoma patients has raised considerable interest because these cells have been proposed as one of the natural defences against the spread of malignant disease via the blood stream. However, a corresponding increase in NK activity was discovered when lymphoid tissue from lymphoma patients was examined. In particular, the highest NK activity was found in splenic tissue involved with HD, and even in uninvolved spleens the NK activity was greater than in normal spleens[47,48]. NK activity is very low in lymph nodes, whether from normal or lymphoma patients. Once again an explanation for the abnormal cell mediated cytotoxicity could be explained by 'ecotaxopathy' with selective accumulation of effector cells in extravascular sites.

EFFECT OF T-CELLS UPON IMMUNOGLOBULIN PRODUCTION BY B-CELLS

This aspect of T-cell function will only be covered briefly, for at present a contradiction exists between *in vitro* and *in vivo* findings thus raising doubts about the validity of *in vitro* results which are based largely upon studying cells isolated from the blood. For example, untreated HD is characterized by hypergammaglobulinaemia, whilst the B-cell types of NHL are often accompanied by hypogammaglobulinaemia. *In vitro* systems for studying immunoglobulin production often use pokeweed mitogen (PWM) as a mixed

T_h and B-cell stimulator. Blood mononuclear cells from both HD and NHL patients produce lower amounts of immunoglobulin in response to PWM than normal controls. Analysis suggested that this was due to a degree of B-cell unresponsiveness in both types of lymphoma. In addition, the deficiency was compounded in HD by a lack of T-cell help and an excess of T-suppressor activity[49,50]. The results are largely due to the conditions of the *in vitro* assay. For the PWM driven system to work there is a requirement for partial B-cell activation *in vivo* and for the elaboration of B-cell stimulatory factors (BSF) by T-cells *in vitro*. In HD there is evidence that there is more than partial activation of B-cells *in vivo* shown by increased spontaneous immunoglobulin production[50]. The altered T-helper/suppressor balance in the blood of HD patients probably accounts for decreased BSF elaboration and subsequent immunoglobulin production. In order to avoid the influence of autologous B-cells, co-culture experiments have been performed in which tonsillar B-cells were mixed with T-cells from lymphoma patients to examine their effect upon immunoglobulin production. In such experiments the T-helper cells from NHL patients with B-cell lymphomas augmented immuno-globulin production whilst, as expected, those from HD and T-cell lymphomas decreased immunoglobulin production[51].

In contrast to the foregoing results immunoglobulin secretion by splenic cells from patients with HD was found to be greatly increased when compared with normal spleens[52], which accords with the clinical hyper-gammaglobulinaemia. All one can infer is that examination of bloodborne cells is an inappropriate method by which to try and examine T-cell/B-cell interactions in lymphomas all of which may be occurring in extravascular sites.

HUMORAL FACTORS INHIBITING T-CELL FUNCTION

It would be a convenient explanation for the progressive lymphopenia and impaired T-cell function found in HD if these were due to autoantibodies specifically cytotoxic for autologous T-cells. Cytotoxic antilymphocyte anti-bodies have been described in HD[53] and refuted[54]. There is no disagreement as to the presence of IgG antibodies able to bind to T-cells in a minority of patients with HD and such antibodies have been detected *in vitro* arising from cultures of spleen cells[52]. However, although these antibodies may be lytic in the presence of rabbit complement[53] they are not lytic with human serum or in the presence of human ADCC effector cells[54]. T-cell reactive antibodies in HD can decrease the lymphocyte PHA response while removal of the antibodies from the lymphocyte membrane can restore it. This phenomenon is not restricted to HD because cold reactive lymphocyotoxic antibodies (which bind at $4°C$) can be found in most patients with mycosis fungoides[55] as well as in a third of patients with HD[56] quite apart from non-malignant diseases such as systemic lupus erythematosus. Although the antibody-containing sera can suppress PHA responses by HD lymphocytes they do not affect lymphocytes from normal healthy individuals. The significance of these antibodies in relation to T-cell function is difficult to assess. They may cause some of the T-cell dysfunction in HD or, more likely, they may reflect the progressive loss of T-cell suppressor control over B-cell function. It is known that as the spread of HD increases there is a concomitant rise in anti-Epstein–Barr virus (EBV) antibody titres without there necessarily being any aetiological connection between EBV and HD[57]. In HD the T-cell reactive antibodies as well as the anti-EBV antibodies are associated with poor prognostic features, such as high spontaneous DNA synthesis, decreased responses to mitogens, low T-cell counts, 'B' symptoms and advanced stage of disease. Cold reactive T-cell antibodies also appear during infectious mononucleosis (IM) in about 25% of patients[58] suggesting that dysregulation of the B-cell system driven by the EBV is responsible for the appearance of a relatively common autoantibody.

Other inhibitors of T-cell function have also been described in HD. A complex consisting of B-lipoprotein, C-reactive protein and C1q has been isolated from spleens of patients with HD which was able to bind to the lymphocytes of a minority of patients with HD causing a decrease in sheep red blood cell rosette formation (E-RFC: a T-cell receptor) and of the PHA response[59]. Ferritin, in its form not containing iron (apoferritin), can also bind to the HD lymphocyte membrane. The HD lymphocytes can be induced to shed ferritin by incubating them overnight in the presence of the immuno-modulating agent, levamisole[60], after which treatment there followed an increase in active E-RFCs and in the response to Con A. An increase in alphafetoprotein associated with the membranes of blood lymphocytes from patients with HD has also been described which may have immuno-suppressive effects.

CONCLUSIONS

An hypothesis which attempts to account for the defective cell-mediated immunity found in patients with lymphomas is portrayed diagramatically in Figures 2 and 3. First of all, the defective interaction between T-helper cells and autologous antigen-presenting cells (APC) leads to an impaired activation of the T-helper cells. This results in a deficiency at this important amplification stage of T-cell immunity (Figure 2). This defective interaction between T-helper cells and APC could come about in a number of ways;

(1) Due to a relative deficiency of T-helper cells of the 'autoreactive' type;
(2) Due to humoral factors which interfere with receptor binding between T-helper cells and APC;
(3) Due to down-regulation of HLA Class II antigens (DR, DP or DQ) on the surface of the APC upon interaction with T-helper cells which could be induced by prostaglandin release by APCs or by immuno-modulatory substances such as alphafetoprotein.

Secondly there is a sequestration of T-helper cells in the lymphoid tissues reacting with autologous HLA Class II antigens (Figure 3). This ecotaxopathy causes a relative deficiency of T-helper cells in the blood and accounts for many of the abnormalities observed in *in vitro* studies using

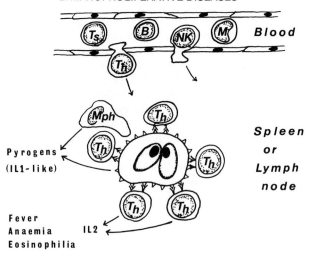

Figure 3 Example of ecotaxopathy in Hodgkin's disease as a cause of distributed lymphocyte function. Legend as for Figure 2. **M:** Monocyte

blood mononuclear cells. It is assumed that the tissue sequestration leads to the death of the lymphocytes involved, for there is a gradual depletion of normal lymphocytes with advanced lymphomatous disease and because lymphocyte turnover is increased in lymphopenic states. In Figure 3 the central cell is depicted as a Reed–Sternberg cell from HD around which T-cell clustering is most clearly observed, but the same may occur in NHL since intense expression of HLA Class II antigens occurs in most of the B-cell, T-cell and true histiocytic lymphomas. However, clustering is not an obvious feature in many types of NHL and, furthermore, assessment of defective CMI is complicated in these diseases by (1) the lack of studies relating CMI to clearly defined types of NHL, (2) the effect that the advanced age of many patients with NHL may have, and (3) the effect that dilution/replacement of normal lymphocytes by malignant lymphocytes has upon *in vitro* and *in vivo* immune responses.

An important question in relation to impaired CMI in lymphomas remains but cannot readily be answered. What relevance does the imparied CMI have to lymphomagenesis or the progress of the lymphoma? There is an increased susceptibility to HD within families and there is some evidence that *in vitro* lymphocytes responses may be impaired within families in which one member has HD[61]. There is also some obliquely relevant information from an animal model of HD. SJL/J mice develop a lymphoreticular tumour which is very similar to human HD. Tumour bearing SJL/J mice develop impaired responses to mitogens, develop humoral factors which impair lymphocyte function and recover lymphocyte function when the tumour is removed[62]. Strains of mice (HRS/J) which have deficient immune responses before developing the tumour show no differences in the age or frequency at which they develop the malignancy nor in the outcome, but the pre-existing immune deficiency does alter the histological appearance of the tumour[63]. This animal model fits with the impression that CMI in lymphomas, especially HD, becomes impaired with increasing tumour burden, but that there are individuals who have impaired CMI even at the earliest stages of disease and in whom the defect may be genetically determined. On the other hand, in the case of the majority of NHL, it seems unlikely that an imperceptible immune deficiency renders patients susceptible to lymphomas so late in life.

There is as yet no evidence that the clustering of T-helper cells around RS or HD cells are involved in the recognition of tumour specific antigens (viral or otherwise). The sequestration and progressive depletion of mature, immunocompetent T-cells from recirculatory pathways leads to immuno-deficiency, but whether this is part of a sustained but unsuccessful attack upon malignant cells or is part of an abnormal immune response is unknown.

References

1. Schier, W. W., Roth, A., Ostroff, G. and Schrift, M. H. (1956). Hodgkin's disease and immunity. *Am. J. Med.*, **20**, 94–9
2. Remington, J. S. (1972). The compromised host. *Hosp. Pract.*, **7**, 59–70
3. Burns, L. J., Westberg, M. W., Burns, C. P., Klassen, L. W., Goeken, N. E., Ray, T. L. and Macfarlane, D. E. (1984). Acute graft-versus-host disease resulting from normal donor blood transfusions. *Acta Haematol.*, **71**, 270–6
4. Kelly, W. D., Lamb, D. L., Varco, R. L. and Good, R. A. (1960). An investigation of Hodgkin's disease with respect to the problem of homotransplantation. *Ann. N. Y. Acad. Sci.*, **87**, 187–202
5. Young, R. C., Corder, M. P., Haynes, H. A. and DeVita, V. T. (1972). Delayed hypersensitivity in Hodgkin's disease. *Am. J. Med.*, **52**, 63–72
6. Kaplan, H. S. (1980). The nature of the immunologic defect. In *Hodgkin's Disease*, 2nd edn, Chapter 6 (Harvard: Harvard University)
7. Amlot, P. L. and Hayes, A. E. (Unpublished observations)
8. Siber, G. R., Weitzman, S. A. and Aisenberg, A. C. (1981). Antibody response of patients with Hodgkin's disease to protein and polysaccharide antigens. *Rev. Infect. Dis.*, **3** (Suppl.), S144–S159
9. Amlot, P. L. and Hayes, A. E. (1985). Impaired human antibody response to the thymus-independent antigen, DNP-Ficoll, after splenectomy. *Lancet*, **1**, 1008–11
10. De Gast, G. C., Halie, M. R. and Nieweg, H. O. (1975). Immunological responsiveness against two primary antigens in untreated patients with Hodgkin's disease. *Eur. J. Cancer*, **11**, 217–24
11. MacLennan, K. A., Vaughan Hudson, B., Jeliffe, A. M., Haybittle, J. L. and Vaughan Hudson, G. (1981). The pretreatment peripheral blood lymphocyte count in 1100 patients with Hodgkin's disease: the prognostic significance and the relationship to the presence of systemic symptoms. *Clin. Oncol.*, **7**, 333–9
12. Herrmann, F., Sieber, G., Jauer, B., Lochner, A., Komischke, B. and Ruhl, H. (1983). Evaluation of the circulating and splenic subpopulations in patients with non-Hodgkin's lymphomas and Hodgkin's disease using monoclonal antibodies. *Blut*, **47**, 41–51
13. Romagnani, S., Del Prete, G. F., Maggi, E., Bosi, A., Bernardi, F., Ponticelli, P., DiLollo, S. and Ricci, M. (1984). Displacement of T-lymphocytes with the 'helper/inducer' phenotype from peripheral blood to lymphoid organs in untreated patients with Hodgkin's disease. *Scand. J. Haematol.*, **31**, 305–14
14. Lauria, F., Foa, R., Gobbi, M., Camaschella, C., Lusso, P., Raspadori, D. and Tura, S. (1983). Increased proportion of suppressor/cytotoxic (OKT8+) cells in patients with Hodgkin's disease in long lasting remission. *Cancer*, **52**, 1385–8
15. Posner, M. R., Reinherz, E., Lane, H., Mauch, P., Hellman, S. and Schlossman, S. F. (1983). Circulating lymphocyte population in Hodgkin's disease after mantle and paraortic irradiation. *Blood*, **61**, 705–8
16. Poppema, S., Bhan, A. K., Reinherz, E. L., Posner, M. R. and Schlossman, S. F. (1982). *In*

situ immunologic characterization of cellular constituents in lymph nodes and spleens involved by Hodgkin's disease. *Blood,* **59**, 226–32

17. Borowitz, M. J., Croker, B. P. and Metzgar, R. S. (1982). Immunohistochemical analysis of the distribution of lymphocyte subpopulations in Hodgkin's disease. *Cancer Treat. Rep.,* **66**, 667–74

18. Aisenberg, A. C. and Wilkes, B. M. (1982). Lymph node T-cells in Hodgkin's disease: Analysis of suspensions with monoclonal antibody and rosetting techniques. *Blood,* **59**, 522–7

19. Dorreen, M. S., Habeshaw, J. A., Wrigley, P. F. and Lister, T. A. (1982). Distribution of T-lymphocyte subsets in Hodgkin's disease characterised by monoclonal antibodies. *Br. J. Cancer,* **45**, 491–9

20. Kvaloy, S., Marton, P. F., Host, H., Solheim, B. G. and Godal, T. (1982). Distribution of T-cell subsets identified by monoclonal antibodies in cell suspensions from lymph node biopsies of human B-cell lymphomas. *Scand. J. Haematol.,* **28**, 293–305

21. de Sousa, M., Yang, M., Lopes-Corrales, E., Tan, C., Dupont, B. and Good, R. A. (1977). Ecotaxis: the principle and its application to the study of Hodgkin's disease. *Clin. Exp. Immunol.,* **27**, 143–59

22. Schick, P., Trepel, F., Theml, H., Benedek, S., Trumpp, P., Kaboth, W., Begemann, H. and Fliedner, T. M. (1973). Kinetics of lymphocytes in Hodgkin's disease. *Blut,* **27**, 223–35

23. Tan, C. T., DeSousa, M. and Good, R. A. (1982). Distinguishing features of the immunology of Hodgkin's disease in children. *Cancer Treat. Rep.,* **66**, 969–75

24. Levy, R. and Kaplan, H. S. (1974). Impaired lymphocyte function in Hodgkin's disease. *N. Engl. J. Med.,* **290**, 181–6

25. Wedelin, C., Bjorkholm, M., Holm, G., Ogenstad, S., Johansson, B. and Mellstedt, H. (1982). Lymphocyte function in untreated Hodgkin's disease: An important predictor of prognosis. *Br. J. Cancer,* **45**, 70–9

26. Engleman, E. G., Benike, C. J., Hoppe, R. T., Kaplan, H. S. and Berberich, F. R. (1980). Autologous mixed lymphocyte reaction in patients with Hodgkin's disease. *J. Clin. Invest.,* **66**, 149–58

27. Smith, J. B., Knowlton, R. P. and Harris, D. T. (1983). Functional aspects of T-cells from patients with non-Hodgkin's lymphoma. Responses to self, TNP-modified self and allo-antigens. *Cancer,* **52**, 1160–4

28. Kaur, J., Spiers, A. S. D., Catovsky, D. and Galton, D. A. G. (1974). Increase of T-lymphocytes in the spleen in Hodgkin's disease. *Lancet,* **2**, 800–2

29. Baroni, C. D., Ruco, L., Uccini, S., Foschi, A., Occhionero, M. and Marcorelli, E. (1982). Tissue T-lymphocytes untreated Hodgkin's disease. Morphologic and functional correlations in spleens and lymph nodes. *Cancer,* **50**, 259–68

30. Goodwin, J. S., Messner, R. P., Bankhurst, A. D., Peake, G. T., Saiki, J. H. and Williams, R. C. (1977). Prostaglandin-producing suppressor cells in Hodgkin's disease. *N. Engl. J. Med.,* **297**, 963–8

31. Bockman, R. S. (1980). Stage dependent reduction in T-colony formation in Hodgkin's disease. *J. Clin. Invest.,* **66**, 523–31

32. Sibbitt, W. L., Bankhurst, A. D. and Williams, R. C. (1978). Studies of cell subpopulations mediating mitogen hyporesponsiveness in patients with Hodgkin's disease. *J. Clin. Invest.,* **61**, 55–63

33. Rosenstreich, D. L., Farrar, J. J. and Dougherty, S. (1976). Absolute macrophage dependency of T-lymphocyte activation by mitogens. *J. Immunol.,* **116**, 131–9

34. Zamkoff, K. W., Dock, N. L., Kurec, A. S. and Davey, F. R. (1982). Diminished autologous mixed lymphocyte reaction in patients with Hodgkin's disease: Evidence for non-T cell dysfunction. *Am. J. Hematol.,* **12**, 327–35

35. Amlot, P. L., Heinzelman, D., Chivers, A. and Youlten, L. J. F. (1980). Stimulation of monocyte prostaglandin production by lymphocytes in Hodgkin's disease. In *Advances in Prostaglandin Research*, (New York: Raven Press)

36. Whisler, R. L., Murray, J. L., Roach, R. W. and Balcerzak, S. P. (1984). Characterisation of multiple immune defects in human malignant lymphoma. *Cancer,* **53**, 2628–34

37. Ford, R. J., Tsao, J., Konttab, N. M., Sahasrabuddhe, C. G. and Metha, S. R. (1984). Association of an interleukin abnormality with the T-cell defect in Hodgkin's disease. *Blood,* **64**, 386–92

38. Hamminga, L., Leijh, P. C., van Oud Alblas, A. B., van Vloten, W. A. and van Furth, R. (1982). Functions of peripheral blood monocytes and granulocytes in cutaneous T-cell lymphoma. *Br. J. Dermatol.*, **107**, 157–64

39. Ward, P. A. and Berenberg, J. L. (1982). Defective regulation of inflammatory mediators in Hodgkin's disease. *N. Engl. J. Med.*, **290**, 76–80

40. Hillinger, S. M. and Herzig, G. P. (1978). Impaired cell mediated immunity in Hodgkin's disease mediated by suppressor lymphocytes and monocytes. *J. Clin. Invest.*, **61**, 1620–7

41. Twomey, J. J., Laughter, A. H., Rice, L. and Ford, R. (1980). Spectrum of immunodeficiencies in Hodgkin's disease. *J. Clin. Invest.*, **66**, 629–37

42. Vanhaelen, C. P. and Fisher, R. I. (1982). Increased sensitivity of T-cells to regulation by normal suppressor cells persists in long term survivors with Hodgkin's disease. *Am. J. Med.*, **72**, 385–90

43. Crowther, D., Fairley, G. H. and Sewell, R. L. (1967). DNA synthesis in the lymphocytes of patients with malignant disease. *Eur. J. Cancer.*, **3**, 417–21

44. Bjorkholm, M., Holm, G., Askergren, J. and Mellstedt, H. (1983). Lymphocyte counts and functions in arterial and venous splenic blood in patients with Hodgkin's disease. *Clin. Exp. Immunol.*, **52**, 485–92

44a. Chassagne, J., Verelle, P., Fonck, Y., Legros, M., Dionet, C., Plagne, R. and Klatzmann, D. (1987). Detection of the lymphadenopathy - associated virus p18 in cells of patients with lymphoid diseases using a monoclonal antibody. In *Acquired Immumodeficiency syndrome.* Gluckman, J. C. and Vilmer, E. (eds.), (Paris: Elsevier)

45. de Mulder, P. H., de Pauw, B. E., van de Ven, E. C., Wagener, T. D. and Haanen, C. (1984). Monocyte mediated antibody dependent cellular cytotoxicity in malignant lymphoma and solid tumours. *Cancer*, **53**, 2444–9

46. Tursz, T., Dokhelar, M. C., Lipinski, M. and Amiel, J. L. (1982). Low natural killer cell activity in patients with malignant lymphoma. *Cancer*, **50**, 2333–5

47. Levy, S., Tempe, J. L., Aleksijevic, A., Giron, C., Oberling, F., Mayer, S. and Lang, J. M. (1984). Depressed NK cell activity of peripheral blood mononuclear cells in untreated Hodgkin's disease: enhancing effect of interferon *in vitro. Scand. J. Haematol.*, **33**, 386–90

48. Ruco, L. P., Procopio, A., Uccini, S., Morcorelli, E. and Baroni, C. D. (1982). Natural killer cell activity in spleens and lymph nodes from patients with Hodgkin's disease. *Cancer Res.*, **42**, 2063–8

49. Ruhl, H., Enders, B., Bur, M. and Sieber, G. (1981). Impaired B-lymphocyte reactivity in patients with Hodgkin's disease and non-Hodgkin's lymphomas. *Blut*, **42**, 271–81

50. Romagnani, S., Del Prete, G. F., Maggi, E., Bellesi, G., Biti, G., Rossi Ferrini, P. L. and Ricci, M. (1983). Abnormalities of *in vitro* immunoglobulin synthesis by peripheral blood mononuclear lymphocytes from untreated patients with Hodgkin's disease. *J. Clin. Invest.*, **71**, 1375–82

51. Gajl-Peczalska, K. J., Chartrand, S. L. and Bloomfield, C. D. (1982). Abnormal immunoregulation in patients with non-Hodgkin's malignant lymphomas. I. Increased helper function of peripheral blood T lymphocytes. *Clin. Immunol. Immunopathol.*, **23**, 366–78

52. Longmire, R. L., McMillan, R., Yelenosky, R., Armstrong, S., Land, J. E. and Craddock, C. G. (1973). *In vitro* splenic IgG synthesis in Hodgkin's disease. *N. Engl. J. Med.*, **289**, 763–7

53. Tognella, S., Mantovani, G., Del Giacco, G. S., Manconi, P. E., Cengiarotti, L., Floris, C. and Grifoni, V. (1975). Effetto del siero citotossico di patienti con malattia di Hodgkin sulla PHA-responsivita *in vitro* di linfociti periferici umani. *Tumori*, **61**, 53–62

54. Jones, D. B., Elliott, E. V., Payne, S. V. and Wright, D. H. (1978). Absence of IgG lymphocytotoxins in untreated Hodgkin's disease patients. *Clin. Exp. Immunol.*, **34**, 100–5

55. Schocket, A. L., Huff, J. C., Carr, R. I. and Norris, D. A. (1982). Humoral immunity in Stage I mycosis fungoides: an increased incidence of lymphocytotoxic antibodies. *Br. J. Dermatol.*, **107**, 285–91

56. Bjorkholm, M., Wedelin, C., Holm, G., Ericsson, H., Nilsson, P. and Mellstedt, H. (1982). Lymphocytotoxic serum factors and lymphocyte functions in Hodgkin's disease. *Cancer*, **50**, 2044–8

57. Levine, P. H., Ablashi, D. V., Berard, C. W., Carbone, P. P., Waggoner, D. E., and Malan, L. (1971). Elevated antibody titres to Epstein–Barr virus in Hodgkin's disease. *Cancer*, **27**, 416–21

58. Thomas, D. B. (1972). Antibodies to membrane antigen(s) common to thymocytes and a subpopulation of lymphocytes in infectious mononucleosis sera. *Lancet*, **1**, 399–403

59. Bieber, M. M., Fuks, Z. and Kaplan, H. S. (1977). E-rosette inhibiting substance in Hodgkin's disease spleen extracts. *Clin. Exp. Immunol.*, **29**, 369–75

60. Moroz, C., Lahat, N., Biniamov, M. and Ramot, B. (1977). Ferritin on the surface of lymphocytes in Hodgkin's disease patients. A possible blocking substance removed by *Clin. Exp. Immunol.*, **29**, 30–5

61. Bjorkholm, M. *et al.* (1978). Immunological family studies in Hodgkin's disease. *Scand. J. Haematol.*, **20**, 297–304

62. Kumar, R. K., Lykke, A. W. and Penny, R. (1981). Immunosuppression associated with SJL/J murine lymphoma. I. Suppression of cell-mediated immune responses after tumor transplantation. *J. Natl. Cancer Inst.*, **67**, 1269–75

63. Johnson, D. A., Shultz, L. D. and Bedigian, H. G., (1982). Immunodeficiency and reticulum cell sarcoma in mice segregating for HRS/J and SJL/J genes. *Leuk. Res.*, **6**, 711–20

7
The Origin of the Reed–Sternberg Cell

D. B. JONES

INTRODUCTION

The 156 years which have elapsed since Thomas Hodgkin first published his paper on some morbid appearances of the lymph nodes[1] have seen major advances in our ability to investigate human cell types. From the development of the most basic techniques in histopathology we have advanced to a stage where genes, or segments of genes responsible for a particular phenotypic expression can be examined in minute detail. Despite considerable effort over this period of time the disease which today bears the name of Thomas Hodgkin remains poorly understood.

The diagnosis of Hodgkin's disease (HD) is based on the recognition of Reed–Sternberg cells (RS)[2,3] in a cellular setting appropriate for one of the subtypes of the disease[4]. Our poor understanding of the complex interactions between cells within the reactive stroma, and the fact that RS cells frequently constitute only a small population of the cells within Hodgkin's tissue have certainly contributed to our failure to comprehend the pathogenesis of HD. It is also now clear that what was once considered to be a single disease entity, containing various histological sub-categories, represents at least two and probably more disease processes, probably evolving within different cell lineages.

EARLY INVESTIGATIONS INTO THE ORIGIN OF THE REED–STERNBERG CELL

The development, in the late 1960s, of rosetting techniques for the identification of lymphocyte lineages and of staining techniques for the identification of immunoglobulins on cells in suspension and in section, allowed the first detailed analyses of the tumour cell populations in HD. Thus, Taylor[5] was able to demonstrate that the neoplastic population in HD contained immunoglobulin and noted that, unlike B-cell lymphoma, both kappa and lambda light chains were present within the same cell. This observation was confirmed by Kadin and colleagues in studies of RS cells isolated from tissue biopsies[6]. At this time, we, and other groups[7-9], undertook phenotypic investigations of dispersed HD lymph node biopsies using the then newly available rosetting techniques. This data can be summarized in the light of our own experience which was that, unlike non-Hodgkin's lymphoma (NHL), where tumour cell populations were identified as being either of T- or B-cell lineage[10], RS cells and mononuclear Hodgkin's cells could not be clearly assigned to either branch of the lymphocyte family, although weak expression of Fc receptors and complement receptors was frequently seen[7]. The general consensus, from these early studies and related investigations of isolated RS cells in short-term culture[11,12], was that the tumour population in Hodgkin's disease was derived from the monocyte/macrophage system. Early studies, employing immuno-histochemistry in formalin fixed, paraffin embedded Hodgkin's tissue, showed that Reed–Sternberg and Hodgkin's cells contained polyclonal immunoglobulin and alpha-1 antitrypsin[13,14]. At the time these studies were undertaken this data was also considered compatible with a histiocytic origin for the Reed–Sternberg cell.

IMMUNOHISTOLOGICAL ANALYSIS OF FROZEN AND FIXED SECTIONS

In recent years, the development of monoclonal antibodies for the identification of cellular phenotypes in both frozen and fixed tissue has greatly enhanced our ability to characterize both neoplastic and reactive lymphoreticular cells. For details of the many monoclonal reagents available, and an explanation of the standardized nomenclature which is recommended for their description, the reader is referred to the most recent proceedings of the *Leucocyte Typing Workshop*[15]. In NHL monoclonal antibodies identifying immunoglobulin light and heavy chains and lineage-related leukocyte markers are an efficient tool for the determination of the cell of origin in the majority of cases[16], although lineage infidelity and heterogeneity of antigen expression can occur, particularly with large pleomorphic tumour cell populations[17,18]. In HD the situation is more complex. Whilst HD cells strongly express major histocompatibility Class II determinants (MHC II) and interleukin-2 (IL-2) receptors, both markers of activation within the lymphoid series[19,20], lineage related epitopes yield equivocal results[19,21-23]. In general, RS cells and their mononuclear counterparts may fail to express antigens characteristic of a specific lymphocyte lineage; show T- or B-cell markers or express both together[23,24]. Detailed investigations of RS cells in fixed, embedded tissue yield equally confusing results. Monoclonal antibodies reactive in fixed, embedded tissue and known to selectively stain cell populations of different lymphocyte lineage are variably expressed in RS cells[23,24]. However, with regard to the routine diagnosis of Hodgkin's lymphoma, immunocytochemical analysis of fixed tissue can yield important diagnostic pointers. Thus, HD cells are strongly positive for MHC Class II with appropriate monoclonal reagents[25]. Further, in some histological sub-types of Hodgkin's disease the carbohydrate antigen, lactofucopentaose III (CD15), and the activation

92

associated glycoprotein designated CD30 under the new nomenclature are frequently positive[23,26,27]. The significance of the expression of CD15 and CD30 will be discussed in the following sections. Immunohistochemical studies of HD have provided convincing evidence that at least two forms of this disease exist[28–33]. The consensus from these studies is that the nodular lymphocyte predominance type of HD exhibits a unique phenotype, showing positivity for J-chain, B-cell markers and the leukocyte common antigen (CD45) and is thus distinguished from the 'conventional' HD phenotype expressing CD15 and CD30 but frequently lacking CD45. Nodular lymphocyte predominant HD can, therefore, be considered as a B-cell proliferation evolving from the germinal centre of the lymph node[34]. This concept is based on studies of fixed and frozen biopsy material[35].

EXPRESSION OF ANTIGENS OF THE MYELOID/MACROPHAGE SERIES

As stated previously the initial interpretation of phenotypic data obtained from early investigations of HD considered that the RS cell could represent a malignant histiocyte. Many of the phenotypic studies described in the preceding section have included monoclonal antibodies reactive with cells of the monocyte/macrophage lineage. None of these studies have provided convincing evidence for a macrophage derivation of RS cells. The monoclonal antibody, MAC 387, reactive with macrophages in routinely processed tissue[36] to a large series of HD biopsies identifies large numbers of reactive macrophages but never stains RS or HD cells (unpublished observations). Not all studies of HD have excluded an origin within this series. Hsu et al.[37] have applied their own monoclonal antibodies to frozen sections of HD tissue and concluded that RS cells share at least some of the antigens expressed by true histiocytic lymphoma. This is, however, a minority view and it is also clear that true histiocytic lymphoma (THL), as defined by these authors, expresses CD30 and IL-2 receptor (CD25). The precise relationship of THL in this study to CD30 positive anaplastic large cell lymphoma (ALC) which is known to lack macrophage antigens and has been shown by gene rearrangement analysis to represent a tumour of lymphoid cells[39] therefore remains to be fully established.

Myeloid reactivity of RS cells was first described by Stein et al.[40] who demonstrated that three monoclonal antibodies, Tü5, Tü6 and Tü9, considered specific to late cells of granulocytic differentiation, frequently stained RS cells. Subsequent investigations have shown that the reactivity described is due to the presence of the carbohydrate antigen lactofucopentaose III (CD15) in the tumour cell population[26,41]. For diagnostic purposes, CD15 is most readily demonstrated with the monoclonal antibody Leu-M1. CD15 is expressed by HD and RS cells in all subtypes of HD except the L&H predominant type. Although this antigen is expressed in cells of the myeloid series it also shows widespread distribution in human tissues and is frequently seen in normal and neoplastic epithelial tissues[30]. Loss of expression in leukocyte populations other than granulocytes and some monocytes is probably due to

Table 1 Carbohydrate sensitivity to glycosyl hydrolases

Enzyme	Substrate
Glycopeptidase-F	N-linked carbohydrate chains
Endoglycosidase-F	high mannose complex saccharides
Endo-beta-galactosidase	linear or branched side chains
Beta-galactosidase	terminal galactoside residues

For detailed descriptions of enzymes and methods see Reference 43

sialylation of the molecule. The lack of expression of CD15 in lymphocyte/ histiocyte predominant HD can be reversed by the application of the enzyme, neuraminidase, to remove sialic acid[31]. The appearance of CD15 in large pleomorphic tumour cells where carbohydrate metabolism may be disturbed, cannot be considered as a lineage specific expression. We have obtained further evidence of the complex expression of CD15 epitopes in relation to varied expression of carbohydrate moieities in HD[42]. Our studies in lymphoma reflect the earlier investigations of Kelly and Fleming[43, 44] in fetal rate skin. These authors employed glycosyl hydrolases to dissect linear, branched, N-linked or fucose-rich carbohydrates from cells (Table 1). This enabled the analysis of the structure of the carbohydrates which are responsible for antigeneicity related to human type II blood group substances in the fetal rat skin. This panel of enzymes was applied to formalin-fixed, paraffin-embedded Hodgkin's tissue in conjunction with a panel of CD15 monoclonal antibodies submitted to the last *Monoclonal Antibody Typing Workshop*[15]. Our first observation was of marked heterogeneity in that different CD15 antibodies identified either granulocytes or RS cells implying that the epitope map for CD15 is different in these two cell types. Secondly, we were able to show that the sensitivity of the CD15 epitopes present in RS cells to glycosyl hydrolase digestion was different from that of the normal granulocyte. This observation provides important evidence that the expression of CD15 in RS cells is a result of abnormal glycosylation, rather than lineage specific expression. Further, analysis of cytogenetic abnormalities in Hodgkin's disease[45] has identified the frequent appearance of structural abnormalities in 11q. It is of interest that certain types of childhood pre-B-cell acute lymphoblastic leukaemia, which show cytogenetic abnormalities in 11q 23, also frequently express aberrant myeloid and monocytic antigens. This evidence would also suggest that CD15 expression in RS cells reflects an abnormal state.

STUDIES OF CARBOHYDRATE METABOLISM IN HD AND RS CELLS

Investigations employing lectin binding also point to abnormalities of carbohydrate metabolism in HD and RS cells. Hsu and Jaffe[26] have demonstrated that the galactose-binding lectin, peanut agglutinin (PNA), binds to RS cells in over 60% of cases investigated. The pattern of PNA staining paralleled that seen with anti-CD15 reagents and suggested reactivity with glycoconjugates in the Golgi region. Detailed analyses of the binding of a panel of lectins have been undertaken in normal lymph nodes and in HD[46]. The pattern identified in HD broadly resembled the pattern in reactive lymph nodes with the exception of clusters of RS cells, where the lectin staining indicates a high concentration of mannosyl residues and a relative deficiency of sialic acid groups. A deficiency in membrane sialic acid residues probably contributes to the many cell adherence phenomena associated with RS cells[47]. We have undertaken detailed analysis of the PNA binding glycoproteins present in cell lines derived from Hodgkin's disease[48]. The probing of nitrocell-ulose membranes from SDS–PAGE separated, detergent solubilized cellular glycoproteins with radio-iodine labelled PNA has revealed heterogenous glycoprotein profiles in which apparently HD restricted glycoprotein bands can be identified[48]. In summary, lectin binding studies parallel observations with CD15 in demonstrating variations in carbohydrate metabolism associa-ted with RS cells.

In addition to studies of the expression of sugars by lectin binding Paietta et al.[49-51] have demonstrated a lectin-like moleculea associated with the plasma membrane of cultured RS cells. The molecule is a galactophilic lectin of Mr 55 000 (p55) and has binding characteristics similar to those of the hepatic asialo glycoprotein receptor to which it is also related antigenically. Antibodies to hepatic binding protein stain the surface of HD cell lines and a proportion of RS cells in immunohistochemical investigations of routine biopsy tissue. Lectin-like activity has been confirmed by the ability of cultured cell lines and purified protein to agglutinate erythrocytes and desialylated T-lymphocytes. The lectin-like activity of this molecule, which shows ectosialyl transferase activity in its purified form, is further demonstrated in studies of neuraminidase treated HD cultured cell lines where the binding of appropriate monoclonal antibodies to surface fucosyl-N-acetyl lactosamine residues is auto-inhibited by their interaction with p55. Molecules of this type could clearly mediate important interactions between tumour cells and reactive stroma in the pathogenesis of HD. However, the universal distribution of p55 in HD has yet to be established.

CD30 AND HODGKIN'S DISEASE

Studies of cellular expression of carbohydrate moieities or the demonstration of abnormal epitope expression with antigenic systems such as CD15 cannot generally contribute to a specific discussion of the relationship of HD cells to a restricted cellular lineage. Similarly, as discussed earlier, attempts at pheno-typing have been generally uninformative in this respect. An alternative approach would be to establish antibodies specifically identifying HD and RS cells and then use these as probes to examine reactive or control tissues for a normal counterpart. This approach was undertaken by Stein and his co-workers who prepared rabbit antisera to a cell line, L428, derived from Hodgkin's disease. After extensive absorption these antisera proved relatively specific for RS cells[52-54]. Subsequently, monoclonal antibodies with a similar reactivity were prepared (CD)[54]. Initial studies[55] showed that the monoclonal antibody, Ki-1 and, to a lesser extent, the antibodies Ki-24 and Ki-27 were

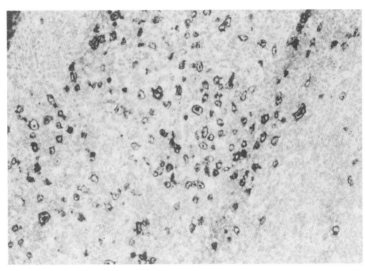

Figure 1 Nodular sclerosing Hodgkin's disease: Ki-1 (CD30) positive RS and mononuclear Hodgkin's cells stained in frozen section. (Alkaline phosphatase reporter system × 200)

almost universally expressed on RS cells and their mononuclear counterparts (Figure 1).

Extensive investigations of a range of normal and reactive tissues using Ki-1 antibody suggested that a normal counterpart of the RS cell existed and that this cell was largely associated with the perifollicular areas of reactive lymph nodes. The antigen, first defined by the antibody Ki-1, was subsequently designated CD30 by the *Third International Leucocyte Typing Workshop*[15]. It is now clear that CD30 is more widely expressed, particularly within the lymphocyte lineage, than was previously thought. CD30 appears on lymphocytes following activation with autologous or allogeneic cells, various mitogens and infectious agents, such as Epstein–Barr virus[39,56,57]. It is also clear that a subset of human NHL designated anaplastic large cell lymphoma can be identified by the strong expression of CD30[39,58,59]. In all these cases the presence of CD30 is associated with the expression of other markers of activation in lymphocytes, an observation which has led to the hypothesis that HD and anaplastic large cell lymphomas represent opposite ends of a spectrum of lymphoproliferative diseases in which lymphokine production by activated neoplastic cells of lymphoid derivation may be low or high. High levels of lymphokine secretion induce extensive reactive stroma formation, resulting in a histology compatible with HD[56].

The concept that RS cells and mononuclear HD cells are related to the lymphocyte lineage is consistent with the bulk of information which we have concerning phenotype and genotype in CD30 positive populations. However, Andreeson *et al.*[60] have described the expression of CD30 on cultured normal human macrophages following specific stimulation and also claimed expression on certain populations of malignant histiocytes. CD30 has also been demonstrated in erythroid precursors and occasional granulocyte precursors in human bone marrow trephines[61]. This data would parallel the observation of Andreeson *et al.*[60] that the erythromyeloid cell line, K562, is positive for CD30. The bone marrow study was undertaken using the paraffin reactive CD30 reagent BER-H2. Questions of lineage aside, monoclonal antibodies to CD15 and CD30 are extremely valuable in the identification of HD in formalin-fixed, paraffin-embedded tissue. Despite its widespread expression on activated lymphocytes, no biological function has yet been attributed to the CD30 molecule. CD30 exists in the cell membrane as a heterodimer consisting of two chains of Mr 120 000 and 105 000. Both appear to be derived from an 84 000 Mr protein present in the cytoplasm[62]. CD30 extracted from lymphocytes often shows a high level of phosphorylation and has, therefore, been considered as a receptor molecule[62]. However, a role for CD30 in signal transmission has not been unequivocally demonstrated and a natural ligand for which CD30 represents the receptor has not yet been identified.

THE ROLE OF HD-DERIVED CELL LINES IN STUDIES OF THE CELLULAR ORIGIN OF HD

It is well established[63] that attempts to grow neoplastic cells from HD or NHL tissues usually result in the appearance of lymphoblastoid cell lines dependent on the Epstein–Barr virus status of the individual patients[64]. The cell lines described by Kadin and Asbury[11] were immunoglobulin positive, whilst other lines in which a minority of cells expressed surface immunoglobulin showed a normal diploid karyotype and uniform expression of the Epstein–Barr virus nuclear antigen (EBNA)[65]. However, a small number of cell lines are now described in the literature which show abnormal karyotype, lack EBNA and are positive for CD30. In this respect, they may be considered as RS cell-derived, although this cannot be proven unequivocally. Currently published CD30 positive HD-derived cell lines are listed in Table 2, together with their phenotypic and genotypic features. This list includes L428, the cell line which was used as the immunogen for the production of the original CD30 antibody[54]. It can clearly be seen that, whilst the phenotype of these cells is very close to that described for RS cells[71], they do not exhibit consistent lineage markers. The phenotypic data obtained from these cell lines demonstrates heterogeneity and parallels that obtained from the frozen section immunophenotyping studies described earlier in this chapter. At best, we can say that investigations of HD-derived cells lend some support to the concept that the RS cell represents a cell which has evolved within the lymphocyte lineage but bears markers characteristic of lymphocyte activation. The genotypic data on these cells will be discussed in the next section in conjunction with genotypic data obtained from HD tissue biopsies. The cell line, SU/RS-HD-1, was established from the spleen of a patient with HD. This aneuploid cell line can be cloned in both liquid and semi-solid media. It is negative for EBNA and is considered histiocytic in its biological characteristics[72]. Insufficient data is available to relate this cell line to the lines described in Table 2.

Studies of the biology of HD cell lines may well prove relevant to the investigation of cell interactions in HD. Thus, L428 cells are potent stimulators

97

Table 2 Cell lines derived from HD tumour biopsies

Designation	Phenotype	Genotype*
Co	T(CD3(c),5,7)	TCR beta, gamma
Ho	T(CD3,4,7)	TCR beta, gamma
L591	B(CD19,22)	Ig genes
L428	B(CD19)	Ig genes, TCR beta
L540	T(CD2,4)	TCR beta, gamma
DEV	B(CD19,20)	Ig genes
Zo	—	Ig genes
HDLM-2	T(CD2)	TCR beta, gamma
KM H-2	CD9,21	Ig genes

Phenotype and genotype of cell lines is often abnormal. All cells positive for CD15, CD30. For detailed analyses see references 66–71, 74.
(c) = cytoplasmic; * = rearranged genes

of human primary mixed lymphocyte cultures and are capable of producing interleukin-1 (IL-1) when appropriately stimulated *in vitro*[73]. Other authors have also described the production of lymphokine by L428 cells[74] and these cells have also been described as releasing transforming growth factor beta (TGF-beta), a molecule which regulates the growth of activated human T-lymphocytes in response to IL-2[75]. Preliminary, and as yet unpublished, studies undertaken by ourselves in conjunction with Dr Johannes Gerdes of the Forschungsinstitut (Borstel, FRG), has shown, tumour necrosis factor (TNF) and interferon (INF-gamma) to be variously released from the cell lines described in Table 2 under conditions of normal or stimulated growth. These findings point to interaction between stromal elements and the tumour cell population in HD. We have also recently applied the monoclonal antibody[76] 10.1 to a range of HD and NHL biopsies[77]. Our studies show that the human Fc receptor (FcR ICD) identified by this antibody and known to be regulated by the action of factors such as IFN-gamma[76], is strongly expressed on macrophages present in both HD and anaplastic large cell lymphoma.

THE CONTRIBUTION OF GENE REARRANGEMENT STUDIES TO LINEAGE INVESTIGATIONS IN HD

The demonstration that gene segments coding for human T-cell receptors and immunoglobulin light and heavy chains undergo random clonal rearrangements during lymphocyte maturation has provided a powerful tool for the analysis of clonal derivation and evolution of NHL of both T-cell and B-cell origin[78]. The reader is referred to chapter 10 and the short review of O'Connor[79] for a detailed explanation of the theory and practice of the evaluation of immunoglobulin gene superfamily rearrangements in lymphoma biopsy tissue. The fact that genotypic investigations can determine lineage in the absence of an identifiable lineage specific phenotype should make gene rearrangement studies the method of choice for investigating the

Table 3 Studies of immunoglobulin gene superfamily rearrangements in Hodgkin's disease

Reference	Case studies			
	n	Germline	T-cell*	B-cell*
Weiss et al.[80]	16	15(1/8)	0(0/8)	1(7/8)
Knowles et al.[81]	15	12(3/3)	1(0/3)	2(0/3)
Griesser et al.[82]	8	4	4	0
Feller et al.[83]	22	4	16	2
O'Conner et al.[84]	35	33	0	2
Raghavachar et al.[85]	35	24	5	6
Sundeen et al.[86]	8	8(2/5)	0(0/5)	0(3/5)
Brinkler et al.[87]	11	6	0	5
Herbst et al.[88]	40	29(4/7)	6(1/7)	5(2/7)

*Rearrangements determined with probes appropriate for various immunoglobulin gene segments or segments of individual T-cell receptor chains. Figures in parentheses represent rearrangements determined on tissue biopsies rich in tumour cells or cell suspensions enriched for tumour cells

RS cell where the phenotypic data is confused. Table 3 summarizes a series of investigations of immunoglobulin and/or T-cell receptor gene rearrangements in HD biopsy tissue. It can be seen that, as with phenotypic investigations and tissue culture studies, the data obtained from HD is not entirely consistent. The first observation is that in many of the studies the majority of cases investigated have not revealed clonal rearrangements of either immunoglobulin or T-cell receptor genes. It is possible that this represents a genuine germline genotype. However, both Weiss et al. and Knowles et al.[80,81] obtained increased frequencies of clonal rearrangements when they specifically investigated cases with a high content of HD and RS cells. Further, Sundeen et al.[86] increased the proportion of cases showing gene rearrangements following enrichment for tumour cells. This data suggests that it is the low frequency of tumour cells, present in biopsies, which accounts for the germline genotype of most cases.

The second set of observations concerns the presence of clonal gene rearrangements related to a particular lymphocyte subset. Cases of HD have been identified which express clonal gene rearrangements characteristic of T- or B-cells and occasional cases show a mixed genotype. It is not clear if these discrepancies are the result of differing experimental procedures or merely reflect small sample size. It is also possible that selection of the histological subtype of cases (for example, tumour cell-rich recurrence) could account for the variation in genotypes shown in different studies.

In a recent investigation in association with colleagues in Berlin[88] we have further investigated immunoglobulin and T-cell receptor gene rearrangements in HD and attempted to compare the gene configurations seen with the phenotypic data in both tissue biopsies and HD cell lines. It is clear that there is some dissociation between phenotype and genotype in the cases examined. Within the B-cell lineage, at least, Gregory et al.[89] have demonstrated an experimental basis for dissociation between genotype and phenotype. Epstein–Barr virus (EBV) transformation of early B-cells leads to a series of B-cell lines with incomplete gene rearrangements but some of the phenotypic characteristics of mature B-cells, implying that transformation during the early stages of immunoglobulin superfamily gene rearrangement can nevertheless lead to cell lines which may variously express mature lymphoid markers. With this experimental investigation in mind it is conceivable that RS cells expressing many lineage-related phenotypic markers, characteristic of mature cells, may actually represent a transformation process which has occurred early during differentiation[90]. As additional support for this theory, Herbst *et al.*[88] cite observations on HD-derived cell lines. At least two cell lines of B-cell lineage have rearranged immunoglobulin heavy chain genes and unusual rearrangements of the kappa chain genes with deletions in either constant or joining regions[90]. Further, the cell line, Co, expresses only the beta chain of the T-cell receptor and this is present in the cytoplasm, rather than on the cell membrane as part of a heterodimer[71]. Both these observations could be considered as indicative of immaturity in the cell line. However, data from cell lines must be interpreted with caution, and it is equally possible that the unusual immunoglobulin gene rearrangements, seen in L428, are aberrant and represent a mature cell with non-productively rearranged immunoglobulin genes. In the cell line Co investigations of messenger RNA have revealed material with a size pattern characteristic of mature, rather than immature, T-cells[67]. Heterogeneity of both phenotype and genotype is seen in peripheral (mature) T-cell lymphomas[91–93] and it is not possible to exclude secondary loss as a reason for the aberrant phenotype in Co. It should be noted, however, that whilst the concept proposed in Herbst *et al.*[88] may place the events leading to neoplastic transformation early in differentiation it does not change our overall concept of the RS cell as a representative of the lymphocyte lineage. The bulk of evidence presented in the preceding sections is broadly, although not unequivocally, supportive of this view.

STUDIES CONCERNING A VIRAL AETIOLOGY FOR HD

Many authors have suggested that HD may have a viral aetiology (reviewed in reference 94). Often these suggestions are intuitive, rather than based on sound biological investigation. Nevertheless, studies of aetiology and epidemiology[95], geographical distribution[94], investigations of social class[96] and the particular histology associated with HD could be interpreted as indicating an infectious agent. Further, the systemic immune derangements associated with HD and discussed by Amlot in this volume could also support a viral aetiology. In view of the presumed B-cell phenotype or genotype of many cases of HD, EBV would be a strong contender as a transforming agent and has previously been suggested as such on epidemiological grounds. Weiss *et al.*[80] were able to identify integrated EBV sequences in 4 of 21 cases of HD, and EBV was also found associated with 5 of 39 HD tissues biopsies by Herbst[88]. It would be tempting to interpret this data as implicating EBV in neoplastic transformation leading to HD. The frequency of EBV sequences in the HD cases investigated is not high and only one of the published HD cell lines listed in Table 2 (L591) is EBNA positive. However, as RS cells are heterogenous in phenotype it is possible that EBV may be involved in the initiation of the neoplastic process in some cases only.

A demonstration by electron microscopy of retroviral particles in HD cells[97] could point to RNA virus as an aetiological agent for HD. However, retrovirus is frequently a symbiont in replicating lymphoid cells and as yet there has been no clear demonstration of transformation of human leukocytes by a retroviral isolate from HD. More recently, human Herpes virus-6 (HHV-6) has been isolated from patients with a variety of lymphoproliferative and immunosuppressive disorders[98] and termed human B-cell lymphotrophic virus (HBLV). Although the precise cellular tropism of HBLV is not known, the virus can be propagated to high titre in human T-cell lines[99]. More recently, HBLV has been isolated from African patients with AIDS[100]. Extensive investigations employing appropriate gene probes have failed to demonstrate an association of HBLV with HD[99]. In summary, the techniques of molecular probing with appropriate gene probes have, as yet, failed to establish a relationship between HD and a single viral isolate.

CONCLUSION

In this chapter we have examined a large volume of data relating to the biology and origin of the RS cell and its mononuclear counterparts. Much of this data supports conflicting views on the cell of origin of the neoplastic population in HD. Part of this confusion originates in the certain fact that the entity previously considered as HD clearly represents at least two different pathological processes, and is compounded by the difficulty in obtaining RS cells or HD cells in sufficient numbers for many detailed biological investigations. It must also be said that there are other cell types (Table 4) which have been suggested as a normal counterpart for the RS cell. These suggestions have usually been made on the grounds of morphological, limited electron microscopic, or limited biological investigations and have not been pursued as rigorously as investigations relating to the lymphocyte/histiocyte series which we have reviewed in this chapter. Despite the wealth of contradictory evidence, it would seem that the most reasonable current interpretation must be that the RS cell represents a transformed derivative of the lymphocyte

Table 4 Other cell types considered as possible progenitors of Hodgkin's tumour cells

	Reference
Interdigitating reticulum cells	101, 102
Dendritic reticulum cells	103, 104
Myeloid lineage	74
Sinus endothelial cells	2

series. It must be stressed, however, that this conclusion reflects a personal interpretation of the information available and, as yet, there is no unequivocal proof of this origin. It seems likely that improvements in our ability to purify minority populations from complex cell mixtures, coupled with the rapid development of techniques of *in situ* hybridization, which will enable detailed investigation of gene expression in minority cell populations in tissue section, will finally provide the conclusive data which is lacking to date. Clearly, however, our ability to fully characterize the Reed–Sternberg cell can only represent the first stage in our understanding of the complex pathological process which leads to the evolution of Hodgkin's disease. Only when we have achieved this can we claim to have solved the complex and interesting intellectual problem posed by Thomas Hodgkin 156 years ago.

References

1. Hodgkin, T. (1832). On some morbid appearance of the absorbent glands and spleen. *Med.-Chir. Trans.* **17**, 68–114
2. Sternberg, C. (1898). Uber erin eigenartige uuter dem Bilde. *Z. Helik.*, **19**, 21–90
3. Reed, D. (1902). On the pathological changes in Hodgkin's disease with special reference to its relationship to tuberculosis. *Johns Hopkins Rep.*, **10**, 133–96
4. Kaplan, H. (1980). *Hodgkin's disease*, 2nd Edn. (Cambridge MA: Harvard University Press)
5. Taylor, C. R. (1976). An immunohistochemical study of follicular lymphoma, reticulum cell sarcoma and Hodgkin's disease. *Eur. J. Cancer,* **12**, 61–75
6. Kadin, M. E., Stiles, D. P., Levy R. and Warnke, R. (1978). Exogenous origin of immunoglobulin in Reed–Sternberg cells of Hodgkin's disease. *N. Engl. J. Med.,* **299**, 1208–14
7. Payne, S. V., Jones, D. B., Haegert, D. G., Smith, J. L. and Wright, D. H. (1977). T- and B-lymphocytes and Reed–Sternberg cells in Hodgkin's disease lymph nodes and spleens. *Clin. Exp. Immunol.,* **2**, 768–9
8. Braylan, R. C., Jaffe, E. and Berard, C. W. (1974). Surface characteristics of Hodgkin's lymphoma cells. *Lancet,* **2**, 1328–9
9. Stuart, A. E., Williams, A. R. W. and Habeshaw, J. A. (1977). Rosetting and other reactions of the Reed-Sternberg cell. *J. Pathol.,* **122**, 81–90
10. Payne, S. V., Smith, J. L., Jones, D. B. and Wright, D. H. (1977). Lymphocyte markers in non-Hodgkin's lymphomas. *Br. J. Cancer,* **36**, 57–64
11. Kadin, M. E. and Asbury, A. K. (1973). Long-term culture of Hodgkin's tissue. *Lab. Invest.,* **28**, 181–4
12. Kaplan, H. and Gartner, S. (1977). Sternberg–Reed giant cells of Hodgkin's disease; cultivation *in vitro*, heterotransplantation and characterisation as neoplastic macrophages. *Int. J. Cancer,* **19**, 511–25
13. Papadimitriou, S., Stein, H. and Lennert, K. (1978). The complexity of immunohistochemical staining pattern of Hodgkin's and Sternberg–Reed cells – Demonstration of immunoglobulin, albumin, alpha-1 antichymotrypsin and lysozyme. *Int. J. Cancer,* **21**, 531–41
14. Payne, S. V., Wright, D. H., Jones, K. J. M. and Judd, M. A. (1982). Macrophage origin of Reed–Sternberg cells: An immunohistochemical study. *J. Clin. Pathol.,* **35**, 159–66
15. McMichael *et al.* (eds). (1988). *Third International Leucocyte Typing Workshop.* (Oxford: Oxford University Press)
16. Smith, J. L., Jones, D. B., Bell, A. J. and Wright, D. H. (1989) Correlation between histology and immunophenotype in a series of 322 cases of non-Hodgkin's lymphoma. *Hematol. Oncol.,* **7**, 37–48
17. Jones, D. B., Wright, D. H., Paul, F. and Smith, J. L. (1986). Phenotypic heterogeneity displayed by T-non-Hodgkin's lymphoma (T-NHL) cells dispersed from diagnostic lymph node biopsies. *Hematol. Oncol.,* **4**, 219–26
18. Jones, D. B., Moore, K. M. and Wright, D. H. (1989). Heterogeneity of antigen expression in B-cell non-Hodgkin's lymphoma. *Adv. Exp. Biol. Med.*, **137**, 139–44
19. Doreen, H. S., Habeshaw, J. A., Stansfeld, A. G. Wrigley, P. M. F. and Lister, T. A. (1984).

Characteristics of Sternberg-Reed and related cells in Hodgkin's disease. *Br. J. Cancer,* **49**, 465–76

20. Pizzolo, G., Chilosi, M., Semenzato, G., Caligaris-Cappio, F., Fiore-Donati, L., Perona, G. and Janossy, G. (1984). Immunohistochemical analysis of Tac antigen expression on tissues involved in Hodgkin's disease. *Br. J. Cancer,* **50**, 415–17

21. Poppema, S., Bhan, A. K., Reinherz, E. L., Posner, M. R. and Schlossman, S. F. (1982). *In situ* immunologic characterisation of cellular constituents in lymph nodes and spleens involved by Hodgkin's disease. *Blood,* **59**, 226–32

22. Stein, H., Gerdes, J., Schwab, U. *et al.* (1983). Evidence for the detection of the normal counterpart of Hodgkin and Sternberg-Reed cells. *Hematol. Oncol.,* **1**, 21–9

23. Angel, C. A., Warford, A., Campbell, A. C., Pringle, J. H. and Lauder, I. (1987). The immunohistology of Hodgkin's disease – Reed-Sternberg cells and their variants. *J. Pathol.,* **153**, 21–30

24. Poppema, S., Hollema, H., Visser, L. and Vos, H. (1987). Monoclonal antibodies (MT1, MT2, MB1, MB2, MB3) reactive with leucocyte subsets in paraffin embedded tissue sections. *Am. J. Pathol.,* **127**, 418–29

25. Norton, A. J. and Isaacson, P. G. (1985). Granulocyte and HLA-D region specific monoclonal antibodies in the diagnosis of Hodgkin's disease. *J. Clin. Pathol.,* **38**, 1241–6

26. Hsu, S. M. and Jaffe, E. S. (1984). Leu-M1 and peanut agglutinin stain the neoplastic cells of Hodgkin's disease. *Am. J. Clin. Pathol.,* **82**, 29–32

27. Pinkus, G. S., Thomas, P. and Said, J. W. (1985). Leu-M1 a marker for Reed-Sternberg cells in Hodgkin's disease. An immunoperoxidase study of paraffin embedded tissues. *Am. J. Pathol.,* **119**, 244–52

28. Poppema, S. (1980). The diversity of the immunohistological staining pattern of Sternberg-Reed cells. *J. Histochem. Cytochem.,* **28**, 788–91

29. Stein, H., Hansmann, M. L., Lennert, K., Brantzaeg, P., Gatter, K. C. and Mason, D. Y. (1986). Reed-Sternberg and Hodgkin cells in lymphocyte predominant Hodgkin's disease of nodular subtype contain J-chain. *Am. J. Clin. Pathol.,* **86**, 292–7

30. Sheibani, K., Battifora, H., Burke, J. S. and Rappaport, H. (1986). Leu-M1 in human neoplasms. An immunohistologic study of 400 cases. *Am. J. Surg. Pathol.,* **10**, 227–36

31. Hsu, S-M., Ho, Y-S., Li, P-J., *et al.* (1986). L and H variants of Reed-Sternberg cells express sialyated Leu-M1 antigen. *Am. J. Pathol.,* **122**, 199–203

32. Jack, A. S., Cunningham, D., Soukop, M., Liddle, C. N. and Lee, F. D. (1986). Use of Leu-M1 and anti-epithelial membrane antigen monoclonal antibodies for the diagnosis of Hodgkin's disease. *J. Clin. Pathol.,* **39**, 267–70

33. Poppema, S., Kaiserling, E. and Lennert, K. (1979). Nodular paragranuloma and progressively transformed germinal centres. Ultrastructural and immunohistologic findings. *Virchows Arch. B (Cell Pathol.),* **31**, 211–25

34. Timens, W., Visser, L. and Poppema, S. (1986). Nodular lymphocyte predominance type of Hodgkin's disease is a germinal center lymphoma. *Lab. Invest.,* **54**, 457–61

35. Abdulaziz, Z., Mason, D. Y., Stein, H., Gatter, K. C. and Nash, J. R. G. (1984). An immunohistochemical study of the cellular constituents of Hodgkin's disease using a monoclonal antibody panel. *Histopathology,* **8**, 1–25

36. Flavell, D. J., Jones, D. B. and Wright, D. H. (1987). Identification of tissue histiocytes on paraffin sections by a new monoclonal antibody. *J. Histochem. Cytochem.,* **35**, 1217–26

37. Hsu, S-M., Pescovitz, M. D. and Hsu, R. L. (1986). Monoclonal antibodies against Su–DHL-1 cells stain the neoplastic cells in true histiocytic lymphoma, malignant histiocytes and Hodgkin's disease. *Blood,* **68**, 213–19

38. Jones, D. B., Gerdes, J., Stein, H., Wright, D. H. (1986). An investigation of Ki-1 positive large cell lymphomas with antibodies reactive with tissue macrophages. *Hematol. Oncol.,* **4**, 315–22

39. Stein, H., Mason, D. Y., Gerdes, J. *et al.* (1985). The expression of the Hodgkin's disease associated antigen Ki-1 in reactive and neoplastic lymphoid tissue, evidence that Reed–Sternberg cells and histiocytic malignancies are derived from activated lymphoid cells. *Blood,* **66**, 848–58

40. Stein, H., Uchanska-Ziegler, B., Gerdes, J., Zeigler, A. and Wernet, P. (1982). Hodgkin and Sternberg-Reed cells contain antigens specific to the late cells of granulopoeisis. *Int. J. Cancer,* **29**, 283–90

41. Dorfman, R. F., Gatter, K. C., Pulford, K. A. F. and Mason, D. Y., (1986). An evaluation

of anti-granulocyte and anti-leucocyte monoclonal antibodies in the diagnosis of Hodgkin's disease. *Am. J. Pathol.,* **123**, 508–19

42. Jones, D. B., Fleming, S. and Wright, D. H. (1988). Heterogeneity of antigen recognition by CD15 antibodies. *J. Pathol.,* **154**, 39A–40A

43. Kelly, S. E. and Fleming, S. (1988). The structure of fucosylated blood group substances in fetal rat skin. The combined use of monoclonal antibodies and glycosyl hydrolases. *Br. J. Dermatol.,* **118**, 765–73

44. Fleming, S. and Brown, G. Distribution of fucosylated n-acetylglycosamine carbohydrate determinants during embryogenesis of the kidney in man. *Histochem. J.,* **18**, 61–6

45. Cabanillas, F. (1988). A review and interpretation of cytogenetic abnormalities identified in Hodgkin's disease. *Hematol. Oncol.,* **6**, 271–4

46. Bramwell, V. H. C., Crowther, D., Gallagher, J. and Stoddart, R. W. (1982). Studies of lectin binding to normal and neoplastic lymphoid tissues. 1. Normal nodes and Hodgkin's disease. *Br. J. Cancer,* **46**, 568–81

47. Payne, S. V., Newell, D. G., Jones, D. B. and Wright, D. H. (1980). The Reed–Sternberg cell/lymphocyte interaction. Ultrastructure and characteristics of binding. *Am. J. Pathol.,* **100**, 7–14

48. Flavell, D. J., Jones, D. B. and Wright, D. H. (1989). Identification of peanut agglutinin binding glycoproteins restricted to Hodgkin's disease-derived cell lines. *Hematol. Oncol.,* 7, 207–17

49. Paietta, E., Stockert, R. J., Morrell, A. G., Diehl, V. and Wiernik, P. H. (1986). Lectin activity as a marker for Hodgkin's disease cells. *Proc. Natl. Acad. Sci. USA,* **83**, 3451–5

50. Paietta, E., Stockert, R. J., Morell, A. G., Diehl, V. and Wiernik, P. (1986). Unique antigen of cultured HD cells. A putative sialyltransferase. *J. Clin. Invest.,* **78**, 349–54

51. Paietta, E., Hubbard, A. L., Wiernik, P., Diehl, V. and Stockert, R. J. (1987). Hodgkin's cell lectin: An ectosialyltransferase and lymphocyte agglutinant related to the hepatic asialoglycoprotein receptor. *Cancer Res.,* **47**, 2461–7

52. Stein, H., Gerdes, J., Kirchner, H., Schaadt, M. and Diehl, V. (1984). Hodgkin and Sternberg–Reed cell antigen(s) directed by an antiserum to a cell line (L428) derived from Hodgkin's disease. *Int. J. Cancer,* **28**, 425–9

53. Schwab, U., Stein, H., Gerdes, J., Lemke, H., Kirchner, H., Schaadt, M. and Diehl, V. (1982). Production of a monoclonal antibody specific for Hodgkin and Sternberg–Reed cells of Hodgkin's lymphoma and a subset of normal lymphoid cells. *Nature,* **299**, 65–7

54. Stein, H., Gerdes, J., Schwab, U., Lemke, H., Mason, D. Y., Ziegler, A., Schenjle, W. and Diehl, V. (1982). Identification of Hodgkin and Sternberg–Reed cells as a unique cell type derived from a newly detected small cell population. *Int. J. Cancer,* **30**, 445–59

55. Stein, H., Gerdes, J., Kirchner, H., Diehl, V., Schaadt, M., Bonk, A. and Steffen, T. (1981). Immunohistological analysis of Hodgkin's and Sternberg–Reed Cells: Detection of a new antigen and evidence of selective IgG uptake in the absence of B-cell and T-cell and histiocytic markers. *J. Cancer Res. Clin. Oncol.,* **101**, 125–34

56. Andreeson, R., Osterholz, J., Löhr, G. W. and Bross, K. J. (1984). A Hodgkin cell-specific antigen is expressed on a subset of auto- and allo-activated T-cells. *Blood,* **63**, 1299–302

57. Drexler, H. G., Jones, D. B., Diehl, V. and Minowada, J. (1989). Is the Hodgkin cell a T- or B-lymphocyte? Recent evidence from geno- and immunophenotypic analysis and *in vitro* cell lines. *Hematol. Oncol.,* 7, 37–48

58. Delsol, G., Stein, H., Pulford, K. A. P., Gatter, K. E., Erber, W. N. and Zinn, K. (1984). Human lymphoid cells express epithelial membrane antigen. *Lancet,* **2**, 1124–8

59. Stein, H. Personal Communication.

60. Andreeson, R., Brugger, W., Lohr, G. and Bross, K. (1989). Human macrophages can express the Hodgkin's cell-associated antigen Ki-l (CD30). *Am. J. Pathol.,* **134**, 187–92

61. Wilkins, B. S. and Jones, D. B. (1989). The use of immunohistochemical techniques with fixed, decalcified, wax-embedded bone marrow trephine biopsies. *Hematol. Rev.,* 3, 149–63

62. Stein, H. and Gerdes, J. (1986). Phänotypische und genotypische Marker bei malignen Lymphomen: Ein Beitrag zum zellulären Ursprung des Morbus Hodgkin und der malignen Histiozytose sowie Implikationen für die Klassification der T-Zell und B-Zell Lymphome. *Verh. Dtsch. Ges. Path.,* **70**, 127–51

63. Nilsson, R. and Pontin, J. (1985). Classification and biological nature of established human haemopoietic cell lines. *Int. J. Cancer,* **5**, 321–41

64. Diehl, V. and Johannson, B. (1977). Establishment of peripheral lymphoid cell cultures from patients with Hodgkin's disease (HD) depending on Epstein–Barr virus (EBV) reactivity and cellular immunity. *Blut,* **34**, 227–36

65. Friend, C., Marovitz, W., Henle, G., Henle, W., Tsuel, D., Hirschorn, K., Holland, J. G. and Cuther, J. (1978). Observations on cell lines derived from patients with Hodgkin's disease. *Cancer Res.,* **38**, 2581–91

66. Rabbitts, T. H., Stinson, A. and Forster, A. (1985). Heterogeneity of T-cell beta-chain gene rearrangements in human leukaemia and lymphomas. *EMBO J.,* **4**, 2217–24

67. Falk, M. H., Tesch, H., Stein, H., Diehl, V., Jones, D. B., Fonatsch, C. and Bornkamm, G. W. (1987). Phenotype versus immunoglobulin and T-cell receptor genotype of Hodgkin-derived cell lines: Activation of immature lymphoid cells in Hodgkin's disease. *Int. J. Cancer,* **40**, 262–9

68. Drexler, H. G., Graedicke, G., Lok, M. S., Diehl, V. and Minowada, J. (1986). Hodgkin's disease cell derived cell lines HDLM-2 and L428: Comparison of morphology, immunology and isoenzyme profiles. *Leuk. Res.,* **10**, 487–500

69. Kamesaki, H., Fukuhara, S., Tatsumi, E., Uchino, H., Yamabe, H., Miwa, H., Shiragawa, S., Hatanaka, M. and Honji, T. (1986). Cytochemical, immunologic, chromosomal and molecular genetic analysis of a novel cell line derived from Hodgkin's disease. *Blood,* **68**, 285–92

70. Drexler, H. G., Amlot, P. L. and Minowada, J. (1987). Hodgkin's disease derived cell lines – Conflicting clues for the origin of Hodgkin's disease. *Leukemia,* **1**, 629–37

71. Jones, D. B., Furley, A. J. W., Gerdes, J., Greaves, M. F., Stein, H. and Wright, D. H. (1989). Phenotypic and genotypic analysis of two cell lines derived from Hodgkin's disease tissue biopsies. *Rec. Res. Cancer Res.,* **117**, 62–6

72. Olsson, L., Bernke, O., Pleibel, N., D'Amore, F., Werldin, O., Fry, K. E. and Kaplan, H. S. (1984). Establishment and characterisation of a cloned giant cell line from a patient with Hodgkin's disease. *J. Natl. Cancer Inst.,* **73**, 809–30

73. Fisher, R. I., Bostick-Bruton, F., Sauder, D. N., Scala, G. and Diehl, V. (1983). Neoplastic cells obtained from Hodgkin's disease are potent stimulators of human primary mixed lymphocyte cultures. *J. Immunol.,* **130**, 2666–70

74. Diehl, V., Burrichter, H., Schaadt, M., Kirchner, H. H., Fonatsch, Chr., Stein, H., Gerdes, J., Heit, W. and Ziegler, A. (1983). Hodgkin's cell lines: Characteristics and possible pathogenetic implications. *Hematol. Oncol.,* **1**, 139–47

75. Newcom, S. R., Kadin, M. and Ansari, A. A. (1988). Production of transforming growth factor-beta activity by Ki-1 positive lymphoma cells and analysis of its role in the regulation of Ki-1 positive lymphoma growth. *Am. J. Pathol.,* **131**, 569–77

76. Dougherty, G. J., Selvendran, Y., Murdoch, S., Palmer, D. G. and Hogg, N. (1989). The human mononuclear phagocyte high-affinity Fc receptor, FcR1, defined by a monoclonal antibody 10.1. *Eur. J. Immunol.,* **17**, 1453–9

77. Jones, D. B., Gerdes, J., Stein, H. and Wright, D. H. Immunohistological evidence for activation of macrophages in Hodgkin's disease (Submitted for publication)

78. Arnold, A., Cossman, J., Bakshi, A., Jaffe, E. S., Waldmann, T. A. and Korsmeyer, S. J. (1983). Immunoglobulin gene rearrangements as unique clonal markers of lymphoid neoplasms. *N. Engl. J. Med.,* **309**, 1593–9

79. O'Connor, N. J. J. (1987). Genotypic analysis of lymph node biopsies. *J. Pathol.,* **151**, 185–90

80. Weiss, L. M., Strickler, J. G., Hu, E., Warnke, R. A. and Sklar, J. (1986). Immunoglobulin and gene rearrangements in Hodgkin's disease. *Hum. Pathol.,* **17**, 1009–19

81. Knowles, D. M., Neri, A., Pellici, P. G., Burke, J. S., Wu, A., Winberg, C. D., Sheibani, K. and Dalla-Favera, R. (1986). Immunoglobulin and T-cell receptor beta-chain gene rearrangement analysis of Hodgkin's disease. *Proc. Natl. Acad. Sci., USA,* **83**, 7942–51

82. Griesser, H., Feller, A., Lennert, K., Tweedale, M., Messner, H. A., Zalcberg, J. Minded, M. D. and Mak, T. W. (1986). The structure of the T-cell gamma chain gene in lympho-proliferative disease and lymphoma cell lines. *Blood,* **68**, 592–4

83. Feller, A. and Griesser, H. (1986). Antigen expression and gene rearrangement studies in anaplastic large cell lymphomas and Hodgkin's disease. In McMichael, A. J. *et al.* (eds) *Leucocyte Typing* III. p.61. (Oxford: Oxford Unviersity Press)

84. O'Connor, N. T. J., Crick, J. A., Gatter, K. C., Mason, D. Y., Falini, B. and Stein, H.

(1987). Cell lineage in Hodgkin's disease. *Lancet,* **1**, 158–9

85. Raghavachar, A., Binder, T. and Bartram, C. R. (1988). Immunoglobulin and T-cell receptor gene rearrangements in Hodgkin's disease. *Cancer Res.*, **48**, 3591–4

85. Raghavachar, A., Binder, T. and Bartram, C. R. (1988). Immunoglobulin and T-cell receptor gene rearrangements in Hodgkin's disease. *Cancer Res.* **48**, 3591–94

86. Sundeen, J., Lipford, E., Uppenkamp, M., Sussman, E., Wahl, L., Raffeld, M. and Cossman, J. Rearranged antigen receptor genes in Hodgkin's disease. *Blood,* **70**, 96–102

87. Brinkler, M. G. L., Poppema, S., Buys, C. H. C. M., Tirrens, W., Osinger, J. and Visser, L. (1987). Clonal immunoglobulin rearrangements in tissue involved by Hodgkin's disease. *Blood,* **70**, 186–91

88. Herbst, H., Tippelmann, G., Anagnostopoulos, I., Gerdes, J., Schwarting, R., Boehm, T., Pileri, S., Jones, D. B. and Stein, H. (1989). Immunoglobulin and T-cell receptor gene rearrangements in Hodgkin's disease and Ki-1 positive anaplastic large cell lymphomas: Dissociation between phenotype and genotype. *Leukemia,* **13**, 103–16

89. Gregory, C. D., Kirchgens, C., Edwards, C. F., Young, L. S., Rowe, M., Forster, A., Rabbitts, T. H. and Rickinson, A. B. (1987). Epstein–Barr virus-transformed human precursor B-cell lines: Altered growth phenotype of lines with germline or rearranged but non-expressed heavy chain genes. *Eur. J. Immunol.,* **17**, 1199–207

90. Falk, M. H., Tesch, H., Stein, H., Diehl, V., Jones, D. B., Fonatsch, C., and Bornkamm, G. W. (1987). Phenotype verus immunoglobulin and T-cell receptor genotype of Hodgkin-derived cell lines: Activation of immature lymphoid cells in Hodgkin's disease. *Int. J. Cancer,* **40**, 262–9

91. Warnke, R. A. and Rouse, R. V. (1985). Limitations encountered in the application of tissue section immunodiagnosis to the study of lymphomas and related disorders. *Hum. Pathol.,* **16**, 326–31

92. Jones, D. B., Wright, D. H., Paul, F. and Smith, J. L. (1986). Phenotypic heterogeneity displayed by T-non-Hodgkin's lymphoma (T-NHL) cells dispersed from diagnostic lymph node biopsies. *Haematol. Oncol.,* **4**, 219–26

93. Smith, J. L., Haegert, D. G., Broadfield, E., Howell, W. M., Wright, D. H. and Jones, D. B. (1988). Phenotypic and genotypic heterogeneity of peripheral T-cell lymphoma. *Br. J. Cancer,* **58**, 723–9

94. Dalglesh, A. G. and McElwain, T. (1986). A viral aetiology for Hodgkin's disease. *Aust. NZ J. Med.,* **16**, 823–7

95. MacMahon, B. (1957). Epidemiological evidence on the nature of Hodgkin's disease. *Cancer,* **10**, 1045–54

96. Gutensohn, N. and Cole, P. (1980). Epidemiology of Hodgkin's disease. *Semin. Oncol.,* **7**, 92–103

97. Olssen, L. and Behnke, O. (1988). Emergence of a retrovirus in a cloned cell line established from a lesion of Hodgkin's disease. *Hematol. Oncol.,* **6**, 213–22

98. Salahuddin, S. Z., Ablashi, D. V., Markham, P. D., Josephs, S. F., Sturzenegger, S., Kaplan, M., Halligan, G., Biberfeld, P., Wongstaal, F., Kramarsky, B. and Gallo, R. C. (1986). Isolation of new virus HBLV in patients with lymphoproliferative disease. *Science,* **234**, 596–601

99. Jarret, R. F., Gledhill, S., Qureshi, F., Crae, S. H., Madhok, R., Brown, I., Evans, I., Krajewski, A., O'Brien, C. J., Cartwright, R. A., Venables, P. and Onions, D. E. (1988). Identification of human herpes virus 6 – Specific DNA sequences in two patients with non-Hodgkin's lymphoma. *Leukemia,* **2**, 496–502

100. Tedder, R. S., Briggs, M., Cameron, C. H., Honess, R., Robertson, D. and Whittle, H. (1987). A novel lymphotropic herpes virus. *Lancet,* **2**, 390–2

101. Kadin, M. E. (1982). Possible origin of the Reed–Sternberg. Cell from and interdigitating reticulum cell. *Cancer Treat. Rep.,* **66**, 601–8

102. Hansmann, M. L. and Kaiserling, E. (1981). Electron microscopic aspects of Hodgkin's disease. *J. Cancer Res. Clin. Oncol.,* **101**, 135–48

103. Curran, R. C. and Jones, E. L. (1978). Hodgkin's disease: An immunohistochemical and histological study. *J. Pathol.,* **125**, 39–51

104. Van Unnik, J. A. M. (1984). The application of the metalophil method for the demonstration of histiocytes. *J. Pathol.,* **144**, 233–9

8
Chronic-type B-lymphocytic Leukaemias

P. RICHARDSON and J. GORDON

CHRONIC LYMPHOCYTIC LEUKAEMIA

With the exception of myeloma, chronic lymphocytic leukaemia (CLL) is, from the fifth decade onward the most common lymphoid malignancy in man[1].

The examination of large series of CLL reveal that the majority of cases represent proliferations of B-lymphocytes[2]. Only 1–2% of reported cases are T-cell in origin[3]. That B-CLL is a clonal expansion is demonstrated by expression on the cell surface of immunoglobulin (SIg) bearing one light chain isotype only[4]. The precise ratio of cases expressing kappa (κ) or lambda (λ) light chain varies considerably among published studies: κ to λ ratios of 0.7[5], 0.9[6], 1.2 (Authors' observation), and 5[7,8] have been reported. The latter figure suggests that the selection of light chain isotype might be a non-random event, possibly influenced by geographical or environmental factors.

Disagreement exists in the literature as to the precise distribution of heavy chain classes in CLL. Virtually all reports, however, agree that IgM is the most commonly expressed, but whether usually alone or co-expressed with IgD is in dispute. Hamblin and colleagues[8] report figures of 39% cases expressing M alone, with 32% M and D, and 22% having no detectable SIg at all. Palestro et al[9] reported 67% having M alone and 17% M and D, while Van der Reijden[6] found that 42% were M alone and an equal number had M and D. One of us (PR, unpublished data) has found that when using the sensitive direct antibody rosette technique[10], in virtually every case where M is expressed, D is also detectable. The SIg on B-CLL is generally weaker in expression than that found with normal peripheral B cells[11]. Variations in reported levels may, therefore, reflect differences in sensitivity of techniques and reagents. A subgroup of CLL expressing IgG alone, accounting for approximately 10% of cases examined, has been defined by several groups (references 6, 8 and PR, unpublished data). An even rarer group expressing IgA alone has also been observed (reference 6 and PR, unpublished data). Triple heavy chain expression, particularly M, D, and G classes has been described for CLL[12]. However, Stevenson and colleagues[13] found differences in idiotype between IgG and other isotypes in such cases, suggesting that the former represented serum-derived material binding to the cell surface.

Several attempts have been made to correlate the SIg phenotype with staging and prognosis in CLL. Ligler and co-workers[14] found that IgG expression was associated with early clinical stages, whilst the clinically more advanced disease was linked to expression of IgM. Berntorp and Zettervall[15] have suggested that a strong expression of SIg is sufficient to auger a poor prognosis, whilst Baldini et al.[16] could find no correlation between SIg phenotype, staging or prognosis. As progress is made in the definition of phenotypic sub-groups using additional markers, this problem should be resolved.

Mouse erythrocyte rosettes

The spontaneous rosetting of mouse erythrocytes with normal and neoplastic B-cells was first described by Stathopoulous and Elliot[17]. Further studies have found the expression of the mouse red cell receptor to be correlated with the clinical diagnosis of CLL[18,19]. However, Abdul-Cader et al.[20] found that the receptor was also present on up to one-third of cases of follicle centre cell tumours exhibiting peripheral blood involvement. This marker, therefore, can no longer be regarded as a strict diagnostic feature, although most cases of CLL are positive[18]. Of 91 cases studied by one of us (PR), only seven were found to lack the mouse red cell receptor entirely (unpublished data). The percentage of neoplastic cells positive varies considerably (10–75% in one study[9]). In general the receptor is weakly expressed, with only occasional examples showing strong expression (PR, unpublished data). Cherchi and Catovsky[21] found a significantly higher percentage of mouse RBC receptor-positive cells in the peripheral blood populations of CLL than in the bone marrow and lymph nodes. They suggested that this might indicate that the receptor has a function in the tissue localization of B cells. It should be stressed that the assay for the receptor is not without its technical problems – for example, the strain of mouse used is said to be important[22]. A thorough review of the technical aspects has been published[23].

CD 5

The surface structures defined by monoclonal antibodies have recently been grouped into Cluster Designations (CD) by the *First and Second International Workshops on Human Leucocyte Differentiation Antigens*[24,25]. Those relevant to the study of B lymphoid malignancies will now be considered. One such antigen of particular relevance to B-CLL is the 65 kilodalton (Kd) glycoprotein, defined by the monoclonal antibodies T101[26], Leu-1[27], OKT 1[28] and RFT1[29] which comprise CD5 by the Workshop designation. Originally described as a marker of T-cells, it was later found expressed both on neoplastic B-cells[26] and on a fraction of normal peripheral B cells[29]. The CD5 molecule is expressed on most cases of CLL[26], although 10% of cases appear to be negative (PR, unpublished observations).

Considering the three markers discussed so far, the CLL cell can be said, typically, to be weakly positive for SIg and to express the mouse red cell receptor and the CD 5 antigen. A minority of cases are mouse red cell receptor-negative and/or CD 5-negative.

MHC Class 2

The expression of class 2 MHC products at the cell surface is an early feature in B-cell differentiation, and is lost only at the terminal stages of antigen-driven differentiation[30]. Thus, most normal peripheral B-cells express MHC Class 2, and, reflecting this, so do the overwhelming majority of B-cell proliferations[31]. Recent studies have shown that the MHC Class 2 locus can be resolved into at least three different loci, given the nomenclature DR, DQ, and DP[32], with gene products similarly labelled. Guy et al.[33], using specific monoclonal antibodies, found that the cells in a proportion of B-CLLs failed to react with an anti-DQ antibody, whilst all were positive for the DR and DP products. MHC Class 2 antigens provide a good marker for defining the neoplastic population of CLL; it must be noted, however, that MHC Class 2 expression is not exclusive to the B-cell compartment, but can be found on activated T-lymphocytes[34], as well as various other cell types.

CD19

One marker that does appear to be specific for B-cells is the CD19 antigen. CD19 is defined by monoclonal antibodies which include B4[35], and HD37[36]. The 95 Kd glycoprotein is to be found on the surface of the earliest identifiable B-lymphocyte, the pre-B-cell, right through the normal differentiation pathway, being lost only at the stage of antibody-secretion. It is not, however, strongly expressed on all CLL cases[36]. CD19 is probably the most reliable pan-B marker currently available.

CD23

Surface markers which are absent on the resting B-lymphocyte, but present on activated cells are, not surprisingly, referred to as 'activation antigens'. The CD23 antigen, a 45 Kd molecule detected with monoclonal antibodies such as MHM6[38] and Blast-2[38] represents such an antigen, absent on resting B-cells, and appearing rapidly upon activation[37]. In lymphoid tissues it is strongly expressed on germinal centre cells[38] and on a few circulating normal peripheral B-cells (Author's unpublished observations). Two-thirds of cases of CLL examined have been found positive for CD23[39]. It appears to be absent or weakly expressed on the mouse red cell receptor-negative/CD5 -negative subgroup of CLL (PR, unpublished observations). A recent report from one of us (JG) suggests that CD23 may focus growth-promoting signals to activated B-cells[4]. Whether CD23 expression on CLL cells is functional remains to be determined.

CD21

A proportion of normal, peripheral B-cells express receptors for the C3d fragment of complement which is also the receptor for the Epstein–Barr virus [EBV][40,41]. The gp140 structure has been designated CD21. It is detected by monoclonal antibodies which include B2[42], BL13[43], and HB5[44], and is expressed on more than 90% of peripheral blood and lymphoid tissue B-cells[45]. It is also expressed on over 80% of B-CLL[39]. The activation of normal, resting B-cells *in vitro* results in a gradual loss of CD21 expression[46]. CD22, a 135 Kd structure bearing epitopes detected with the monoclonal antibodies HD39[47] and TO15[48], is a B-lineage specific marker, strongly expressed on 75% of normal, peripheral B-cells, but rather poorly represented on B-CLL. Less than 25% of cases express this marker[39]. There is a suggestion that CD22 is an example of a 'resting' B-cell antigen, as its expression is gradually lost following *in vitro* activation of normal B-cells.

CD20

Yet another B-lineage restricted antigen is found in the CD20 cluster. CD20 antisera detect a 35 Kd non-glycosylated phosphoprotein, originally defined by B1[49]. CD20 is often described as a Pan-B antigen, but, unlike CD19, it is not as widely represented throughout differentiation. It is present on $> 90\%$ of normal, peripheral B-cells and over 95% of CLL tested, but is absent on at least 50% of normal pre-B-cells in the bone marrow[39]. As with the B-lineage restricted antigens discussed so far, CD20 is lost in the terminal stages of differentiation. Thus, it is an adequate marker of B-cells, but its value is restricted to the more 'mature' B-lymphoid malignancies, as exemplified by B-CLL.

Non-lineage-restricted antigens

Several groups of monoclonal antibodies have been produced which have reactivities not only with B-cells, but also with other cell types. CD24 is such an example and is a 42 Kd chain glycoprotein[116]. It was originally defined by the antibody BA-1[51], and is present on nearly all normal, peripheral B-cells as well as granulocytes and some monocytes. Most cases of CLL show significant expression of this antigen[52].

CD9 is another example, being a 24 Kd antigen detectable by the monoclonal antibody BA-2[53]. It has a similar pattern of positivity to the CD24 antigen, in that it is present on normal, peripheral B-cells, granulocytes and monocytes[53]. It has an interesting distribution on CLL, however, being present on approximately 35% of cases in one series (PR, unpublished observations).

The CD10 antigen, probably better known as the common acute lymphoblastic leukaemia antigen (CALLA), is a 100 Kd structure originally described as being found on the majority of cases of childhood acute lymphoblastic leukaemias[54]. Monoclonal antibodies such as AL2[55] and J5[56] have now been raised against CD10. The antigen has also been found on normal pre-B-cells[57] and on some granulocytes[58]. In a large series of B-CLL examined, only an occasional case was found with 10% or more of the neoplastic cells expressing CD10. The significance of this finding is not clear.

Plasma cell antigens

Monoclonal antibodies are available which recognize determinants on the surface of both normal and neoplastic plasma cells. In general such reagents fail to react with B-CLL[60], which is perhaps not entirely unexpected since CLL is only rarely associated with a serum paraprotein[59]. Antibodies in this group include OKT10[60], PCA-1[61], and BU11[62]. A single case of CLL positive for plasma cell antigens has been reported[62]. This case, however, displayed morphological lymphoplasmacytoid differentiation.

Mixed phenotypes

Occasional reports appear in the literature regarding the phenomenon of 'mixed' markers – that is, B-lymphoproliferations apparently co-expressing T-cell markers or antigens usually associated with the monocyte/granulocyte series. Spontaneous rosetting with sheep erythrocytes, normally a feature of T-cells, has been described in cases of B-CLL[63,65] and the sheep red cell receptor (CD2) has been detected with specific antibodies[64]. There is evidence, however, that some of these cases may be reflecting an antibody activity of the SIg against a determinant on sheep erythrocytes, perhaps the Forssmann antigen[63]. At least two cases of B-CLL apparently expressing the T8 (CD8) antigen have been found (PR, unpublished observations).

The antibody OKM1[66] originally described as having reactivity against an epitope on the granulocyte complement receptor (C3bi-receptor or CR3) has been reported to be expressed on B-CLL[67] and one of us (PR) has obtained results in broad agreement with this finding (unpublished observations). It has recently been shown that the OKM1 antigen (CD11) has some structural similarity to the LFA-1/CD18 antigen[68], a molecule found on the surface of most lymphocytes, granulocytes and monocytes, and thought to be important in cytolytic T-cell-mediated killing and in the activities of the natural killer cell[69]. It is possible, therefore, that OKM1 cross-reacts with a CD18-related structure.

PROLYMPHOCYTIC LEUKAEMIA

Prolymphocytic leukaemia (PLL) was originally described as a rare variant of CLL, on the grounds of its clinical profile and characteristic morphology[70]. It is now, however, generally regarded as a separate clinical entity. Compared to the CLL cell, the typical PLL cell is larger, with a prominent central nucleolus and peripherally condensed nuclear chromatin. Reflecting its low incidence, relatively few studies have been undertaken on the surface characteristics of PLL.

Most PLL cases are of the B-cell lineage, with occasional T-cell variants[71]. An examination of SIg in 17 cases of PLL was undertaken by Costello et al.[72] who found little difference from CLL SIg profiles. Scott et al.[73] found a kappa to lambda ratio of 4.2, in 28 cases of PLL, compared with 1.5 for 295 cases of CLL. SIg expression is stronger on PLL than on[74] CLL and the receptor for the mouse RBC receptor is absent in nearly all cases studied[19] as also is the

111

CD5 antigen[57], so that a typical marker profile for B-PLL appears to be strongly expressed SIg, with both the mouse RBC receptor and CD5 being negative.

The monoclonal antibodies FMC.7[75] and RFA.4[57] have been reported to be positive in most cases of B-PLL, whilst unreactive with the majority of B-CLLs[76]. FMC.7 has been shown to bind to about 50% of normal, peripheral B-cells[75], and to all SIg-positive cells in human cord blood[77]. In addition, the entire B-cell population in some cases of immunodeficiency is FMC.7-positive[115]. As with all B-cell malignancies, B-PLL expresses MHC class 2 antigens strongly[78] and also the CD19, pan-B antigen[36]. One interesting difference between the B-CLL and B-PLL is that whereas fewer than 25% of B-CLLs express CD22, and then only weakly, eight out of nine cases of PLL showed a strong expression of this antigen[47]. Den Ottolander et al.[79] reported that B-PLL had a lower expression of the CD24 and CD9 antigens compared with B-CLL, and made the additional observation that PLL cells appear to express the OKM-1 antigen to a greater degree than CLL.

HAIRY CELL LEUKAEMIA

For many years, it was considered that the neoplastic cell of hairy cell leukaemia (HCL) had affinity more with the monocyte/macrophage lineage than the lymphocyte[80]. This was attributed to its monocytoid appearance in Romanowsky-stained preparations, and the phagocytic ability exhibited by the cells in most (but not all) cases[81]. However, the availability of good heteroantisera and, subsequently, of monoclonal antibodies, demonstrated, unequivocally, the expression of monotypic SIg on the majority of cases[82]. The demonstration by Korsmeyer et al.[83] that HCL cells have rearranged and expressed their immunoglobulin genes has put the issue beyond doubt that HCL is a malignant proliferation of B-cells.

A striking characteristic of HCL is that in the majority of cases, the neoplastic cells bear IgG on the cell surface, either alone or in association with other Ig classes. Jansen et al.[84], in a series of 62 patients found that 31% of cases had G alone, 25% expressed G and A, and 12% MD and GA. Golomb et al.[85] examined the SIg profiles of 37 patients, and reported that 27 had neoplastic populations expressing either G alone or with another isotype, including the triple expression of M, D, G or D, G, A in three cases. The finding of this distinct phenotypic bias toward IgG expression in HCL is an interesting contrast to B-CLL, where the predominant expression is of the IgM class. As for the distribution of light chain type, kappa to lambda ratios of 1.1[84], 2[82], 4[85] and up to 4.6[86] have been reported. As with CLL, some as yet undefined factors may work on selection (or detection) of light chain type by the neoplastic cell in some of these series. The possibility that patient survival may be influenced by phenotypic profile has been examined by at least two groups. Jansen et al.[84] found that while heavy chain type had no apparent influence on survival, light chain class may have done, with kappa expressors faring better than cases bearing lambda. Golomb et al.[86] found no difference in survival among heavy chain groups, but in their study kappa expressors did worse.

In common with B-CLL, but unlike B-PLL, HCL cells have a tendency to exhibit the mouse RBC receptor. Burns and Cawley[87] reported eight, out of 15 cases studied, expressing the receptor, and went on to show that, within affected spleens, the neoplastic cells had a stronger affinity for the mouse erythrocytes than those in the peripheral circulation. In addition, they found an apparent correlation between this phenotype and the SIg profile, with cases expressing IgG alone being largely mouse RBC receptor-negative. Similar findings of approximately equal numbers of mouse RBC receptor-positive and -negative cases were recorded by Catovsky et al.[18]. The above finding by Burns and Cawley[87], of stronger receptor expression on the splenic population is in interesting comparison with the data of Cherchi and Catovsky[21], who found the converse for CLL, with circulating cells having stronger receptor expression than those infiltrating bone marrow and lymph nodes.

The CD5 antigen appears to be absent on the majority of HCL cases so far studied, a finding in common with B-PLL. Herrman et al.[88] found only one clearly positive case in 14 studied, and Caligaris-Cappio et al.[89] demonstrated CD5 on three of nine cases examined, although it was rather weakly expressed compared with that found on the typical B-CLL cell.

HCL cells have clearly been shown to express the common B-cell features of MHC class 2 products[89,90], the CD20 antigen[89,91], and the receptor for the Fc portion of IgG[82]. The FcIgG receptor is said to be particularly strongly expressed on HCL cells, compared with B-CLL[92].

The 'activation' antigen, CD23, has not been intensively studied on HCL cells. Pallesen[93] found it strongly expressed on two cases, whilst Steel et al.[52] recorded a weak positivity on one case. One of us (PR) has examined ten cytochemically-proven cases of HCL and found five CD23-negative, four weakly positive and only one case with a reasonably convincing positivity (unpublished observations). The conclusion would seem to be that approximately half the cases may be positive for CD23 antigen.

There seems to be good agreement between the various studies undertaken, that most, if not all HCL cases express the CD22 antigen quite strongly[47,94]. This contrasts with B-CLL, but is similar to B-PLL[47]. Ten cases examined by one of us (PR) all had moderate-to-strong CD22 expression (unpublished observations).

Expression of the CD21 antigen would seem to be deficient on HCL cells. Using the EAC rosette assay for C3 receptor, Jansen et al.[92] could find no evidence of expression on 28 cases studied. Pallesen[93] reported negative findings on two cases, and weak positives and negatives were recorded by steel et al.[52] and Mason et al.[95]. Using the BL13 monoclonal antibody one of us (PR) found three positives out of ten examined, the remainder being either negative or only weakly reactive (unpublished observations).

The B-cell associated antigen CD24 is found on a minority of HCL cases. Meijer et al.[90] found seven out of ten cases negative, whilst Jansen et al.[96] failed to detect any significant CD24 positivity, using antibody BA-1. Herrmann et al.[88] found three out of 14 cases were reactive with BA-1, so the conclusion would be that most cases are not significantly positive for the CD24 molecular complex.

113

The CD9 B-cell associated marker was found to be expressed in only one of 14 cases examined by Herrmann et al.[88]. Using the antibody BA-2, one of us (PR) has found weakly positive neoplastic cells in three cases (unpublished observations). CD10, the common acute lymphoblastic leukaemia antigen, has not been detected in a series of ten cases investigated (PR, unpublished observations).

The two antibodies which tend to distinguish B-PLL from B-CLL, FMC.7 and RFA.4, are positive for most, if not all, cases of HCL[88,89,97] although the affinity is claimed to be greater for B-PLL than for HCL, in the case of FMC.7[76]. Other antibodies have been described which appear to exhibit an even more discriminatory pattern of reactivity for HCL. Posnett et al.[98] have prepared two monoclonal antibodies, alpha-HC1 and alpha-HC2, which appear to define antigenic determinants on the surface of HCL cells only, and a third antibody, S-HCL3 (Leu-M5) which is HCL-reactive but not lymphoid-lineage specific[99].

The receptor for Interleukin-2 (CD25), also known as 'Tac'[100], has been found to be expressed on HCL cells[83,88]. The CD25/Tac antigen has, subsequently, been found on B-CLL cells, but at a lower level of expression[101] than seen with HCL.

Reactivity with monoclonal antibodies directed against plasma cell surface determinants, have been reported for HCL. Anderson et al.[91] described a series of 22 HCL cases, of which 16 expressed significant positivity for the PCA-1 antigen[102], although another well-defined antibody, PC-1[103] was unreactive. Of the two antibodies, PC-1 is considered the more specific for the plasma cell, as PCA-1 also cross-reacts with granulocytes and monocytes. Anderson's group[91] interpreted their findings as suggesting that HCL represents a neoplastic transformation of a 'near-terminally differentiated' B-cell[91]. In another study, Nathan et al.[62] reported one case of HCL, out of three studied, which expressed both PCA-1 and BU11, the latter an antigen expressed on plasma cells, and weakly expressed on some normal, peripheral B-cells.

The presence of the OKM-1 antigen on the surface of B-CLL cells has already been described[67], but a demonstration of this marker of monocyte/macrophage lineage on HCL has proved difficult. Herrmann et al.[88] found two weakly positive cases out of 14, and Tubbs et al.[104] found no positives amongst ten HCL spleens, examined with immunohistochemistry. Ruco et al.[105] recorded OKM-1 positivity in three affected spleens. It is an interesting technical point that immunohistochemistry failed to detect OKM-1 antigen in ten spleens examined by Meijer's group[90], but the antigen was detectable in cell suspensions suggesting differing sensitivities of the two techniques. Worman et al.[97] failed to find OKM-1 on 11 cases studied, and additionally, could not detect five other monocyte/macrophage lineage-specific markers. The image of the HCL cell as a neoplastic lymphocyte, and not a macrophage, would appear to be intact.

It seems almost an inevitability with B-lymphoproliferative disorders that T-cell variants, and cases expressing mixed T- and B-phenotypes should be reported in the literature. HCL proves no exception, and rare examples of HCL have been cited, which have the clinicopathological features of the disease and yet express a T-cell surface phenotype[106]. Armitage *et al.*[107] describe three cases of E-rosette-positive, SIg-positive HCL, the E-rosette positivity being supported by reactivity with OKT-11 monoclonal antibody (CD2 reactive).

With the typical morphology, of a monocytoid cell with microfilamentous surface processes, and the characteristic strong positivity for the tartrate-stable isoenzyme of acid phosphatase[108], HCL does not usually provide any diagnostic problems for the haematologist. As has been shown, surface pheno-typic differences exist between B-CLL and B-HCL that distinguish between these entities, but the similarities between B-PLL and HCL, in terms of clinical features and surface phenotype, may make this task a little more difficult.

CONCLUDING REMARKS

Having considered the differing patterns of reactivity to be found in the chronic-type B-cell leukaemias, it is worthwhile examining the possible inter-relationships of the three groups in addition to the relationship they bear to normal counterparts. Addressing the latter question, various groups have attempted to locate normal counterparts of the neoplastic cells of CLL, PLL and HCL, with interesting and sometimes controversial results. The rationale of these studies is that the normal counterpart would be expected to possess most of the morphological and phenotypic characteristics of the neoplastic cell.

Commonly found in fetal lymph node, but rarer in adult tissue, is a weak SIg-positive, mouse RBC receptor-positive, CD5-positive B-cell population, located at the edge of the germinal centres. Caligaris-Cappio *et al.*[29] have postulated that this population is the normal progenitor of the B-CLL cell, which has an identical phenotype. It is often remarked that the B-CLL cell has features of a somewhat immature B-cell, largely because of the weak SIg expression, compared with the normal, circulating B-cell. It has been suggested that the CLL cell is 'frozen' at a stage of differentiation somewhere between a pre-B-cell and a mature, peripheral B-cell[109]. Evidence for this might include the observation that most CLL appear to express IgM only[8,9], which would agree with the known acquisition of SIg in antigen-independent development of the normal cell. However, one of us (PR), using a sensitive assay has found IgM and IgD co-expressed on most B-CLLs, with IgM alone a very rare finding (unpublished observation). IgG is thought to be acquired late in B-cell differentiation, and yet 10% of CLL express IgG, usually alone (unpublished observation). The finding of the 'B-CLL-like' cell in association with germinal centres in lymph nodes has provoked some speculation that the B-CLL cell might have a 'memory' cell origin, as it is thought the germinal centre may be the generative tissue of such cells[110]. The arguments used by all schools of thought are, essentially, based upon circumstantial evidence, and a direct demonstration of the true derivation of the B-CLL cell is lacking, at the time of writing.

Robinson *et al.*[111], using immunoelectron microscopy, found possible

115

candidates for normal counterparts of PLL and HCL cells, in normal peripheral blood, where 40% of a B-enriched population were found to have the morphological features of 'prolymphocytes'. In addition, these cells were MHC class 2-positive and a proportion expressed FMC.7. The same group also identified another fraction of the B-population (about 10%), the cells of which had a villous outline, similar to HCL cells, and showed some positivity for MHC Class 2, FMC.7, and the putative HCL-specific antibodies alpha-HC1 and alpha-HC2. It would be interesting to know whether these 'normal hairy cells' displayed any positivity for tartrate-stable acid phosphatase and the IL-2 receptor (CD25). Occasional tartrate-stable acid phosphatase-positive cells can be observed in preparations of normal peripheral blood cells and have also been noted in normal bone marrow, lymph nodes and spleen by Mover et al.[112]. With reference to the phenotypic bias of HCL cells toward IgG expression, Machii and co-workers[113] observed that normal peripheral B-cells expressing IgG, tended to have microfilamentous surface projections and tartrate-stable acid phosphatase activity.

A possible inter-relationship of CLL, PLL, and HCL has been suggested by a series of experiments involving the exposure in vitro of B-CLL cells to the tumour promoting agent, 12-o-tetradecanoyl-phorbol-13-acetate (TPA)[88,89]. After 72 hours incubation, the CLL cells underwent a morphological transformation, from small lymphocytes with relativly smooth surface topography, to larger cells, having surface projections, reminiscent of HCL cells. More remarkable was the change in surface antigenic phenotype, from a typical B-CLL profile, of SIg-positive, mouse RBC receptor-positive, FMC.7/RFA.4-negative, to one of mouse RBC receptor-negative, FMC.7/RFA.4-positive. In addition, these 'transformed' cells acquire positivity for tartrate-stable acid phosphatase, and, hence, an apparent progression, from CLL to HCL has been achieved. This transformation is not entirely satisfactory, however, as the HCL-like cells produced still retain CD5-positivity. They also lose SIg expression and acquire significant cytoplasmic immunoglobulin, features of the terminally-differentiated B-cell, bringing to mind the suggestion of Anderson's group[91], that HCL cells have features in common with the antibody-secreting cell. Caligaris-Cappio et al.[89] looked at the response to TPA of purified mouse RBC receptor-positive, CD5-positive B-cells from normal, peripheral blood, a fraction often equated with the normal counterpart of the CLL cell, and found loss of SIg and mouse RBC receptor, and acquisition of cytoplasmic immunoglobulin. However, in spite of tartrate-stable acid phosphatase acquisition, there was no significant increase in RFA.4-positivity and none of the morphological changes observed with the CLL response.

In a similar experiment, Robert et al.[114] incubated B-CLL cells with Escherichia coli lipopolysaccharide, a known B-cell mitogen, and examined the resulting 'blast' cells, finding an acquisition of FMC.7 positivity, loss of mouse RBC receptor, and stronger SIg expression, particularly of the IgM type, as well as an accumulation of cytoplasmic immunoglobulin. The suggestion was made that the CLL cells had acquired the characteristics of B-PLL cells. These are important and impressive experiments, but the results must be interpreted with caution, raising, as they do, the possibility that HCL

116

and PLL are conditioned closely related to CLL, and to each other.

Cases of CLL with 'prolymphocytoid' transformation are occasionally seen[50]. This rather provocative nomenclature requires some clarification. Most cases of classical CLL show the familiar morphology of the small lymphocyte, on Romanowsky-stained blood films, but occasional examples occur where this population is accompanied by larger, blast-like cells, and it is these cases that are categorized as 'prolymphocytoid'. These cells are not entirely the same in appearance as a typical PLL cell, and usually show no difference in phenotype from CLL cells retaining weak SIg and mouse RBC receptor-positivity. However, cases where CD5 and mouse RBC-positivity are lost, and FMC.7/RFA.4-positivity are acquired, have been reported[76]. Thus it seems some drift towards a PLL-like state may occur, although no complete transformation of a CLL to an unequivocal PLL has been reported. Further-more, there is no record of a case of CLL in which the spontaneous appear-ance of HCL-like cells has occured, along the lines of the prolymphocytoid transformation. One of us (PR) has observed the occasional HCL-like cell in wet preparations of CLL cells, and has also found strongly tartrate-stable acid phosphatase-positive cells in CLL populations, albeit numerically insignificant ($< 1\%$); unpublished observation).

References

1. Rundles, R. W. and Moore, J. O. (1978). Chronic lymphocytic leukemia. *Cancer*, **42**, 941–5
2. Aisenberg, A. C., Block, K. J. and Long, J. C. (1973). Cell surface immunoglobulin in chronic lymphocytic leukemia. *Am. J. Med.*, **55**, 184–91
3. Lille, I., Desplaces, A., Meeus, L., Saracino, R. T. and Brouet, J. C. (1973). Thymus-derived proliferating lymphocytes in chronic lymphocytic leukemia. *Lancet*, **1**, 263
4. Gordon, J., Webb, A. J., Walker, L., Guy, G. R. and Rowe, M. (1986). Evidence for an association between CD23 and the receptor for a low molecular weight B cell growth factor. *Eur. J. Immunol.*, **16**, 1627–30
5. Han, T., Ozer, H., Henderson, E. S., Dadey, B., Nussbaum-Blumenson, A. and Barcos, M. (1981). Defective immunoregulatory T-cell function in chronic lymphocytic leukemia. *Blood*, **58**, 1182–9
6. Van der Reijden, H. J., Van der Gaag, R., Pinkster, J., Rumke, H. C., Van, T. Veer, M. B., Melief, C. J. M. and Von dem Borne, A. E. J. K. (1982). Chronic lymphocytic leukemia: Immunologic markers and functional properties of leukemic cells. *Cancer*, **50**, 2826–33
7. Rudders, R. A. and Howard, J. P. (1978). Clinical and cell surface marker characterisation of the early phase of chronic lymphocytic leukemia. *Blood*, **52**, 25–35
8. Hamblin, T. J., Oscier, D. G., Gregg, E. O. and Smith, J. L. (1985). Cell markers in a large single centre series of chronic lymphocytic leukemia: The relationship between CLL and PLL. *Br. J. Haematol.*, **61**, 556 (Meeting Abstract)
9. Palestro, G., Botto Mica, F., Valente, G., Novero, D. and Stramignomi, A. (1983). Heterogeneity of chronic lymphocytic leukemias (CLL). *Path. Res. Pract.*, **178**, 153–4 (Meeting Abstract)
10. Ling, N. R. and Richardson, P. R. (1981). A critical appraisal of the direct antibody-rosette test for the detection of cell surface antigens. *J. Immunol. Meth.*, **47**, 265–74
11. Slease, R. B., Wistar, R. and Scher, I. (1979). Surface immunoglobulin density on human peripheral blood mononuclear cells. *Blood*, **54**, 72–87
12. Dhaliwal, H. S., Ling, N. R., Bishop, S. and Chapel, H. (1978). Expression of immunoglobulin G blood lymphocytes in chronic lymphocytic leukemia. *Clin. Exp. Immunol.*, **4**, 226–36
13. Stevenson, F. K., Hamblin, T. J. and Stevenson, G. T. (1981). The nature of immunoglobulin G on the surface of B lymphocytes in chronic lymphocytic leukemia. *J.*

Exp. Med., **154**, 1965–9

14. Ligler, F. S., Kettman, J. R., Graham Smith, R. and Frenkel, E. P. (1983). Immunoglobulin phenotype on B cells correlates with clinical stage of chronic lymphocytic leukemia. *Blood,* **62**, 256–63
15. Berntorp, E. and Zettervall, O. (1985). High expression of lymphocyte surface immunoglobulin in chronic lymphocytic leukemia may be a bad prognostic sign. *Scand. J. Haematol.,* **34**, 213–18
16. Baldini, L., Mozzara, R., Cortelezzi, A., Neri, A., Radaelli, F., Cesena, B., Maiola, A. T. and Polli, E. E. (1985). Prognostic significance of immunoglobulin phenotype in B cell chronic lymphocytic leukemia. *Blood,* **65**, 340–4
17. Stathopoulous, G. and Elliot, E. V. (1974). Formation of mouse and sheep red blood cell rosettes by lymphocytes from normal and leukemic individuals. *Lancet,* **1**, 600
18. Catovsky, D., Cherchi, M., Okos, A., Hegde, U. and Galton, D. A. G. (1976). Mouse RBC rosettes in B lymphoproliferative disorders. *Br. J. Haematol.,* **33**, 173–7
19. Gupta, S. and Grieco, M. H. (1975). Rosette formation with mouse erythrocytes: Probable marker for human B-lymphocytes. *Int. Arch. Allergy. Appl. Immun.,* **49**, 734–42
20. Abdul-Cader, Richardson, P. R., Walsh, L., Ling, N. R., MacLennon, I. C. M., Jones, E. L. and Leyland, M. (1983). The incidence of B-cell leukemia and lymphopenia in B-cell neoplasia in adults: A study using the Kiel classification of non-Hodgkin's lymphomas. *Br. J. Cancer,* **48**, 185–93
21. Cherchi, M. and Catovsky, D. (1980). Mouse red cell rosettes in CLL: Different expression in blood and tissues. *Clin. Exp. Immunol.,* **39**, 411–16
22. McGraw, D. J., Kurec, A. S. and Davey, F. R. (1982). Mouse erythrocyte formation: A marker for resting B lymphocytes. *Am. J. Clin. Pathol.,* **77**, 177–83
23. Irving, W. L., Youinou, P. Y., Walker, P. R. and Lydyard, P. M. (1984). Receptors for mouse erythrocytes on human lymphocytes: Technical aspects. *J. Immunol. Meth.,* **69**, 137–47
24. Bernard, A., Boumsell, L., Dausset, J., Milstein, C. and Schlossman, S. F. (eds) (1984). *Leucocyte Typing.* (Berlin, Heidelberg: Springer-Verlag)
25. (1986). *Leucocyte Typing 2* (three volumes). (New York, Berlin, Heidelberg, Tokyo: Springer-Verlag)
26. Royston, I., Maijda, J. A., Baird, S. M., Meserve, B. L. and Griffiths, J. C. (1980). Human T cell antigen defined by monoclonal antibodies: The 65,000-Dalton antigen of T cells (T65) is also found on chronic lymphocytic leukemia cells bearing surface immunoglobulins. *J. Immunol.,* **125**, 725–31
27. Wang, C. Y., Good, R. A., Ammirati, P., Dymbort, G. and Evans, R. L. (1980). Identification of a p69, 71 complex expressed on human T cells sharing determinants with B-type chronic lymphocytic leukemia cells. *J. Exp. Med.,* **151**, 1539–44
28. Rheinherz, E. L., Kung, P. C., Goldstein, G., Levey, R. H. and Schlossman, S. F. (1980). Discrete stages of human intrathymic differentiation: Analysis of normal thymocytes and leukemic blasts of T lineage. *Proc. Natl. Acad. Sci. USA.,* **77**, 1588–92
29. Caligaris-Cappio, F., Gobbi, M., Bofill, M. and Janossy, G. (1982). Infrequent normal B lymphocytes express features of B chronic lymphocytic leukemia. *J. Exp. Med.,* **155**, 623–8
30. Halper, J., Fu, S. M., Wang, C. Y., Winchester, R. and Kunkel, H. G. (1978). Patterns of expression of human 'Ia-like' antigens during the terminal stages of B-cell development. *J. Immunol.,* **120**, 1480–4
31. Pizzolo, G., Chilosi, M., Ambrosetti, A., Semenzato, G., Fiore-Donati, L. and Perona, G. (1983). Immunohistologic study of bone marrow involvement in B-chronic lymphocytic leukemia. *Blood,* **62**, 1289–96
32. Bach, F. H. (1985). The HLA Class 2 genes and products: The HLA-D region. *Immunol. Today,* **6**, 89–94
33. Guy, K., Van Heyningen, V., Ziegler, A. and Steel, C. M. (1984). Disparity in HLA-DC antigen expression on chronic lymphocytic leukemia cells. *Dis. Mark.,* **2**, 287–93
34. Brown, G., Walker, L., Ling, N. R., Richardson, P., Johnson, G. D., Guy, K. and Steel, C. M. (1984). T cell proliferation and expression of MHC class 2 antigens. *Scand. J. Immunol.,* **19**, 373–7
35. Nadler, L. M., Andersson, K. C., Marti, H., Bates, M., Park, E., Daley, J. F. and Schlossman, S. F. (1983). B4, a human B lymphocyte-associated antigen expressed on normal, mitogen-activated, and malignant B lymphocytes. *J. Immunol.,* **131**, 244–50

36. Pezzutto, A., Dorken, B., Feller, A., Moldenhauer, G., Schwartz, R., Wernet, P., Thiel, E. and Hunstein, W. (1986). HD37 monoclonal antibody: A useful reagent for further characterisation of 'non-T, non-B' lymphoid malignancies. In Reinherz, E. L., Haynes, B. F., Nadler, L. M. and Bernstein, I. D. (eds) *Leucocyte Typing 2: Volume 2, Human B Lymphocytes*, pp. 69–77 (New York, Berlin, Heidelberg, Tokyo: Springer-Verlag)

37. Rowe, M., Hildreth, E. K., Rickinson, A. B. and Epstein, M. A. (1982). Monoclonal antibodies to Epstein–Barr virus-induced transformation-associated cell surface antigen: Binding patterns and effect upon virus specific T-cell cytotoxicity. *Int. J. Cancer*, **29**, 373–81

38. Thorly-Lawson, D. A., Schooley, R. T., Bhan, A. K. and Nadler, L. M. (1982). Epstein–Barr virus superinduces a new human B cell differentiation antigen (B1-ast-1) expressed on transformed lymphoblasts. *Cell*, **30**, 415–25

39. Nadler, L. M. (1986). B cell/leukemia panel workshop: Summary and comments. In Reinherz, E. L., Haynes, B. F., Nadler, L. M. and Bernstein, I. D. (eds) *Leucocyte Typing 2. Volume 2, Human B lymphocytes*, pp. 3–43. (New York, Berlin, Heidelberg, Tokyo: Springer-Verlag)

40. Weiss, J. J., Tedder, T. F. and Fearon, D. T. (1984). Identification of a 145,000 Mr membrane protein as the C3d receptor (CR2) of human B lymphocytes. *Proc. Natl. Acad. Sci. USA.*, **81**, 881–8

41. Jondal, M. and Klein, G. (1973). Surface markers on Human B and T Lymphocytes 2: Presence of Epstein–Barr virus receptors on B lymphocytes. *J. Exp. Med.*, **138**, 1365–78

42. Nadler, L. M., Stashenko, P., Hardy, R., Van Aghthoven, A., Terhorst, C. and Schlossman, S. F. (1981). Characterisation of a human B cell-specific antigen (B2) distinct from B1. *J. Immunol.*, **126**, 1941–7

43. Cohen, J. H. M., Fischer, E., Kazatchkine, M. D., Brochier, J. and Revillard, J. P. (1986). Characterisation of monoclonal anti-human B-cell antibody BL13 as an anti-C3d-receptor (CR2) antibody. *Scand. J. Immunol.*, **23**, 279–85

44. Tedder, T. F., Clement, L. T. and Cooper, M. D. (1983). Use of monoclonal antibodies to examine differentiation antigens on human B cells. *Fed. Proc.*, **42**, 415 (Meeting Abstract)

45. Hsu, S. M. and Jaffe, E. S. (1984). Phenotypic expression of B-lymphocytes: 1. Identification with monoclonal antibodies in normal lymphoid tissue. *Am. J. Pathol.*, **114**, 387–95

46. Freedman, A. S., Boyd, A. W., Fisher, D. C., Schlossman, S. F. and Nadler, L. M. (1986). Changes with *in vitro* activation of the B cell panel antigens. In Reinherz, E. L., Haynes, B. F., Nadler, L. M. and Bernstein, I. D. (eds) *Leucocyte Typing 2. Volume 2, Human B Lymphocytes*, pp. 443–454. (New York, Berlin, Heidelberg, Tokyo: Springer-Verlag)

47. Moldenhauer, G., Dorken, B., Schwartz, R., Pezzutto, A. and Hammerling, G. J. (1986). Characterisation of a human B-lymphocyte antigen defined by monoclonal antibodies HD6 and HD39. In Reinherz, E. L., Haynes, B. F., Nadler, L. M. and Bernstein, I. D. (eds) *Leucocyte Typing 2: Volume 2, Human B Lymphocytes*, pp. 97–108. (New York, Berlin, Heidelberg, Tokyo: Springer-Verlag)

48. Stein, H., Gerdes, J. and Mason, D. Y. (1982). The normal and malignant germinal center. *Clin. Haematol.*, **11**, 531–59

49. Stashenko, P., Nadler, L. M., Hardy, R. and Sclossman, S. F. (1980). Characterisation of a human B lymphocyte-specific antigen. *J. Immunol.*, **125**, 1678–85

50. Enno, A., Catovsky, D., O'Brien, M., Cherchi, M. Kumaran, T. O. and Galton, D. A. G. (1979). 'Prolymphocytoid' transformation of chronic lymphocytic leukemia. *Br. J. Haematol.*, **41**, 9–18

51. Abramson, C. S., Kersey, J. H. and LeBien, T. W. (1981). A monoclonal antibody (BA-1) reactive with cells of human B lymphocyte lineage. *J. Immunol.*, **126**, 83–8

52. Steel, C. M., Elder, P. and Guy, K. (1986). Screening of Workshop 'B' series antibodies by radioimmunobinding to human leukocyte cell lines and to cells from human lymphoid tumours. In Reinherz, E. L., Haynes, B. F., Nadler, L. M. and Bernstein, I. D. (eds) *Leukocyte Typing 2. Volume 2, Human B Lymphocytes*, pp. 69–77. (New York, Berlin, Heidelberg, Tokyo: Springer-Verlag)

53. Kersey, J. H., LeBien, T. W., Abramson, C. S., Newman, R., Sutherland, R. and Greaves, M. (1981). A human hemopoietic progenitor and acute lymphoblastic leukemia -associated cell surface structure identified with monoclonal antibody. *J. Exp. Med.*, **153**, 726–31

54. Greaves, M. F., Brown, G., Rapson, N. T. and Lister, T. A. (1975). Antisera to acute lymphoblastic leukemia cells. *Clin. Immunol. Immunopathol.*, **4**, 67–84

55. LeBacq, A. M., Ravoet, A. M., Bazin, H., De Bruyere, M. and Sokal, G. (1984). Complementary anti-Calla like monoclonal antibodies. In Bernard, A., Boumsell, L., Dausset, J., Milstein, C. and Schlossman, S. F. (eds) *Leucocyte Typing*, p. 680. (Berlin, Heidelberg, New York, Tokyo: Springer-Verlag)

56. Ritz, J., Pesando, J. M., Notis-McConarty, J., Lazarus, H. and Schlossman, S. F. (1980). A monoclonal antibody to human acute lymphoblastic leukaemia antigen. *Nature* (London), **283**, 583–5

57. Gobbi, M., Caligaris-Cappio, F. and Janssy, G. (1983). Normal equivalent cells of B cell malignancies: Analysis with monoclonal antibodies. *Br. J. Haematol.*, **54**, 393–403

58. Pesando, J. M., Hoffman, P., Martin, N. and Conrad, T. (1986). Anti-Calla antibodies identify unique antigens on lymphoid cells and granulocytes. *Blood*, **67**, 588–91

59. Alexanian, R. (1975). Monoclonal gammopathies in lymphoma. *Arch. Intern. Med.*, **135**, 62–6

60. Van Camp, B., Thielmans, C., Dehou, M. F., De May, J. and De Waele, M. (1982). Two monoclonal antibodies (OKIa1 and OKT10) for the study of the final B cell maturation. *J. Clin. Immunol.*, **2**, 67

61. Anderson, K. C., Park, S. K., Bates, M. P., Leonard, R. C. F., Hardy, R. Schlossman, S. F. and Nadler, L. M. (1983). Antigens on human plasma cells identified by monoclonal antibodies. *J. Immunol.*, **130**, 1132–8

62. Nathan, P. D., Walker, L., Hardie, D., Richardson, P., Khan, M., Johnson, G. D. and Ling, N. R. (1986). An antigenic study of human plasma cells in normal tissue and in myeloma: Identification of a novel plasma cell-associated antigen. *Cell. Exp. Immunol.*, **65**, 112–19

63. Beck, J. D., Koziner, B., Mertelsman, R., Platsoueas, C. D., Clarkson, B. and Good, R. A. (1980). B cells from a patient with chronic lymphocytic leukemia bind to sheep erythrocytes: An immunologic analysis. *Clin. Immunol. Immunopathol.*, **16**, 233–7

64. Aisenberg, A. C., Bloch, K. C. and Wilkes, B. M. (1981). Malignant lymphoma with dual B and T cell markers. Analysis of the neoplastic cells with monoclonal antibodies directed against T cell subsets. *J. Exp. Med.*, **154**, 1709–14

65. Mitrou, P. S., Bergmann, L., Holloway, K. and Zerth, G. (1981). E-Rosette formation in B-cell lymphatic leukemias induced by binding activity of monoclonal surface immunoglobulins to sheep red blood cells. *Clin. Immunol. Immunopathol.*, **20**, 346–53

66. Breard, J., Reinherz, E. L., Kung, P. C., Goldstein, G. and Schlossman, S. F. (1980). A monoclonal antibody reactive with human peripheral blood monocytes. *J. Immunol.*, **124**, 1943–8

67. Ligler, F. S., Schlam, M. L., Curley, R., Brodskey, I. and Benzel, J. E. (1983). Monocyte markers and the common acute lymphoblastic antigen on chronic lymphocytic leukemia cells. *Am. J. Hematol.*, **15**, 335–42

68. Cosgrove, L. J., Sandrin, M. S., Rajasekariah, P. and McKenzie, I. F. C. (1986). A genomic clone encoding the alpha chain of the OKM1, LFA-1, and platelet glycoprotein IIb-IIIa molecules. *Proc. Natl. Acad. Sci. USA.*, **83**, 752–6

69. Krensky, A. M., Sanchez-Madrid, F., Robbins, E., Nagy, J. A., Springer, T. A. and Burakoff, S. J. (1983). The functional significance, distribution and structure of LFA-2, LFA-2, and LFA-3: Cell surface antigens associated with CTL-target interactions. *J. Immunol.*, **131**, 611–16

70. Galton, D. A. G., Goldman, J. N., Wiltshaw, E., Catovsky, D., Henry, K. and Goldenberg, G. J. (1974). Prolymphocytic leukemia. *Br. J. Haematol.*, **27**, 7–23

71. Catovsky, D., Lynch, D. C. and Beverley, P. C. L. (1982). T cell disorders in hematological disease. *Clin. Hematol.*, **11**, 661–96

72. Costello, C., Catovsky, D., O'Brien, M. and Galton, D. A. G. (1980). Prolymphocytic leukemia: An ultrastructural study of 22 cases. *Br. J. Haematol.*, **44**, 389–94

73. Scott, C. S., Limbert, H. J., Mackarill, I. D. and Roberts, B. E. (1985). Membrane phenotypic studies in B cell lymphoproliferative disorders. *J. Clin. Pathol.*, **38**, 995–1001

74. Kjeldsberg, M. D. and Marty, J. (1981). Prolymphocytic transformation of chronic lymphocytic leukemia. *Cancer*, **48**, 2447–57

75. Brooks, D. A., Beckman, I. G. R., Bradley, J., McNamara, P. J., Thomas, M. E. and Zola, H. (1981). Human lymphocyte markers defined by antibodies derived from somatic cell hybrids: 4.A monoclonal antibody reacting specifically with a subpopulation of human B lymphocytes. *J. Immunol.*, **126**, 1373–7

76. Catovsky, D., Cherchi, M., Brooks, D., Bradley, J. and Zola, H. (1981). Heterogeneity of B cell leukemias demonstrated by the monoclonal antibody FMC.7. *Blood,* **58**, 406–8

77. Zola, H., Moore, H. A., Bradley, J., Need, J. A. and Beverley, P. C. L. (1983). Lymphocyte subpopulations in human cord blood: Analysis with monoclonal antibodies. *J. Reproductive Immunol.,* **5**, 311–17

78. Bergmann, L., Mitrou, P. S., Cherdron, T., Holloway, K., Jost, J., Timm, V. and Zerth, G. (1982). Expression of Ia-like antigen in lymphatic leukemia and non-Hodgkin lymphomas in correlation with other markers. *Scand. J. Haematol.,* **29**, 224–34

79. Den Ottolander, G. J., Schuitt, H. R., Waayer, J. L., Huibregsten, L., Hijmans, W. and Jansen, J. (1985). Chronic B-cell Leukemias: Relation between the immunological features. *Clin. Immunol. Immunopathol.,* **35**, 92–102

80. Mitus, W. J., Mednicoff, I. B., Wittels, B. and Dameshek, W. (1971). Neoplastic lymphoid reticulum cells in the peripheral blood: A histochemical study. *Blood,* **17**, 206–15

81. Utsinger, P. D., Yount, W. J., Fuller, C. R., Logue, M. J. and Orringer, E. P. (1977). Hairy cell leukemia: B lymphocyte and phagocytic properties. *Blood,* **49**, 19–27

82. Burns, G. F., Cawley, J. C., Worman, C. P., Karpas, A., Barker, C. R., Goldstone, A. H. and Hayhoe, F. G. J. (1978). Multiple heavy chain isotypes on the surface of the cells of hairy cell leukemias. *Blood,* **52**, 1132–47

83. Korsmeyer, S. J., Greene, W. C., Cossman, J., Hsu, S. M., Jensen, J. P., Neckers, L. M., Marshall, S. L., Bakhshi, A., Depper, J. M., Leonard, W. T., Jaffe, E. S. and Waldman, T. A. (1983). Rearrangement and expression of immunoglobulin genes and expression of Tac antigen in hairy cell leukemia. *Proc. Natl. Acad. Sci. USA.,* **80**, 4521–6

84. Jansen, J., Schuit, H. R. E., Herrman, J. and Hijmans, W. (1984). Prognostic significance of immunoglobulin phenotype in hairy cell leukemia. *Blood,* **63**, 1241–4

85. Golomb, H. M., Davis, S., Wilson, C. and Vardiman, J. (1982). Surface immunoglobulins on hairy cells in 55 patients with hairy cell leukemia. *Am. J. Hematol.,* **12**, 397–401

86. Golomb, H., Strehl, S., Oleske, D. and Vardiman, J. (1985). Prognostic significance of immunoglobulin phenotype in hairy cell leukemia: Does it exist? *Blood,* **66**, 1358–61

87. Burns, G. F. and Cawley, J. C. (1980). Spontaneous mouse erythrocyte-rosette formation: Correlation with surface immunoglobulin phenotype in hairy cell leukaemia. *Clin. Exp. Immunol.,* **39**, 83–9

88. Herrmann, F., Dorken, B., Ludwig, W. D. and Schwarting, R. (1985). A comparison of membrane marker phenotypes in hairy cell leukemia and phorbol-ester induced B-CLL cells using monoclonal antibodies. *Leuk. Res.,* **9**, 529–36

89. Caligaris-Cappio, F., Janossy, G., Campana, D., Chilosi, M., Bergui, L., Foa, R., Delia, D., Giubellino, M. C., Preda, P. and Gobbi, M. (1984). Lineage relationship of chronic lymphocytic leukemia and hairy cell leukemia: Studies with TPA. *Leuk. Res.,* **8**, 567–78

90. Meijer, C. J. L. M., Albeda, F., Van der Walk, P., Spaander, P. J. and Jansen, J. (1984). Immunohistochemical analysis of the spleen in hairy cell leukaemia. *Am. J. Pathol.,* **115**, 266–74

91. Anderson, K. C., Boyd, A. W., Fisher, D. C., Leslie, D., Schlossman, S. F. and Nadler, L. M. (1985). Hairy cell leukemia: A tumour of pre-plasma cells. *Blood,* **65**, 620–9

92. Jansen, J., Schuitt, H. R. E., Meijer, C. J. L. M., Van Nieuwenkoop, J. A. and Hijmans, W. (1982). Cell markers in hairy cell leukemia studied in cells from 51 patients. *Blood,* **59**, 52–60

93. Pallesen, G. (1986). Immunohistological analysis of tissue specificity of the fifty-two workshop anti-B lymphocyte monoclonal antibodies. In Reinherz, E. L., Haynes, B. F., Nadler, L. M. and Bernstein, I. D. (eds) *Leukocyte Typing 2, Volume 2, Human B Lymphocytes*, pp. 277–288. (New York, Berlin, Heidelberg, Tokyo: Springer-Verlag)

94. Dorken, B., Feller, A., Pezzutto, A., Ho, A. D. and Hunstein, W. (1984). Monoclonal antibodies against B cell differentiation antigens (HD6, HD28, HD37, and HD39) – Immunodiagnostic reagents for B cell leukemias and lymphomas. *2nd International Conference on Malignant Lymphoma,* p 75. June, Lugano, Switzerland. Swiss League against Cancer and Swiss Group For Clinical Cancer Research

95. Mason, D. Y., Ladyman, H. and Gatter, K. C. (1986). Immunohistochemical analysis of monoclonal anti-B cell antibodies. In Reinherz, E. L., Haynes, B. F., Nadler, L. M. and Bernstein, I. D. (eds) *Leucocyte Typing 2, Volume 2, Human B Lymphocytes,* pp. 69–77. (New York, Berlin, Heidelberg, Tokyo: Springer-Verlag)

96. Jansen, J., Den Ottolander, G. J., Schuit, H. R. E., Waayer, J. L., Hijmans, W. and Cohen,

J. A. (1984). Hairy cell leukemia: Its place among the chronic B cell leukemias. *Semin. Oncol.*, **11**, 386–93

97. Worman, C. P., Brooks, D. A., Hogg, N., Zola, H., Beverley, P. C. L. and Cawley, J. C. (1983). The nature of hairy cells: A study with a panel of monoclonal antibodies. *Scand. J. Haematol.*, **30**, 223–6

98. Posnett, D. N., Chiorazzi, N. and Kunkel, H. G. (1982). Monoclonal antibodies with specificity for hairy cell leukemia cells. *J. Clin. Invest.*, **70**, 254–61

99. Schwarting, R., Stein, H. and Wang, C. Y. (1985). The monoclonal antibodies alpha S-HCL1 (alpha Leu 14) and alpha S-HCL3 (alpha Leu M5) allow the diagnosis of Hairy Cell Leukemia. *Blood*, **65**, 974–83

100. Uchiyama, T., Border, S. and Waldmann, H. (1981). A monoclonal antibody (anti-Tac) reactive with activated and functionally mature human T cells: 1.Production of anti-Tac monoclonal antibody and distribution of Tac-positive cells. *J. Immunol.*, **126**, 1393–7

101. Foa, R., Gioverelli, M., Jemma, C., Fierro, M. T., Lusso, P., Ferrando, M. L., Lauria, F. and Forni, G. (1985). Interleukin 2 (IL-2) and interferon-gamma production by T lymphocytes from patients with B-chronic lymphocytic leukemia: Evidence that normally released IL-2 is absorbed by the neoplastic B-cell population. *Blood*, **66**, 614–19

102. Anderson, K. C., Bates, M. P., Slauglerhoupt, B., Schlossman, S. F. and Nadler, L. M. (1983). Antigens on human plasma cells identified by monoclonal antibodies. *J. Immunol.*, **130**, 1132–8

103. Anderson, K. C., Bates, M. P., Slauglerhoupt, B., Schlossman, S. F. and Nadler, L. M. (1984). A monoclonal antibody with reactivity restricted to normal and neoplastic plasma cells. *J. Immunol.*, **132**, 3172–9

104. Tubbs, R. R., Savage, R. A., Sebek, B. A., Fishleder, A., and Weick, J. K. (1984). Antigenic phenotype of splenic hairy cells. *Am. J. Med.*, **76**, 199–205

105. Ruco, L. P., Stoppacciaro, A., Valtieri, M., Procopio, A. and Uccini, S. (1983). Hairy cell leukemia: Absence of natural killer activity and of Interleukin-1 release in OKM1 positive spleen hairy cells. *Clin. Immunol. Immunopathol.*, **26**, 47–55

106. Cawley, J. C., Burns, G. F. and Hayhoe, F. G. J. (1980). Hairy cell leukemia. *Recent Results in Cancer Research*, Vol. 72, pp. 82–83. (New York, Berlin, Heidelberg, Tokyo: Springer-Verlag)

107. Armitage, R. J., Worman, C. P., Galvin, M. C. and Cawley, J. C. (1985). Hairy cell leukemia with hybrid B–T features: A study with a panel of monoclonal antibodies. *Am. J. Hematol.*, **18**, 335–44

108. Yam, L. T., Li, C. Y. and Lam, K. W. (1971). Tartrate-resistant acid phosphatase isoenzyme in the reticulum cells of leukemic reticuloendotheliosis. *N. Engl. J. Med.*, **284**, 357–60

109. Johnstone, A. P. (1982). Chronic lymphocytic leukemia and its relationship to normal B lymphopoiesis. *Immunol. Today*, **3**, 343–8

110. Klaus, G. G. B. and Kunkel, A. (1981). The role of germinal centres in the generation of immunological memory. In *Microenvironments in Haemapoietic and Lymphoid Differentiation*, CIBA Foundation Symposium No. 84, pp. 265–280. (London: Pitman Medical)

111. Robinson, D. S. E., Posnett, D. N., Zola, H. and Catovsky, D. (1985). Normal counterparts of hairy cells and B-prolymphocytes in the peripheral blood: An ultrastructural study with monoclonal antibodies and the immunogold method. *Leuk. Res.*, **9**, 335–48

112. Mover, S., Li, C. Y. and Yam, L. Y. (1972). Semiquantitative evaluation of tartrate-resistant acid phosphatase activity in human blood cells. *J. Clin. Lab. Med.*, **80**, 711–17

113. Machii, T. and Kitani, T. (1984). Similarities between IgG-bearing lymphocytes and hairy cells: Cytologic and cytochemical studies. *Blood*, **64**, 166–72

114. Robert, K. H., Juliusson, G. and Biberfeld, P. (1983). Chronic lymphocytic leukemia cells activated *in vitro* reveal cellular changes that characterise B-prolymphocytic leukemia and immunocytoma. *Scand. J. Immunol.*, **17**, 397–401

115. Gupta, S., Brooks, D. A., Bradley, J. and Zola, H. (1985). Monoclonal antibody-defined B lymphocyte subpopulations in primary immune deficiency disorders. *J. Clin. Lab. Immunol.*, **16**, 59

116. Pirruccello, S. J., and LeBien, T. W. (1986). The human B cell-associated antigen CD24 is a single chain sialoglycoprotein. *J. Immunol.*, **136**, 3779–84

9
Malignant Lymphoma of Mucosa Associated Lymphoid Tissue (Malt)

P. G. ISAACSON and J. SPENCER

The majority of extranodal non-Hodgkin's lymphomas occur in the gastro-intestinal tract and other mucosal organs where the tumours arise from mucosa associated lymphoid tissue (MALT). This lymphoid tissue may be a normal tissue component as in the mucosa of the intestine and bronchi, or acquired, usually as the result of an 'autoimmune' disorder as in the stomach, salivary glands and thyroid. In either case, the organization and histological features of the lymphoid tissue are distinctive and differ from that of peripheral lymph nodes. As a consequence, the clinicopathological features of the lymphomas derived from MALT are equally distinctive, differing from the much more common nodal lymphomas[1]. At present, studies of MALT derived lymphomas have principally been confined to those of B-cell origin. These appear to account for the great majority of this group of lymphomas. It is conceivable that an equally distinctive group of T-cell lymphomas arises from MALT, and the recent characterization of coeliac associated lymphoma as a T-cell neoplasm[2] suggests that this is indeed the case. The clinicopathological features of MALT derived lymphomas can only be fully comprehended in relation to the histology and physiologic behaviour of MALT. Thus the cells of these lymphomas share the homing patterns of MALT lymphocytes and this may account for the slow evolution of the lymphomas and their tendency to remain localized. Certain specific and diagnostically useful histological features common to these lymphomas can also be explained in relation to their origin from MALT.

CHARACTERISTICS OF NORMAL MALT

Immune responses to antigens from the lumen of the gut are initiated in lymphoid nodules distributed throughout the small and large intestine. They are macroscopically invisible in untreated human intestine and are concentrated in the Peyer's patches of the terminal ileum[3]. These nodules, which consist of B-cell follicles with intervening T-cell areas, are in intimate contact with the overlying epithelium and are the major component of gut-associated lymphoid tissue (GALT). GALT is present in the human small intestine from early in fetal life and does not, therefore, accumulate in response to dietary or microbial antigens[4]. Similar concentrations of lymphoid tissue have been described in the bronchi, where they are known as bronchus-associated lymphoid tissue (BALT). Lymphoid nodules in the stomach, salivary gland and thyroid, are acquired either as a natural consequence of ageing, or in the course of putative autoimmune disease and bear certain similarities to GALT and BALT, but have not yet been characterized in any detail, especially with respect to their generation of a mucosal type of immune response.

Antigen from the lumen of mucosal organs is transported across the epithelium covering lymphoid nodules (so called dome epithelium) via specialized cells (M cells)[5-7], and animal studies have shown that it interacts with the underlying lymphoid tissue[8,9]. B-cells, activated as a result of antigenic challenge, then leave the follicles by the efferent lymphatics and enter the bloodstream via the mesenteric lymph nodes and the thoracic duct. They then 'home' back to the mucosa by a mechanism not fully understood, where they appear as plasma cells[10,11]. The majority of these plasma cells synthesize IgA[12,13]. IgA dimers are able to bind to secretory component (SC), a glycoprotein synthesized by mucosal epithelium[14]. The complex of dimeric IgA and SC is actively transported across the epithelium to the mucosal surface[15,16], where the IgA presumably interacts with lumenal antigens[17]. Some of the IgA enters the mucosal lymphatics and thence the systemic circulation[18]. This intravascular dimeric IgA is available for uptake and transport by SC synthesizing cells at other mucosal sites which may or may not possess MALT, and in this way the mucosae are united by a common mucosal immune system. It has been postulated that the mucosae are also united by lymphoid cells that migrate between them and there is some experimental evidence for this in rodents[19,20]. In other animals however, such as the sheep, there is evidence against such a mechanism[21]. The extent of interspecies differences in mucosal immunity is thus not fully understood, and it is important to bear this in mind when extrapolating from animals to man.

Antibodies of the IgA isotype are not confined to the human mucosae, and they exist as two sub-classes A_1 and A_2 in both monomeric and dimeric forms[22]. There is a predominance of cells producing dimeric IgA and the proportion of IgA_2 is greater at mucosal sites compared to peripheral lymph nodes[23,24]. The epithelium in human gut, bronchi, salivary and lachrymal glands together with that of many other mucosal organs, including the genitourinary tract, expresses SC enabling transport of dimeric IgA to the lumenal surface in each case whether or not MALT is present[25].

Detailed morphological and immunohistochemical studies of human GALT have shown important differences from laboratory animals and highlighted features of direct relevance to MALT derived lymphomas[26-28]. The most obvious component of human Peyer's patches is the B-cell follicle consisting of a reactive follicle centre surrounded by a mantle of small lymphocytes (Figure 1). Sheets of lymphocytes are distributed around and between the

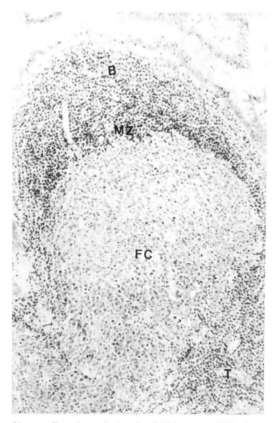

Figure 1 Section of human Peyer's patch showing follicle centre (FC) with surrounding mantle zone (MZ). B-cells (B) are distributed between the mantle zone and surface epithelium. T-cell zone (T) is seen below the follicle centre and contains high endothelial venules. H & E × 110

follicles and immunohistochemical studies have shown that most of these are B-cells. The smaller distinct T-zone containing high endothelial venules is situated between the B-cell follicle and the muscularis mucosae. The mantle zone around the follicle centre merges with a broader zone of B-cells which extends up to the dome epithelium. The mantle zone B-cells express both surface (S) IgM and SIgD in contrast to the surrounding B-cells which lack SIgD, but express SIgM or $SIgA_1$. These extrafollicular B-cells are further distinguished by their size and nuclear morphology. They are larger than mantle zone cells and contain irregular heterochromatic nuclei resembling those of centrocytes. An important feature of these centrocyte like extrafollicular B-cells is their invariable presence in the dome epithelium over each lymphoid follicle, but not the epithelium of the surrounding crypts (Figure 2)[29]. This intraepithelial population of B-cells is to be distinguished from intraepithelial T-cells which form the major intraepithelial lymphocyte component throughout the gut[30]. Like mantle zone cells, but in contrast to follicle centre cells, the centrocyte like cells react with the monoclonal antibody KB61[31], but not with MHM6[32], which can be used to label follicle centre cells. The phenotype of these newly recognized B-cells bears a close resemblance to that of marginal zone B-lymphocytes of the spleen to which they also bear a strong morphological resemblance. Centrocyte like B-cells with the phenotype described above do not exist in fetal GALT. At 16 weeks gestation B- and T-cells are present in human GALT, but with no distinct zonation. At 19 weeks however, B- and T-cell zones are clearly present. B-cells at this time express surface IgM and IgD and the antigen CD5 which is present on the majority of T-cells, but not on adult B-cells. Follicle centres, centrocyte like B-cells and plasma cells are all absent from fetal GALT at 19 weeks, suggesting that these three cell types are dependent upon antigen for their generation or they may mature later in fetal life[4].

Cells with centrocyte like morphology are present in the dome region of the Peyer's patches of rats and mice, but in these species the SIgD-ve B-cell population is not present. Centrocyte like cells as described in man have, however, been identified in baboons[28]. Another important difference between

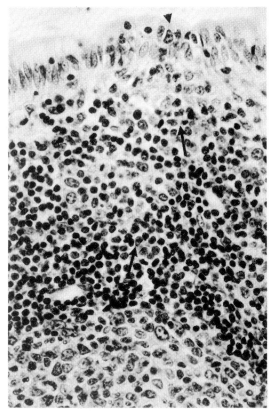

Figure 2 Higher power of human Peyer's patch showing portion of follicle centre at the bottom of the picture. Above this the mantle zone merges with perifollicular centrocyte like cells (arrows) which can be seen to infiltrate the surface epithelium (arrow heads). H & E × 320

rodent and primate GALT relates to the distribution of plasma cells and their precursors. In rodent Peyer's patches, immunoblasts and plasma cells containing cytoplasmic (C) IgA have been observed within and around high endothelial venules, presumably representing a 'homing' population[33]. In humans, on the other hand, plasma cells with CIgA are seen in the dome region and not in the zone of cells containing high endothelial venules[27]. This calls into question the similarity between homing mechanisms of rodents and humans. There is as yet no direct evidence in man for migration of antibody forming cells generated in GALT via the lymphatics regional lymph nodes and blood, to seed the lamina propria.

GENERAL FEATURES OF MALT DERIVED B-CELL LYMPHOMAS

The clinical features of this group of lymphomas are distinguished by a long history frequently suggesting a reactive or inflammatory disorder, rather than a neoplasm. This, coupled with a good response to local therapy, has resulted in the term 'pseudolymphoma' being applied to many of these mucosal lesions. These features, however, can be explained in the context of the circulation patterns of MALT and it is thus of some importance to establish the existence of these properties in humans. The term pseudolymphoma is an unfortunate one that no doubt includes both non-neoplastic reactive lymphoid proliferations and lymphomas. The use of immunohistochemical techniques to establish whether light chain restriction is present, should almost always permit distinction between the two and, it is hoped, result in the abandonment of the term 'pseudolymphoma'. The tendency of MALT derived lymphomas, when they spread, to involve other mucosal sites, has been noted especially with respect to salivary gland, lung[34] and thyroid tumours[35]. An association between lymphomas of MALT and involvement of Waldeyers ring, has also been documented particularly with regard to gastric lymphoma[36]. Waldeyers ring is sometimes considered to be an example of MALT, although it also shows features of peripheral lymphoid tissue. These observations provide indirect evidence that circulating B-cells with mucosal homing properties may well be responsible for a degree of common mucosal immunity in humans.

The histological features of MALT derived lymphomas bear a direct resemblance to that of their parent tissue[1]. Reactive follicle centres are usually abundant, although they may be almost completely obscured by the other elements, or there may be loss of a follicular arrangement of the follicle centre cells. A diffuse infiltrate of centrocyte like cells is another constant feature. It is this population that forms lymphoepithelial lesions which characterize lymphomas of MALT. These lesions appear to be a neoplastic expression of the specific association that has been demonstrated between centrocyte like cells and the dome epithelium of normal MALT. The number of lesions depends on the degree to which the tumour is constituted by centrocyte like cells. Mature plasma cells are also frequently seen in lymphomas of MALT. They may make up the bulk of the tumour, or be relatively inconspicuous and even absent. Since plasma cells are invariably present at mucosal sites as a reactive population, immunohistochemistry is necessary in order to identify neoplastic (monoclonal) plasma cells.

In some cases of lymphoma derived from MALT efferent mucosal lymphatics distended with immunoblasts may be present. These CIg synthesizing blasts can be shown to be monotypic (i.e. part of the neoplastic clone), and it is presumably these cells that are destined to enter the circulation and return to the mucosa. Since these blasts are destined to become non-dividing plasma cells, this may explain why MALT associated lymphomas following the physiological circulation pathways, are slow to disseminate from their primary site.

Immunohistochemical studies have shown that there is close similarity between MALT and the lymphomas derived from them. Thus, while all the components of a lymphoma show the same light chain restriction, indicative of a common clonal origin, the individual cellular components (centrocyte like cell and plasma cell) show phenotypic differences similar to those seen in non-neoplastic tissue. These findings indicate that there is a hierarchical relationship between the two cell types, but the role of this relationship in the generation of an immune response is not yet clear. Many of the concepts relating to MALT derived lymphomas are based on the two most intensively studied tumours, namely gastric lymphoma and the variety of small bowel lymphoma known as Mediterranean lymphoma or immunoproliferative small intestinal disease (IPSID). Data relating to lung, salivary gland and thyroid lymphoma are less complete, but their similarity to GALT lymphomas is striking.

Gastric lymphoma

The normal stomach is devoid of lymphoid tissue. Mucosal lymphoid nodules almost invariably appear with age, either as part of a natural process, or due to chronic gastritis, a disease which in some cases appears to have an immune basis. It is uncertain whether there is any connection between chronic gastritis and lymphoma and there have been no studies on the incidence of auto-antibodies to parietal cells or intrinsic factor in patients with gastric lymphoma. Patients with gastric lymphoma are usually over 50, but the disease is increasingly being recognized at an earlier age[37]. The symptoms are those of gastritis and peptic ulcer, often with an intermittent response to anti-ulcer therapy. Abdominal pain and weight loss are symptoms of advanced disease. Endoscopy usually reveals antral lesions (although the tumour may occur elsewhere in the stomach) suggesting inflammation or peptic ulcer disease, rather than a neoplasm. Unless the pathologist is aware of the condition, endoscopic biopsies are frequently interpreted as showing gastritis, perhaps with an unusually heavy lymphocytic infiltrate and a history of repeated endoscopic biopsies is not unusual.

The histological features of gastric lymphoma closely resemble those of normal MALT[37]. Follicle centres, are often identifiable and these are surrounded by a variable, usually poorly formed mantle zone. Extending mucosally is an infiltrate of centrocyte like cells which forms lympho-epithelial lesions (Figures 3 and 4). This infiltrate may mix with plasma cells

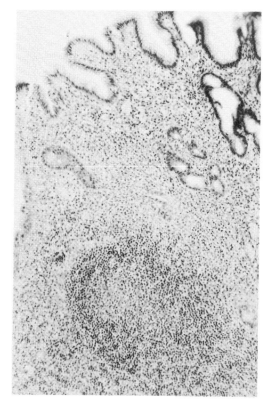

Figure 3 Section of gastric lymphoma showing a follicle above which there is an infiltrate of centrocyte like cells destroying glands. H & E × 80

and a dense zone of plasma cells may be present superficially. These are usually reactive, but in approximately one-third of cases, light chain restriction can be shown in the plasma cells by immunohistochemistry, indicating that they are part of the neoplastic clone. The infiltrate of centrocyte like cells also extends into the sub-mucosa, where it is often accompanied by dense sclerosis. Efferent lymphatics distended with immunoblasts are a feature of many gastric lymphomas. Cytoplasmic Ig can be demonstrated in these cells and is of the same isotype as the rest of the tumour (Figures 5 and 6). Gastric lymphomas are usually associated with superficial erosions or a defined ulcer, but the muscularis propria is almost always intact. In more advanced lesions, the centrocyte like elements appear more obviously neoplastic and invasive and the diagnosis presents less difficulty. Lymphoepithelial lesions are an important diagnostic feature, but in large advanced tumours there may be overgrowth by neoplastic follicle centre cells, usually centroblasts and in the absence of centrocyte like cells, lymphoepithelial lesions may not be seen.

Immunocytochemistry performed on cryostat sections confirms the expression of monotypic SIg by the centrocyte like cells (Figure 7).

129

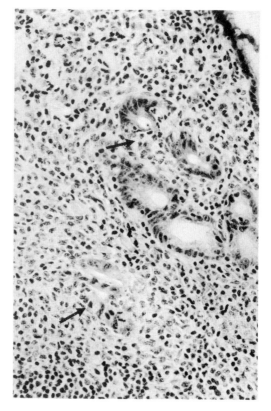

Figure 4 High power of mucosa shown in Figure 3. Invasion of glands by centrocyte like cells forming characteristic lymphoepithelial lesions is well shown (arrows). H & E × 200

Antibodies to dendritic reticulum cells can help to identify follicular structures. Neoplastic plasma cells when present are best shown in paraffin sections by demonstrating monotypic CIg (Figure 8). A combined morphological and immunocytochemical approach is especially important in interpreting gastric biopsies where the presence of a diffuse infiltrate of centrocyte like cells forming lymphoepithelial lesions in diagnostic.

Lymph node spread occurs late in gastric lymphoma and is usually restricted to the gastric lymph nodes. The nodes are infiltrated by centrocyte like cells in a perifollicular distribution (Figure 9).

Mediterranean lymphoma (MTL)

This type of lymphoma, occurs principally in the Middle East and is in many ways the prototype of MALT derived lymphomas[38]. The tumour occurs in young adults and is preceded by a history of malabsorption, which is then complicated by tumour masses usually in the jejunum. In over one-third of

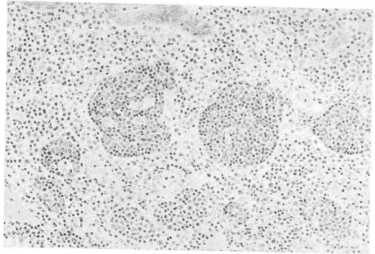

Figure 5 Section of mucosa from gastric lymphoma showing lymphatics distended with immunoblasts. H & E × 110

cases an abnormal alpha heavy chain paraprotein can be identified in the blood or duodenal juice.

Histologically, plasma cells infiltrate the lamina propria throughout the upper small intestine and sometimes beyond (Figure 10). There are infiltrates of centrocyte like cells which form prominent lymphoepithelial lesions; in later stages these may undergo blast transformation and be cytologically bizarre. As larger tumour masses form with associated mesenteric lymph node involvement, the cytological elements tend to be mixed together.

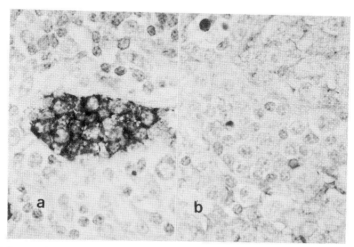

Figure 6 Immunoblasts within lymphatics in a case of gastric lymphoma stained for kappa light chain (a) and lambda light chain (b). There is kappa light chain restriction in common with the rest of the lymphoma. Immunoperoxidase × 420

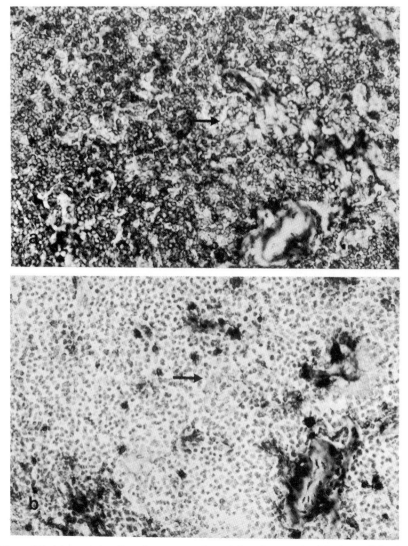

Figure 7 Serial cryostat sections from a case of gastric lymphoma stained for kappa light chain (**a**) and for lambda light chain (**b**). Centrocyte like cells show kappa light chain restriction. Immunoperoxidase × 200

Immunohistochemical studies[39,40] demonstrate synthesis of CIg of α 1 heavy chain subclass in the plasma cells (Figure 11) which distinguishes them from the CIg-ve follicle centre cells and centrocyte like cells (Figure 12). The absence of light chains in the plasma cells has given rise to considerable debate as to the clonal (neoplastic) nature of the plasma cell infiltrate, especially when it is the sole element of the disease. Light chain restriction has, however, recently been demonstrated in a few cases, a finding which

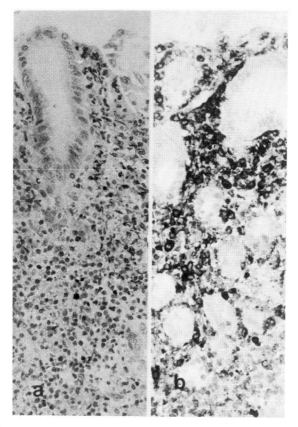

Figure 8 Serial paraffin sections from a case of gastric lymphoma stained for kappa light chain (**a**) and lambda light chain (**b**). Plasma cells are synthesizing monotypic cytoplasmic immunoglobulin (lambda light chain restriction). Immunoperoxidase × 210

supports the neoplastic nature of the plasma cell[41]. Mediterranean lymphoma thus contains the same clonally related B-cell variants common to MALT derived lymphomas, but it is distinguished by its strange pattern of immunoglobulin synthesis. The basis for this is not known, but the geographic and racial distribution of MTL suggests that genetic factors are responsible.

Intestinal lymphoma

Localized B-cell lymphomas of the small and large intestine also occur with increased frequency in the Middle East[42], but unlike MTL this variant is also well recognized in western countries. There is no associated malabsorption or synthesis of abnormal alpha chain and a neoplastic plasma cell infiltrate, when present, is localized to the region of the tumour. These tumours resemble the gastric lymphomas described above, except that lympho-

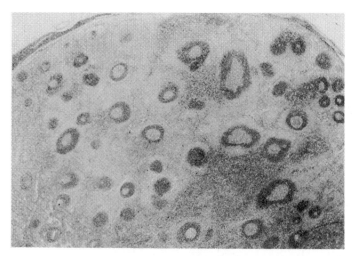

Figure 9 Lymph node involvement in a case of gastric lymphoma. The node is infiltrated by centrocyte like cells distributed in a perifollicular pattern. H & E × 10

epithelial lesions may be hard to find, In other ways these tumours share the characteristics of other lymphomas derived from MALT.

Pulmonary lymphoma

MALT is well recognized in the lung where it is known as bronchus associated lymphoid tissue (BALT). There are close similarities between primary B-cell lymphoma of the lung and gastric lymphoma as described above[1,34]. The lymphomas have a long history, and remain localized for prolonged periods.

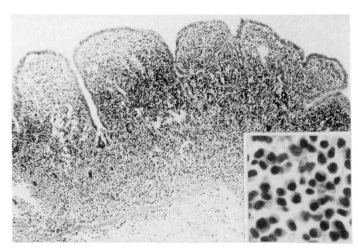

Figure 10 Small intestinal mucosa from a case of Mediterranean lymphoma. Intestinal villi are broadened and stunted and there is a diffuse infiltrate of plasma cells as seen in the inset. H & E × 50; inset × 480

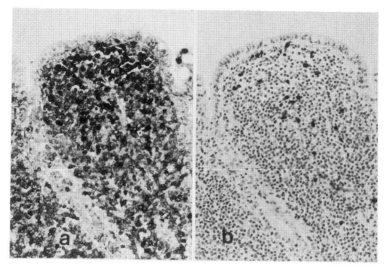

Figure 11 Mucosa from a case of Mediterranean lymphoma stained for alpha-1 heavy chain (**a**) and kappa and lambda light chains (**b**). Only a few reactive plasma cells express cytoplasmic light chain. Immunoperoxidase × 140

A proportion of cases evolve in a setting of a lymphoproliferative, possibly autoimmune disorder, known as lymphocytic interstitial pneumonia (LIP)[43]. Because of the uncertainty regarding the histology of pulmonary lymphoma and its relation to LIP, the term pseudolymphoma is often used. As in the stomach, this term has now been shown to be without foundation since most cases show light chain restriction.

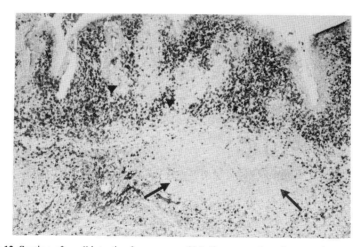

Figure 12 Section of small intestine from a case of Mediterranean lymphoma stained for alpha-1 heavy chain. A CIg negative lymphoid follicle is seen in the submucosa (arrows). CIg negative centrocyte like cells forming lymphoepithelial lesions (arrowheads) stand out in contrast with the plasma cell infiltrate in the mucosa. Immunoperoxidase × 50

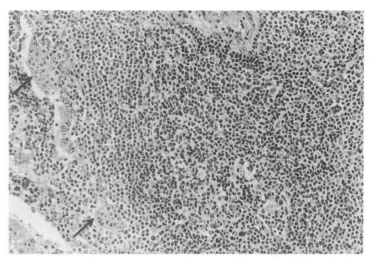

Figure 13 Section from a case of pulmonary lymphoma showing a reactive follicle in the centre with surrounding centrocyte like cells invading lymphoepithelial structures (arrows). H & E × 110.

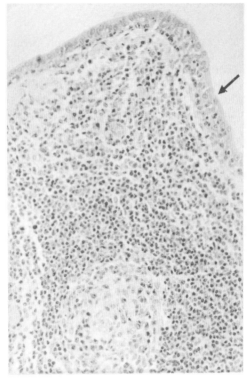

Figure 14 Section of salivary gland from a case of Sjögren's syndrome showing a follicle centre with an ill-defined mantle zone merging with the centrocyte like cells. These can be seen infiltrating the duct epithelium (arrow). Note the marked similarity to Figure 1. H & E × 110

The histology of pulmonary lymphoma is strikingly similar to that of gastric lymphoma. The same two components, namely centrocyte like cells and more rarely, plasma cells are seen (Figure 13). The centrocyte like cells form lymphoepithelial lesions with bronchiolar epithelium.

Immunocytochemical studies on lung lymphomas[34] have confirmed the monotypic nature of the lymphoid infiltrate. Morphological criteria alone are insufficient to distinguish between reactive and neoplastic infiltrates.

Salivary gland lymphoma

Like the stomach, the normal salivary gland does not contain MALT. However, in Sjögrens syndrome and related conditions, tissue showing the characteristics of MALT accumulates around ducts (Figure 14). The association of centrocyte like cells with duct epithelium is more exaggerated than in the intestine and results in the formation of prominent lymphoepithelial lesions; the so-called myoepithelial lesions. The majority of lymphocytes in these lesions are B-cells (centrocyte like cells), but T-cells are also present (Hyjek and Isaacson; unpublished observations). It is against the background of this lymphoid infiltrate, sometimes known as 'myoepithelial sialadenitis', that lymphoma evolves[44]. Once again, in salivary gland lymphomas centrocyte like cells and in some cases, plasma cells can be recognized (Figure 15). The centrocyte like cells may form large sheets around typical lymphoepithelial lesions, or may be less conspicuous. The evolution of lymphoma in myoepithelial sialadenitis is slow and can be recognized in its early stages as focal proliferations of lymphoid cells showing light chain restriction[44]. Without immunohistochemical identification of light chain restriction, it is often impossible to be certain whether or not the lymphoid infiltrate is neoplastic.

Lymphoma of the thyroid

Although it shares its embryonic origin with the gut, the thyroid gland is not usually considered to be a mucosal organ. When lymphoid tissue accumulates in the thyroid, however, as in Hashimoto's disease, it resembles MALT[45], with the formation of lymphoepithelial structures, which, unlike the salivary gland are inconspicuous and may be difficult to identify. Unlike true mucosal organs, such as the salivary gland, the thyroid cells do not produce secretory component so that a true mucosal immune response is not generated, even in the presence of acquired MALT like structures. Thyroid lymphomas arise in the setting of lymphoid infiltration of the gland, usually Hashimoto's diseas , and their histology is entirely characteristic of the MALT group of tumours[35]. This is especially true of lymphoepithelial lesions, which may be strikingly prominent (Figure 16).

OTHER LYMPHOMAS OF PUTATIVE MALT ORIGIN

Lymphomas of orbit and breast

Lymphomas of the orbit and breast have, in the past, presented the same diagnostic difficulties as those of the mucosal organs described above.

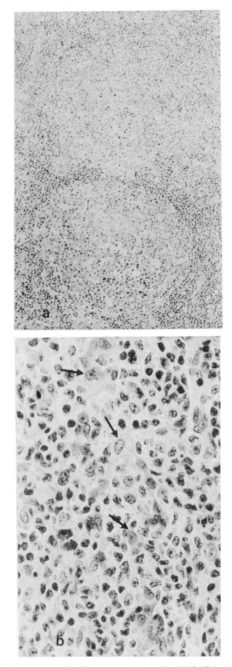

Figure 15 Malignant lymphoma of salivary gland showing (**a**) follicle centre below surrounded by a narrow mantle zone. Above there is an infiltrate of centrocyte like cells mixed with remnants of duct epithelium. A higher power view (**b**) shows the characteristic nuclear irregularity of these cells. Duct epithelial cells are arrowed, H & E top × 80; bottom × 280

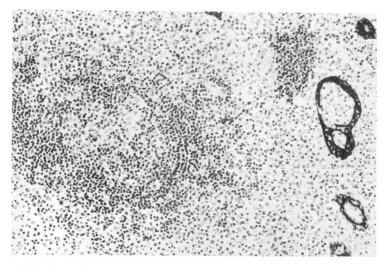

Figure 16 Malignant lymphoma of thyroid gland showing a follicle centre with surrounding mantle zone merging into an infiltrate of centrocyte like cells which form prominent lymphoepithelial lesions. Section has been stained with an anti-cytokeratin to highlight the lymphoepithelial lesions. Immunoperoxidase × 110

Although not as thoroughly studied as other MALT lymphomas it is possible that they too belong to this group of diseases.

Burkitts lymphoma

Wright[46] has raised the intriguing possibility that Burkitts lymphoma (BL) arises in the jaws in specialized MALT which is associated with the development of teeth. The pattern of spread of BL is quite different from that of peripheral nodal lymphomas and spread to mucosal sites, especially to lactating breast, is characteristic. Furthermore, a tumour indistinguishable from BL occurs as a primary small intestinal lymphoma in children, especially in the Middle East. The main difference between BL and the MALT lymphomas is the rapid dissemination of the former and its distinctive histological appearance. Burkitts lymphoma may, nevertheless, be a tumour arising from MALT follicle centre cells (small centroblasts), which unlike other MALT lymphomas is frozen in its differentiation pathway due to its association with Epstein–Barr (EB) virus. This, too, would explain its more aggressive behaviour.

Multiple lymphomatous polyposis

A distinctive type of lymphoma forming multiple polyps in the intestine was first described by Cornes[47]. Isaacson et al.[48] later characterized this disease as a B-cell lymphoma which both morphologically and phenotypically was of the centrocytic type[49]. Malignant lymphoma, centrocytic, occurs as a peripheral nodal disorder which although often widely disseminated, shows no predilection for the gastrointestinal tract. Multiple lymphomatous polypsis, on the other hand, appears to arise in the intestine, where the initial and principal focus of disease appears to be in the ileocaecal region. However, here too unlike the more common types of MALT associated B-cell lymphoma described above, widespread dissemination outside the gastrointestinal tract commonly occurs.

Histologically, the tumour is composed of a uniform population of centrocytes. On occasion, these surround pre-existing follicle centres giving rise to so-called mantle zone lymphoma[48], and replacement of these follicles by tumour cells may result in a nodular pattern, although it is not strictly a follicular lymphoma. An important distinction from the more common gastrointestinal B-cell lymphomas lies in the absence of lymphoepithelial lesions. The centrocytes of centrocytic lymphoma differ phenotypically from both the centrocytes of follicle centres and the centrocyte like cells described above. The cells usually express surface IgM and IgD, are C3b receptor positive and, importantly, usually express the T-cell antigen CD5. B-cells with this phenotype cannot be identified in normal lymphoid tissue, but are characteristically seen in fetal ileal Peyer's patches[4]. It is thus conceivable that MLP arises from nests of these fetal lymphocytes and that this accounts for the ileocaecal localization of the disease. On this basis too, MLP might be considered as a tumour of MALT.

T-cell lymphoma of MALT

Recent evidence that the distinctive type of intestinal lymphoma complicating coeliac disease is of T-cell rather than macrophage origin[2,50,51] raises the possibility that this lymphoma arises from the T-cell component of MALT. The clinical and histopathological features of this tumour have been exhaustively described[52] and will not be repeated here. Malignant intra-epithelial lymphocytes are present in some cases, and this raises the interesting possibility that these tumours may arise from specialized T-lymphocytes which populate the gut epithelium and which are seen to be increased in coeliac disease.

CONCLUSIONS

Since the early 1970s remarkable advances have been made in the understanding of non-Hodgkin's lymphoma. Work on these tumours has, however, been concentrated almost exclusively on peripheral nodal disease whilst extranodal lymphoma has received relatively little attention. Furthermore, much of the work on lymphoma has been concerned with immunological phenotyping as a means of rationalizing the morphology and clinical behaviour in the form of reproducable classifications. Little attention has been paid to the relationship between behavioural properties of benign and malignant lymphoid cells. The behaviour of cells of the B-cell compartment of the gastrointestinal tract has been thoroughly studied in animals, and the clinical features of gut lymphomas in humans suggest that this is an important factor in these tumours and lymphomas arising in other mucosal sites. Our studies confirm this, and, furthermore, suggest that the study of malignant lymphoma can provide a useful window on the biology of normal lymphoid tissue.

References

1. Isaacson, P. and Wright, D. H. (1984). Extranodal malignant lymphoma arising from mucosa-associated lymphoid tissue. *Cancer,* 53, 2515–24
2. Isaacson, P. G., O'Connor, N. T. J., Spencer, J., Bevan, D. H., Connolly, C. E., Kirkham, N., Pollock, D. J., Wainscoat, J. S., Stein, H. and Mason, D. Y. (1985). Malignant histiocytosis of the intestine – a T cell lymphoma. *Lancet,* 2, 688–91
3. Cornes, J. S. (1965). Number size and distribution of Peyer's patches in the human small intestine. Part 1. The development of Peyer's patches. *Gut,* 6, 225–9
4. Spencer, J., MacDonald, T. T., Finn, T. and Isaacson, P. G. (1986). The development of gut-associated lymphoid tissue in the terminal ileum of fetal human intestine. *Clin. Exp. Immunol.,* 64, 536–43
5. Owen, R. L. and Jones, A. L. (1974). Epithelial cell specialisation within human Peyer's patches: an ultrastructural study of intestinal lymphoid follicles. *Gastroeenterology,* 66, 189–203
6. Owen, R. L. (1977). Sequential uptake of horseradish peroxidase by lymphoid follicle epithelium of Peyer's patches in the normal unobstructed mouse intestine: an ultrastructural study. *Gastroenterology,* 72, 440–51
7. Bockman, D. E., Boydston, W. R. and Beezhold, D. H. (1983). The role of epithelial cells in gut-associated immune reactivity. In McGhee, J. R. and Mestecky, J. (eds) *The Secretory Immune System.* vol. 409, pp. 129-144. (New York: New York Academy of Sciences)
8. Richman, L. K., Graeff, A. S. and Strober, W. (1981). Antigen presentation by macrophage-enriched cells from mouse Peyer's patch. *Cell. Immunol.,* 62, 110–18
9. MacDonald, T. T. and Carter, P. B. (1982). Isolation and functional characterisation of adherent phagocytic cells from mouse Peyer's patches. *Immunology,* 45, 769–74
10. Griscelli, G., Vasalli, P. and McCluskey, R. T. (1969). The distribution of large dividing lymph node cells in syngeneic recipient rats after intravenous injection. *J. Exp. Med.,* 130, 1427–51
11. Hall, J. G., Parry, D. M. and Smith, M. E. (1972). The distribution and differentiation of lymph–borne immunoblasts after intravenous injection into syngeneic recipients. *Cell Tiss. Kin.,* 5, 269–81
12. Crabbe, P. A., Baxin, H., Eyssen, H. and Heremans, J. F. (1968). The normal microbial flora as a major stimulus for proliferation of plasma cells synthesising IgA in the gut. *Int. Arch. Allergy Appl. Immunol.,* 34, 362–75
13. Nash, D. R., Vaerman, J. P., Bazin, H. and Heremans, J. F. (1969). Identification of IgA in rat serum and secretions. *J. Immunol.,* 103, 145–8
14. South, M. A., Cooper, M. D., Wollheim, F. A., Hong, R. and Good, R. A. (1966). The IgA system. I. studies on the transport and immunocytochemistry of IgA in the saliva. *J. Exp. Med.,* 123, 615–27
15. Porter, P., Noakes, D. E. and Allen, W. D. (1972). Intestinal secretions in pre-ruminant calf. *Immunology,* 23, 299–312
16. Orlans, E., Peppard, J. V., Reynolds, J. and Hall, J. G. (1978). Rapid active transport of immunoglobulin A from blood to bile. *J. Exp. Med.,* 147, 588–92
17. Walker, W. A. and Isselbacher, K. J. (1977). Intestinal antibodies. *N. Engl. J. Med.,* 297, 767–73
18. Vaerman, J. P., Andre, C., Bazin, H. and Heremans, J. F. (1973). Mesenteric lymph as a major source of serum IgA in guinea pigs and rats. *Eur. J. Immunol.,* 3, 580–4
19. Bienenstock, J., McDermott, M., Befus, D. and O'Neill, M. (1978). A common mucosal immunologic system involving bronchus breast and bowel. *Adv. Exp. Med. Biol.,* 107, 53–9
20. Montgomery, P. C., Ayyildiz, A., Lemaitre-Coelho, I. M., Vaerman, J-P. and Rockey, J. H. (1983). Induction and expression antibodies in secretions: The occular immune system. In McGhee, J. R. and Mestecky, J. (eds). *The Secretory Immune System,* vol. 409, pp. 428–440. (New York: New York Academy of Sciences)

21. Spencer, J. and Hall, J. G. (1984). Studies on the lymphocytes of sheep. IV Migration patterns of lung-associated lymphocytes efferent from the caudal mediastinal lymph node. *Immunology*, **52**, 1–5

22. Vaerman, J. P. and Heremans, J. F. (1966). Subclasses of human IgA based on differences in the alpha polypeptide chains. *Science*, **153**, 647–9

23. Andre, C., Andre, F. and Fargier, M. C. (1978) Distribution of IgA$_1$ and IgA$_2$ plasma cells in various normal human tissues and in the jejunum of plasma IgA-deficient patients. *Clin. Exp. Immunol.*, **33**, 327–31

24. Crago, S. S., Kutteh, N. H., Moro, I., Allansmith, M. R., Radl, J., Haaijman, J. J. and Mestecky, J. (1984). Distribution of IgA$_1$-, IgA$_2$- and J chain-containing cells in human tissue. *J. Immunol.*, **132**, 16–18

25. Tourville, D. R., Adler, R. H., Bienenstock, J. and Tomasi, T. B. (1969). The human secretory immunoglobulin system: immunohistochemical localisation of σA, secretory 'piece' and lactoferrin in normal human tissues. *J. Exp. Med.*, **129**, 411–29

26. Spencer, J., Finn, T., Pulford, K. A. F., Mason, D. Y. and Isaacson, P. G. (1985). The human gut contains a novel population of B lymphocytes which resemble marginal zone cells. *Clin. Exp. Immunol.*, **62**, 607–12

27. Spencer, J., Finn, T. and Isaacson, P. G. (1986). Human Peyer's patches – an immunohistochemical study. *Gut*, **27**, 405–10

28. Spencer, J., Finn, T. and Isaacson, P. G. (1986). A comparative study of the gut-associated lymphoid tissue in primates and rodents. *Virch. Arch.*, **51**, 509–19

29. Spencer, J., Finn, T. and Isaacson, P. G. (1985). Gut-associated lymphoid tissue: a morphological and immunocytochemical study of the human appendix. *Gut*, **26**, 672–9

30. Fergusson, A. (1977). Progress report. Intraepithelial lymphocytes of the small intestine. *Gut*, **18**, 921–37

31. Pulford, K. A. F., Ralfkiaer, E., MacDonald, S. N., Erber, W. N., Falini, B., Gatter, K. C. and Mason, D. Y. A. (1986). A new monoclonal antibody (KB61) recognising an antigen of 40,000 molecular weight which is selectively expressed on a subpopulation of human lymphocytes. *Immunology*, **57**, 71–6

32. Rowe, M., Hildreth, J. E. K., Rickinson, A. B. and Epstein, M. A. (1982). Monoclonal antibodies to Epstein–Barr virus-induced, transformation-associated cell surface antigens: binding patterns and effect upon virus-specific T-cell cytotoxicity. *Int. J. Cancer*, **29**, 373–80

33. Sminia, T. and Plesch, B. E. C. (1982). An immunohistochemical study of cells with surface and cytoplasmic immunoglobulins *in situ* in Peyer's patches and lamina propria of rat small intestine. *Virch. Arch.*, **40**, 181–9

34. Herbert, A., Wright, D. H., Isaacson, P. G. and Smith, J. L. (1984). Primary malignant lymphoma of the lung: Histopathologic and immunologic evaluation of nine cases. *Hum. Pathol.*, **15**, 415–22

35. Anscombe, A. M. and Wright, D. H. (1985). Primary malignant lymphoma of the thyroid – a tumour of mucosa-associated lymphoid tissue: review of seventy-six cases. *Histopathology*, **9**, 81–97

36. Ree, H. J., Rege, V. B., Knisley, R. E., Thayer, W. R., D'amico, R. P., Song, J. Y. and Crowley, J. P. (1980). Malignant lymphoma of Waldeyer's ring following gastrointestinal lymphoma. *Cancer*, **46**, 1528–35

37. Isaacson, P. G., Spencer, Jo. and Finn, T. (1986). Primary B-cell gastric lymphoma. *Hum. Pathol.*, **17**, 72–82

38. World Health Organisation. (1976). Alpha-chain disease and related small intestinal lymphoma: A memorandum. *Bull. WHO*, **54**, 615–24

39. Isaacson, P. (1979). Middle East lymphoma and α-chain disease. An immunohistochemical study. *Am. J. Surg. Pathol.*, **3**, 431–41

40. Asselah, F., Slavin, G., Sowter, G. and Assehah, H. (1983). Immunoproliferative small intestinal disease in Algerians. 1. Light microscopic and immuno-chemical studies. *Cancer*, **52**, 227–37

41. Isaacson, P. G. and Price, S. K. (1985). Light chains in Mediterranean lymphoma. *J. Clin. Pathol.*, **38**, 601–7

42. Al-Bahrani, Z. R., Al-Mondhiry, H., Bakir, F. and Al-Saleem, T. (1983). Clinical and pathological subtypes of primary intestinal lymphoma. Experience with 132 patients over a 14 year period. *Cancer*, **52**, 1666–72

43. Banerjee, D. and Ahmad, D. (1982). Malignant lymphoma complicating lymphocytic interstitial pneumonia: A monoclonal B-cell neoplasm arising in a polyclonal lymphoproliferative disorder. *Hum. Pathol.,* **13**(8), 780–4

44. Schmid, U., Helbron, D. and Lennert, K. (1982). Development of malignant lymphoma in myeopithelial sialadenitis (Sjörgren's syndrome). *Virch. Arch. (Pathol. Anat.),* **395**, 11–43

45. Wilkin, T. J. and Casey, C. (1984). The distribution of immunoglobulin-containing cells in human autoimmune thyroiditis. *Acta Endocrinol.,* **106**, 490–8

46. Wright, D. H. (1985). Histogenesis of Burkitt's lymphoma: a B-cell tumour of mucosa-associated lymphoid tissue. pp. 37–45. Presented at the *WHO Symposium on Burkitt's Lymphoma: A Human Cancer Model.* December 26–29, Lyon

47. Cornes, J. S. (1961). Multiple lymphomatous polyposis of the gastrointestinal tract. *Cancer,* **14**, 249–57

48. Isaacson, P. G., Maclennan, K. A. and Subbuswamy, S. G. (1984). Multiple lymphomatous polyposis of the gastrointestinal tract. *Histopathology,* **8**, 641–56

49. Stein, H., Gerdes, J. and Mason, D. Y. (1982). The normal and malignant germinal centre. *Clin. Haematol.,* **11**, 531–59

50. Salter, D. M., Krajewski, A. S. and Dewar, A. E. (1986). Immunophenotype analysis of malignant histiocytosis of the intestine. *J. Clin. Pathol.,* **39**, 8–15

51. Loughran, T. P., Kadin, M. E. and Deek, H. J. (1986). T-cell intestinal lymphoma associated with celiac sprue. *Ann. of Int. Med.,* **104**, 44–7

52. Isaacson, P. and Wright, D. H. (1978). Malignant histiocytosis of the intestine: its relationship to malabsorption and ulcerative jejunitis. *Hum. Pathol.* **9**, 661–77

10
T-cell Neoplasia

A. D. RAMSAY and W. J. SMITH

INTRODUCTION

The T-cell arises from an undifferentiated mesenchymal precursor cell probably originating in the bone marrow, and undergoes processing in the thymus. It is unclear whether the stem cell is committed to becoming a T-cell before this processing, or if the thymus itself induces T-cell differentiation. During development, at around 8 weeks gestation, the thymus gland, which is initially epithelial in nature, becomes filled with lymphoid cells. Lymphopoiesis then commences and continues until infancy when the thymus reaches its maximum size (around 70 g), and subsequently decreases with age as the gland involutes[1].

Histologically, the thymus gland is divided into lobules by fibrous septa, and within these there is a division into outer cortex and inner medulla. Development proceeds from cortex to medulla, the mature cells then entering the bloodstream. The cortex is more densely cellular, and contains actively dividing lymphoid cells. Various stages of T-cell development are seen in the cortex, including precursor cells, immature thymic blasts and more mature thymocytes. As the cells enter the medulla division stops, and the mature T-cells pass into the blood vessels to be carried to peripheral lymphoid tissue. The process of T-cell differentiation can be followed by the changes in thymocyte surface antigens, with eventual development of the final mature helper or suppressor T-cell phenotype. Figure 1 shows a schematic diagram of this differentiation, indicating the cluster antigen expression at each stage. The epithelial cells of the thymus produce several peptide hormones that are important in the development of the T-cells[2]. Specialized dendritic macrophages in the thymus also play a role in T-cell production, probably being involved in the generation of self-tolerance[3].

At the molecular level T-cells recognize antigen in association with the host's major histocompatability complex (self-MHC). Only T-cells capable of such recognition are able to leave the thymus. The T-cell receptor (TCR) is the structure responsible for interaction with the antigen/MHC complex. Two heterodimeric TCRs have been identified; the α:ß complex on functional

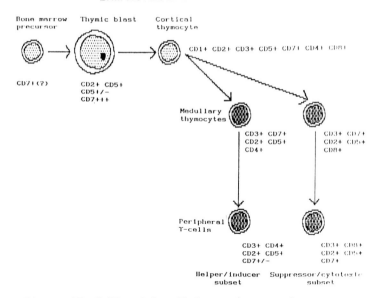

Figure 1 Diagram of T-cell differentiation with cluster antigen expression

helper and cytotoxic T-cells and the γ:δ heterodimer present on immature (CD4– CD8–) lymphocytes. The genes encoding the α, ß and γ chains have been isolated and shown to have homology with immunoglobulin genes[4]. The genetic mechanisms responsible for the generation of receptor heterogeneity are discussed in the final section of this chapter.

In peripheral lymph nodes T-cells are predominantly seen in the paracortical region, although a small number are seen in the B-cell follicle centres. The paracortex is characterized by a rich network of vessels having a prominent endothelial lining, the high endothelial venules (HEVs). These vessels are important in T-cell transport between the bloodstream and lymph nodes. Within the paracortex T-cells encounter antigen (presented by specialized macrophages termed interdigitating reticulum cells), and undergo proliferative changes in response to this stimulation. So the paracortex contains a mixed population of T-cells ranging from small mature forms through intermediate-sized cells to large T-immunoblasts with prominent nucleoli. Many of these normal paracortical features are recapitulated in T-cell neoplasms.

CATEGORIES OF T-CELL NEOPLASMS

Cutaneous T-cell lymphoma (CTCL)

The National Cancer Institute Workshop in 1978 recommended that the term *cutaneous T-cell lymphoma* (CTCL) should be used to encompass T-cell neoplasms of adults that exhibit skin involvement[6]. This includes mycosis fungoides in its various forms and the Sézary syndrome, with its leukaemic and erythrodermic patterns. Other related entities include lymphomatoid papulosis[6] and regressing atypical histiocytosis[7].

T-lymphoblastic lymphoma

This is a highly aggressive tumour composed of primitive 'T-lymphoblasts' that are variously categorized as prothymocytes or thymocytes. The clinical and morphological features overlap with those of the T-cell variety of acute lymphoblastic leukaemia. Such neoplasms may be referred to as thymic or immature T-cell lymphomas[8].

Peripheral T-cell lymphoma (PTCL)
(Adult, post-thymic or pleomorphic T-cell lymphoma)

This is the hardest group of T-cell neoplasms to define, these tumours make up the bulk of nodal T-cell lymphomas in adults. They may be termed 'adult', 'pleomorphic', 'peripheral' or 'post-thymic' tumours[9,10], although none of these terms is completely satisfactory. Into this group falls the lymphoma associated with the human T-cell leukaemia/lymphoma virus (HTLV)[11].

CLINICOPATHOLOGICAL ASPECTS

CTCL

The CTCL make up the commonest pattern of T-cell lymphoma, with a reported incidence similar to that of Hodgkin's disease. The disease is commoner in men (with a male:female ratio of approximately 2:1) and over 80% of cases are seen in patients over 45 years of age[12].

Clinically, CTCL is separated into three stages, the patch stage, the plaque stage and the tumour stage. Patients in the former category often have a long history of erythematous macular patches, usually on the trunk and extremities. These patches may wax and wane, and are not infrequently diagnosed as forms of psoriasis or eczematous dermatitis. Plaques are irregular or annular scaling lesions, pink to purple-brown in colour, can involve any part of the skin surface and may be associated with pruritus. Patients with the plaque stage are grouped into Stage 1A or 1B, depending upon whether greater or less than 10% of the skin surface is involved. The plaques stage may follow the patch stage, or arise *de novo*.

The tumour stage occurs late in the course of the disease, with firm dome-shaped ('mushroom-like') nodules usually on the face, scalp and body folds. It is frequently associated with a rapid progression of the disease, with lymph node and visceral involvement (spleen, lungs, liver, kidney and gastrointestinal tract). Rarely the tumour stage presents *de novo* in a form termed 'tumuer d'emblée'.

Erythroderma may occur at any stage of the disease, but in the Sézary variant it is associated with circulating cells which have hyperchromatic convoluted nuclei, the Sézary–Lutzner cells. The lymph nodes are inevitably involved in this form of CTCL[13].

147

Histologically CTCL may be epidermotropic or non-epidermotropic. The epidermotropic form, usually seen in patch and plaque stages, shows a band-like mononuclear cell infiltrate at the junction of papillary and reticular dermis. The infiltrate is initially polymorphous, containing morphologically normal lymphocytes and macrophages, larger mononuclear cells with hyperchromatic nuclei, and lymphoid cells with markedly convoluted nuclei. As the disease progresses the infiltrate becomes increasingly monomorphous, the large hyperchromatic mononuclear cells predominating. Characteristically the epidermis is infiltrated by convoluted cells, either singly or in clusters forming Pautrier microabscesses. The extent of epidermal involvement varies, with more severe cases showing microabscesses in the skin appendages. Figure 2 shows the histological features of a typical case of mycosis fungoides.

In the non-epidermotropic form the epidermis and upper papillary dermis are often totally uninvolved. This variant is usually seen in the tumour stage of CTCL, and the histology may change from epidermotropic to non-epidermotropic with the development of tumours. Histologically, there is a slowly progressive increase in large atypical lymphoid cells in the dermis, these stretching the overlying epidermis to produce the clinically-apparent lesions. These lymphoid cells show marked nuclear pleomorphism, and many have irregular nuclei. They are not immediately identifiable as CTCL cells, and may be confused with other lymphomas or non-lymphoid tumours including melanoma.

CTCL is most often a relatively indolent disease, and is best classed as a low-grade T-cell neoplasm. The early patch and plaque stages may last for years, and the overall median survival is reported as 9–10 years. Development of the non-epidermotropic form is associated with a poorer prognosis[14].

TLL

These fairly rare tumours are most often seen in children or young adults, and there is a 2:1 male predominance[9]. Classically the presentation is with a mediastinal mass, in keeping with the thymic nature of the neoplastic cells, and there may be accompanying pleural effusions and enlarged lymph nodes. Although the peripheral blood and bone marrow are frequently initially normal, the disease rapidly becomes leukaemic, with numerous T-lympho-blasts invading these sites. With the onset of the leukaemic phase other extra-nodal sites may be involved, in particular the CNS. T-lymphoblastic lymphoma, therefore, forms a spectrum with T-acute lymphoblastic leukaemia. The leukaemia may present concurrently with the mediastinal mass, or the disease may remain as a pure leukaemia with no solid tumour formed.

Pathologically the tumour is composed of sheets of immature cells showing a high mitotic rate, and frequent individual cell necrosis (Figure 3). In many cases macrophages are prominent, producing a 'starry sky' pattern that resembles Burkitt's lymphoma. Individual cells show a relatively large nucleus with a small amount of cytoplasm. Although there is usually nuclear pleomor-phism, with many of the nuclei being convoluted, this feature is variable, and it is unwise to exclude a T-cell origin if the nuclei are round or oval. Lymph

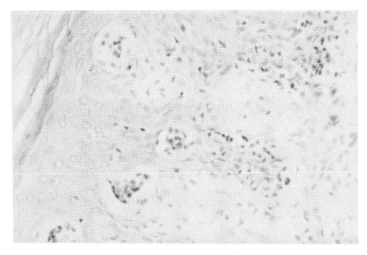

Figure 2 Medium power photomicrograph of skin involved in a cutaneous T-cell lymphoma. Groups of lymphocytes in the epidermis constitute Pautrier microabscesses

nodes often show a characteristic pattern of involvement, the B-cell follicles being spared initially, and the underlying nodal architecture being preserved. As the tumour cells spread into surrounding fat and connective tissue, they often adopt an 'Indian file' pattern, with rows of single cells infiltrating between collagen bundles.

PTCL

The incidence of the PTCL is difficult to define, as in the past many cases have been diagnosed either as Hodgkin's disease or as histiocytic lymphoma. All studies of this group show a wide range, with patients presenting from the third decade onwards[15–17]. Although these neoplasms are node-based diseases, the sites involved show tremendous variation. We have encountered cases where the initial disease was detected in bladder, testis, soft tissue, bone and skin, but all progressed to involve lymph nodes[18]. There is clearly a relationship with CTCL, as some of the PTCL arise in patients with a history of MF, and many show a predilection for skin and subcutis. Epidermotropism, however, is usually absent.

The retrovirus known as human T-cell leukaemia/lymphoma virus (HTLV)-1 is associated with clusters of T-cell lymphomas in Japan and the Caribbean[19]. These tumours are diseases of adults and have a chronic course with a fulminant terminal phase. Patients show widespread lymphadenopathy, hepatosplenomegaly, frequent hypercalcaemia (with or without skeletal lesions) and skin manifestations[11]. In some cases focal epidermotropism with Pautrier microabscess formation is seen, and the disease may be confused with forms of CTCL. Figure 4 illustrates the histology of an HTLV-1 associated T-cell lymphoma.

The histology of the PTCL is extremely variable, and there is no good method of subclassification. Stansfeld divides T-cell lymphomas according to

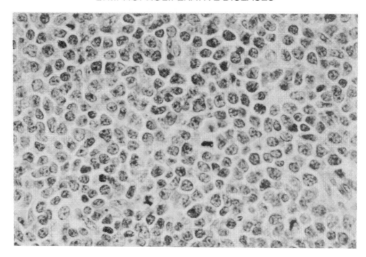

Figure 3 High power photomicrograph of T-lymphoblastic lymphoma showing a sheet of primitive cells (Reprinted from the *Journal of Pathology* by kind permission of Editor-in-chief)

the cell size and whether the nuclei are pleomorphic or monomorphic[20]. Others use the terms immunoblastic, diffuse large-cell, mixed small and large cell, monomorphic medium-sized cell, etc[16,21]. In addition, there are the categories of angio-immunoblastic lymphadenopathy (AIL)-like T-cell lymphoma, T-zone lymphoma, and lymphoepithelioid (Lennert's) lymphoma.

General histological features of T-cell lymphomas include the presence of prominent high endothelial venules, an eosinophil infiltrate, convoluted or

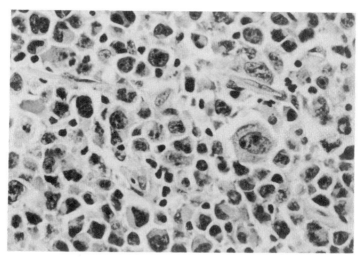

Figure 4 High power photomicrograph of a pleomorphic T-cell lymphoma associated with HTLV-1 infection (Reprinted from the *Journal of Pathology* by kind permission of the Editor-in-Chief)

irregular nuclear outline of the malignant cells, cells with large nucleoli resembling Reed–Sternberg cells, restriction of the disease to the paracortex, and a wide range in neoplastic cell size. Additional pointers to the T-cell nature of a lymphoma are clear cytoplasm of the tumour cells, a large number of reactive macrophages and a tendency for lymph node architecture, in particular the sinus structure, to be preserved in the early stages of involvement. Despite these numerous features, it is often difficult to diagnose a lymphoma as being of T-cell lineage on histological grounds alone. Some T-cell lymphomas may show none of the histological features described.

Falling into the PTCL category are certain histological varieties of T-cell lymphoma that merit separate discussion. The condition, variously termed angio-immunoblastic lymphadenopathy (AIL), angio-immunoblastic lymphadenopathy with dysproteinaemia (AILD) or immunoblastic lymphadenopathy, (IBL) was described in 1974 (AILD)[22] and 1975 (IBL)[23] in elderly patients with generalized lymphadenopathy, skin rash, fever, anaemia, hepatosplenomegaly and raised immunoglobulins. Histology of the lymph nodes showed an obliteration of the normal architecture with a marked proliferation of small blood vessels and a mixed cellular infiltrate composed of large immunoblasts and plasma cells in a background of small lymphocytes. Many of the latter show nuclear irregularity and have clear 'halo-like' cytoplasm, indicating their T-cell nature (Figure 5). Although a percentage of patients died of intercurrent infection, the disease initially appeared relatively indolent, but there were soon reports of a high incidence of malignant lymphoma arising within AIL. Some were B-cell lymphomas, but many appeared to be T-cell derived[24]. In addition, a group of T-cell lymphomas were reported that had the histological and clinical features described in AIL[25]. Thus the relationship between T-cell lymphoma and AIL has become blurred, and genetic analysis of cases of AIL have detected clonal

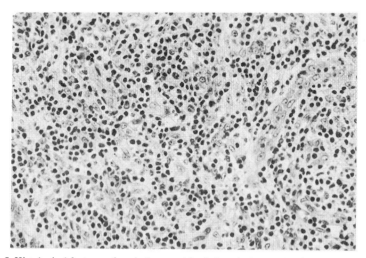

Figure 5 Histological features of angio-immunoblastic lymphadenopathy-like T-cell lymphoma showing prominent vessels and numerous cells with clear cytoplasmic 'haloes'

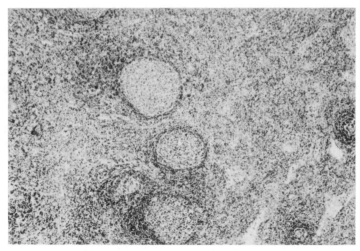

Figure 6 T-zone lymphoma. Low power photomicrograph showing residual follicles separated by a cellular infiltrate (Reprinted from the *Journal of Pathology* by kind permission of the Editor-in-Chief)

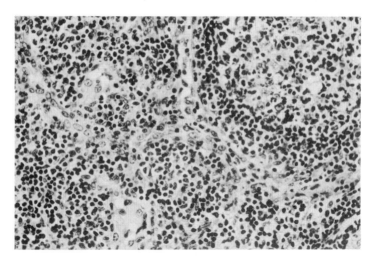

Figure 7 T-zone lymphoma. High power view showing a residual follicle (top right) and the surrounding infiltrate. The latter contains prominent vessels and cells with clear cytoplasm, and resembles Figure 5

T-cell populations[26]. The term AIL-like T-cell lymphoma is used for the lymphoma with the features of AIL. It remains to be seen whether all cases of AIL are in fact early lymphomas, and whether all the cases classed as AIL-like lymphoma are true neoplasms.

In 1978 Lennert described a form of T-cell lymphoma in which the neoplastic infiltrate tended to involve the paracortex of affected lymph nodes, and was composed of T-lymphocytes of varying size, interdigitating reticulum cells and high endothelial venules[27]. The tumour thus occupied the T-zone, and contained all the elements seen in the normal T-zones of lymph nodes. The term T-zone lymphoma was applied to this tumour, and it was considered to be the T-cell analogue of follicular B-cell lymphoma. Histologically, T-zone lymphoma is characterized by surviving follicles that are widely separated by the pleomorphic infiltrate. Within the infiltrate are large and small T-cells, with immunoblastic forms and smaller forms (often having a plasmacytoid appearance), and arborizing high endothelial vessels. In our experience the infiltrate is identical to that seen in AIL-like T-cell lymphoma, and the diagnosis is made by examining the lymph node architecture. Figures 6 and 7 are low and high power photomicrographs showing the histological features of a case of T-zone lymphoma.

The final type of T-cell lymphoma to be considered separately is termed lymphoepithelioid T-cell lymphoma or Lennert's lymphoma[28]. In this condition numerous epithelioid histiocytes are seen throughout a lymph node in which the normal architecture has been effaced. The histiocytes may lie singly or in clusters forming small granulomas. Between the histiocytes the malignant T-cells can be seen, often with large blastic forms that can resemble Reed–Sternberg cells.

Although the lymphoepithelioid pattern is described in T-cell lymphomas, it may be seen in other disorders including Hodgkin's disease, B-cell lymphomas and inflammatory lesions such as toxoplasmosis. The concern in such cases is the T-cell lymphoma, and although the epithelioid histiocytic infiltrate is an interesting feature, it is of somewhat secondary importance.

The prognosis of PTCL is difficult to assess, since they are not a uniform group, and are only now being correctly identified. There is evidence that they behave in aggressive fashion in many instances[9,10,16], but some cases may have an indolent course[29]. Specifically, T-cell lymphomas involving nasopharynx and pharynx seem to have a long natural history, with local recurrence being more of a problem than disseminated disease[30]. Hopefully as the PTCL are more readily recognized and the clinical patterns defined, it will become possible to separate them into prognostic categories in a manner analogous to that used for B-cell lymphomas.

IMMUNOHISTOCHEMISTRY

Antibodies

A wide range of monoclonal antibodies is available for the detection of T-cells and their subsets in frozen section. Table 1 lists the most useful cluster antigens together with the antibodies used in our establishment, their specificity and source reference.

More recently a range of monoclonal antibodies that are useful in detecting the lineage of lymphoid cells in paraffin section has become available[38,39]. These mainly recognize portions of the leukocyte common antigen (CD45, CD45R), and have been termed lineage-related antibodies. In particular the antibodies UCHL1[40] and MT1[41] are of value in the identification of T-cells in

153

Table 1 Antibodies used on frozen section

Cluster antigen	Antibody used	Type	Source	Details and reference
CD1a	NA134	M	a	recognizes cortical thymocytes and Langerhans cells[31]
CD2	Leu 5	M	b	recognizes the E-rosetting antigen. A pan-T marker[32]
CD3	UCHT1	M	c	IgG$_1$ antibody against the 20 kD chains on the T-cell surface. Pan-T marker[33]
CD5	UCHT2	M	c	detects a 41 kD antigen on T-cells and a subset of B-cells[34]
CD7	3A1	M	c	IgG$_2$ antibody directed against a 41 kD antigen on T-cells. Pan-T[35]
CD4	Leu 3a	M	b	IgG$_1$ antibody recognizing the 55 kD antigen on the T-helper/inducer subset[36]
CD8	UCHT4	M	c	IgG$_1$ antibody recognizing the 32 kD antigen on the T-suppressor/cytotoxic subset[37]

M = murine monoclonal antibody; P = polyclonal antibody;
a: Professor A. J. McMichael, Oxford; b: Becton–Dickinson Ltd; c: Dr P. Beverley, ICRF

paraffin section. Although some cross-reactions with B-cells have been noted[42], in general positive staining with both of these antibodies, combined with negative staining with B-cell markers, is good evidence of a T-cell lineage. Studies of T-cell lymphomas carried out on paraffin section material have also shown that certain non-lineage markers are useful in helping to identify neoplastic T-cells[42]. The latter may show expression of α-1-anti-trypsin, epithelial membrane antigen (EMA), the CD15 granulocyte/Reed–Sternberg cell antigen, and the CD30 cellular activation antigen. Details of these paraffin section antibodies, both lineage-related and non-lineage, are given in Table 2.

Immunophenotype

Cutaneous T-cell lymphoma is, in general, a disease of CD4+ helper T-cells[49]. The usual immune phenotype is CD3+, CD2+, CD5+, CD4+, CD7+/−, CD8−, CD1−. There is some variability in phenotype, however, and loss of pan-T markers can be seen. Very occasional cases have a CD8+ phenotype[49]. In the tumour form expression of T-cell antigens may be extremely limited, and unless there is a good history of pre-existing CTCL, it can be difficult to confirm the T-cell nature of the malignant cells. In paraffin section CTCL will usually stain with the lineage-related T-cell antibodies UCHL1 and MT1, and some cases also express the CD15 marker seen in Reed–Sternberg cells[50]. Lymphomatoid papulosis shares the CD4 and CD15 expression of the CTCL[51].

T-lymphoblastic lymphoma has a characteristic phenotype, being the only T-cell neoplasm that expresses CD1a[52]. There is usually associated expression of CD3, CD5, CD2 and CD7 antigens, with CD7 being a particularly useful

Table 2 Antibodies used on paraffin section

Cluster antigen	Antibody used	Type	Source	Details and reference
CD45R0	UCHL1	M	c	IgG2a antibody against a 190 kD determinant of the leukocyte common antigen on T-cells, some macrophages and neutrophils[40]
CD43	MT1	M	f	a commercial antibody reacting with 100, 110 and 190 kD antigens probably related to the leukocyte common antigen, and present on T-cells, myeloid cells, and macrophages[41]
CD45RB	PD7/26	M	d	IgG₁ antibody recognizing the T200 leukocyte common antigen[43]
—	α1AT	P	e	alpha-1-antitrypsin[44]
CD15	Leu M1	M	b	IgMκ antibody detecting a conjugated polysaccharide (lacto-N-fuco-pentaosyl III) on the cell surface of granulocytes and Reed–Sternberg cells[45]
CD30	Ber H2	M	g	detects the Ki-1 cellular activation antigen (molecular weight approx. 110 kD)[46]
—	HMFG2	M	h	IgG₁ antibody raised against human milk fat globule membrane. Recognizes epithelial membrane antigen[47]
—	TAL-1B5	M	h	IgG₁ antibody that recognizes the alpha chain subunit of the human HLA-D locus[48]

M = murine monoclonal antibody; P = polyclonal antibody;
b: Becton–Dickinson Ltd; c: Dr P. Beverley, ICRF; d: Dr D. Y. Mason, Oxford; e: Dakopatts Ltd; f: Eurodiagnostics; g: Prof. H. Stein, Freie Universität, Berlin; h: Imperial Cancer Research Fund, London

marker[53]. A high degree of variability is seen with TLL, however, and abnormal phenotypes are not uncommon. The subset markers may also show almost any combination, including CD4+/CD8+ and CD4–/CD8–. Enzyme histochemistry, with detection of terminal deoxynucleotidyl transferase and dot-like acid phosphatase staining, may be helpful in the diagnosis of TLL. In general the leukaemic form (T-ALL) expresses a less mature phenotype, and it is reported that cases expressing CD1a and/or CD4 and CD8 (resembling mature cortical thymocytes) tend not to show bone marrow infiltration at an early stage in the disease[54]. In paraffin section these tumours usually stain with the lineage-related antibodies UCHL1 and MT1, although a proportion of cases are positive with only one of these markers. (A. J. Norton, personal communication)

PTCL show extreme variability in their immune phenotype, and loss of T-cell antigens is a common feature. The majority of cases express CD3, but this marker is absent in some neoplasms. Similarly, a given tumour may fail to express CD2, CD5 or CD7 and one study has shown that CD7 is the pan-T antigen most commonly lost in the PTCL[17]. It is, therefore, clear that a panel of antibodies must be used when studying these tumours, as no one antibody can detect all T-cell lymphomas. T-subset cluster antigen expression is also

Table 3 Immunostaining of peripheral T-cell lymphomas

Cluster antigen	Cases of PTCL showing positive staining
CD3	28/32
CD2	23/31
CD5	19/32
CD7	30/32
CD4	17/23
CD8	15/23

heterogeneous. There may be expression of CD4, CD8, CD4 and CD8, or neither subset marker[18]. In general the lymphomas associated with HTLV-1 express a helper phenotype, and are CD4 positive in a manner similar to the CTCL[55]. A summary of the results of using a panel of antibodies on 32 PTCL is given in Table 3.

The more recent lineage-related antibodies are of value in the diagnosis of PTCL, with most cases showing positivity with UCHL1 and MT1. In addition many cases, in particular those composed of large immunoblast-like or Reed–Sternberg-like pleomorphic cells, will show granular cytoplasmic expression of α_1-antitrypsin, CD15 positivity, CD30 positivity, and surface staining with epithelial membrane antigen[42]. The α_1-antitrypsin positivity is probably responsible for many such cases having been diagnosed as histiocytic lymphoma in the past, and it is now clear that α_1-antitrypsin is not a useful marker for cells of histiocytic lineage. Anti-lysozyme, in contrast, appears to be a valid marker of histiocytes since T-cell lymphomas are uniformly negative for lysozyme[18,42].

GENETIC ANALYSIS

Methods

Sequencing of the cloned TCR genes has shown that they are organized in a manner analogous to immunoglobulin genes on the germline chromosome[4]. DNA encoding variable (V), diversity (D), joining (J) and constant (C) segments (exons) are separated by intervening DNA (introns). During lymphocyte differentiation segments of the V, D (ß chain locus) and J regions are combined to form a functional variable region exon which is transcribed together with the constant (C) region. This process of somatic recombination produces a specific V–(D)–J gene rearrangement which is unique to each cell (Figure 8). The large number of possible combinations facilitates the generation of numerous receptors, each of which recognizes a specific antigen/MHC combination. If a T-cell undergoes clonal expansion as a result of neoplastic transformation, each daughter cell will carry the genetic configuration unique to that clone. This provides the basis for the identification of clonality by genotypic analysis using Southern blotting[56].

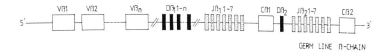

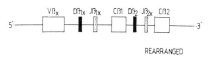

Figure 8 Diagrammatic representation of genetic rearrangement in the T-cell receptor ß chain. V = joining segments, D = diversity segments, J = joining segments, C = constant segments. Selected variable, diversity and joining segments are combined with the two constant segments in the rearranged genome

High molecular weight genomic DNA is purified from the sample and digested with restriction endonucleases. These enzymes, originally obtained from bacteria, digest DNA at specific sites within characteristic nucleotide sequences. Restriction digests of DNA are composed of DNA fragments of various lengths. DNA fragments are separated by agarose gel electrophoresis and then transferred to a nitrocellulose filter, forming a replica of the gel (Southern blotting). A radioactive plasmid containing the appropriate cloned gene segment, (for example, the TCR ß-chain constant region) is incubated with the filter under defined conditions. During this process, the probe (the cloned segment) hybridizes to the immobilized homologous DNA. An auto-radiograph is obtained by exposing the filter, after removing the excess probe by washing, to X-ray film, thus providing a permanent record of the data.

The process of genetic rearrangement alters the distance (in terms of DNA base pairs) between the endonuclease cleavage sites. Digestion of DNA purified from a differentiated lymphocyte will generate a fragment from the rearranged region that differs in size from that produced by digestion of germline (non-rearranged) DNA. If a cell which has undergone gene rearrangement subsequently undergoes clonal expansion, then digestion of DNA from that clone will produce large numbers of these non-germline fragments. Comparison of the sizes of restriction fragments binding to the probe from the sample and from control DNA facilitates the detection of a clone of lymphoid cells. Novel fragment(s) that are homologous to the probe may also be generated by the presence of genetic polymorphisms (i.e. alterations in the DNA sequence) in a restriction enzyme recognition sequence. It is statistically unlikely that polymorphisms would affect more than one recognition sequence within the region of interest. Consequently, digestion of the sample DNA is carried out with more than one enzyme in order to confirm that gene rearrangement rather than DNA polymorphism is responsible for the novel fragments.

Hybridization of the probe to control (non-rearranged) DNA produces a germline pattern of bands on autoradiography. Hybridization to DNA from a clone of lymphoid cells will produce a different pattern of bands due to the difference in size (and hence electrophoretic mobility) of the fragments. Each T-cell (and B-cell) possesses its own unique genetic configuration, consequently DNA purified from a reactive (polyclonal) lymphoid population will generate fragments of various sizes which are homologous to the probe. No distinct bands will be seen on the autoradiograph, since the signal generated by each individual fragment/probe hybrid will be undetectable. Genetic analysis, therefore, facilitates the identification of a clonal B- or T-cell population. A sample of the results of this method of analysis are shown in Figure 9.

Rearrangement of the TCR genes occurs in a hierarchical fashion: the γ locus undergoing rearrangement early in T-cell differentiation, followed by the ß gene and finally the α locus[4]. Rearrangement of the Cß locus can occur in a variety of ways: one or two of the Cß1 or Cß2 alleles can be rearranged,

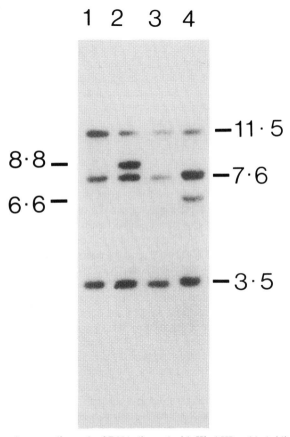

Figure 9 Sample autoradiograph of DNA digested with Hind III and hybridized with the T-cell receptor ß-chain probe. The band sizes are given in kilobases of DNA. Track 1 contains DNA from normal neutrophils, and tracks 2, 3 and 4 contain DNA purified from putative T-cell lymphomas. In tracks 2 and 4 the presence of additional bands (at 8.8 and 6.6 kilobases, respectively) indicates that rearrangement has occurred. Only germline fragments are present in track 3, with no evidence of rearrangement. (Courtesy of Dr N. T. J. O'Connor)

158

or one or both Cß1 alleles may be deleted. This rearrangement occurs prior to the co-ordinate translation of the mRNAs for the α:ß heterodimer. A functional T-cell receptor consists of this heterodimer in association with the CD3 molecule. Consequently, clonal expansions of T-cells can be detected by gene rearrangement studies even in the absence of CD3 expression[57]. The large size of the Jα region complicates the analysis of α gene rearrangement by conventional methods, but the use of pulsed field gel electrophoresis, which resolves DNA fragments greater than 20 kilobases, will overcome this[58].

Results of genetic analysis

Until the TCR probes were available, cytogenetic abnormalities or the detection of enzymes encoded by genes located on the X-chromosomes were used to distinguish clonal and reactive T-cell proliferations. These methods were not always satisfactory, and distinguishing between, for example, lymph node involvement in advanced mycosis fungoides (MF) and reactive derma-topathic lymphadenopathy (a benign change in lymph nodes associated with any long-standing skin condition) was problematical. Studies on DNA extracted from lymph node and skin biopsies from patients with MF have confirmed the clonal nature of T-cells in both skin and lymph nodes, even in cases where the nodal histology was apparently reactive[59]. Lymphocytes from patients with Sézary's syndrome have been analysed by several groups: in all cases Cß rearrangement was detected[60]. The clonality of lymphomatoid papulosis has been shown by molecular methods[61].

Rearranged Cß with germline immunoglobulin (Ig) genes have been observed in 90% of childhood T-acute lymphoblastic leukaemias (T-ALLs) analysed[62]. In the remaining 10% of cases the immunoglobulin heavy chain (IgH) genes had also undergone recombination. Genetic analysis of T-cell chronic lymphocytic leukaemia (T-CLL) and prolymphocytic leukaemia (T-PLL) also confirm that they are monoclonal proliferations of T-cells[63].

The majority of cases of adult peripheral T-cell lymphoma (PTCL) studied exhibit at least two rearranged Cß alleles, while the immunoglobulin genes retain a germline configuration[18,60,64]. Dual rearrangement of Ig and TCR genes occasionally occurs[60].

Immunophenotyping and genotyping of cases of Lennert's lymphoma have confirmed its T-cell nature[65]. Determination of T-cell clonality by immunolog-ical and genetic methods in malignant histiocytosis of the intestine (MHI – coeliac associated lymphoma) has shown that it is of T-cell rather than histiocytic origin[66].

Chromosomal translocations associated with particular T-cell neoplasms have been identified[67]. It is noteworthy that many of these involve chromo-somes on which the TCR genes are located. The α chain locus is at 14q11–12, the ß locus at 7q32 and the γ chain is at 7p15[67]. The inversion of chromosome 14 [t(14;14) (q11;q32)] is associated with T cell lymphomas and chronic leukaemias. Molecular analysis of one case has shown that complex rearrange-ments of the genes encoding the TCR α chain and IgH chain have generated a hybrid gene (IgT)[68]. Chromosome 14 abnormalities are also associated with childhood ALL, adult T-cell leukaemia and T-cell malignancies arising in patients with ataxia telangectasia[67]. The translocation [t(8;14) (q24; q11)] seen in 10% of T-ALLs consists of the transposition of the α chain locus to a region immediately distal to the *c-myc* oncogene[67].

The ß chain locus is also implicated in T-lymphoblastic associated translocations involving chromosomes 7 and 9[67]. Abnormal recombination events between the ß chain gene and 9q34 have resulted in DNA which is transcribed, although no protein product has been identified.

It is hoped that a detailed molecular analysis of these genetic events will eventually aid our understanding of these neoplasms.

CONCLUSIONS

In conclusion, the T-cell neoplasms may be divided into cutaneous, lymphoblastic and peripheral categories. The first two have distinct clinical features, whereas the latter group is clinically heterogeneous, including cases related to HTLV infection, angio-immunoblastic lymphadenopathy-like T-cell lymphoma, and lymphoepithelioid T-cell lymphoma. Immunologically, the cutaneous neoplasms mark predominantly as T-helper cells, the lymphoblastic lymphomas have a phenotype resembling cortical thymocytes, and the peripheral tumours may show almost any variation of the mature T-cell phenotype. Because of this variability panels of anti-T-cell antibodies should be used to study these tumours in frozen section, and both lineage-related and non-lineage antibodies should be used in paraffin section. Genotypic analysis provides a valuable means of confirming the clonality and lineage of the T-cell lymphomas, and the cytogenetics of these neoplasms will be a fertile field for future study.

References

1. Rosen, F. S., Cooper, M. D. and Wedgwood, R. J. (1984). The primary immunodeficiencies (part 1). *N. Engl. J. Med.,* **311**, 235–42
2. Trainin, N., Pecht, M. and Handzel, Z. T. (1983). Thymic hormones; inducer and regulators of the T-cell system. *Immunol. Today,* **4**, 16–21
3. Kyewski, B. A., Rouse, R. V. and Kaplan, H.S. (1982). Thymocyte rosettes: Multicellular complexes of lymphocytes and bone marrow-derived stromal cells in the mouse thymus. *Proc. Natl. Acad. Sci. USA,* **79**, 5646–50
4. Hood, L. Kronenberg, M. and Hunkapiller, T. (1985). T-cell antigen receptors and the immunoglobulin supergene family. *Cell,* **40**, 225–9
5. Lamberg, S. I. and Bunn, P. A. (eds). (1979). Proceedings of the Workshop on cutaneous T-cell lymphomas (Mycosis fungoides and Sézary syndrome). *Cancer Treat. Rep.,* **63**, 561–736
6. Willemze, R., Meyer, C. J. L. M., VanVloten, W. A. and Scheffer, E. (1982). The clinical and histological spectrum of lymphomatoid papulosis. *Br. J. Dermatol.,* **107**, 131–44
7. Flynn, K. J., Dehner, L. P., Gajl-Peczalska, K. J., Dahl, M. V., Ramsay, N. and Wang, N. (1982). Regressing Atypical Histiocytosis: a cutaneous proliferation of atypical neoplastic histiocytes with unexpectedly indolent behaviour. *Cancer,* **49**, 959–70
8. Nathwani, B. N., Kim, H. and Rappaport, H. (1976). Malignant lymphoma, lymphoblastic. *Cancer,* **38**, 964–83
9. Brisbane, Ju, Berman, L. D. and Neimann, R. S. (1983). Peripheral T-cell lymphoma: a clinicopathologic study of nine cases. *Am. J. Clin. Pathol.,* **79**, 285–93

10. Grogan, T. M., Fielder, K., Rangel, C., Jolley, C. J., Wirt, D. P., Hicks, M. J., Miller, T. P., Brooks, R., Greenberg, B. and Jones, S. (1985). Peripheral T-cell lymphoma: aggressive disease with heterogeneous immunotypes. *Am. J. Clin. Pathol.*, **83**, 279–88

11. Knowles, D. M. II. (1986). The human T-cell leukaemias: clinical, cytomorphologic, immunophenotypic and genotypic considerations. *Hum. Pathol.*, **17**, 14–33

12. Edelson, R. L. (1983). Cutaneous T-cell lymphomas. *J. Dermatol. Surg. Oncol.*, **9**, 641–4

13. Scheffer, E., Meijer, C. J. L. M., VanVloten, W. A. and Willemze, R. (1986). A histological study on lymph nodes from patients with Sézary's syndrome. *Cancer*, **57**, 2375–80

14. Yamamura, T., Aozasa, K. and Sano, S. (1984). The cutaneous lymphomas with convoluted nucleus. *J. Am. Acad. Dermatol.*, **10**, 796–803

15. Van der Valk, P., Willemze, R. and Meijer, C. J. L. M. (1986). Peripheral T-cell lymphomas: a clinicopathological and immunological study of 10 cases. *Histopathology*, **10**, 235–49

16. Jack, A. S. and Lee, F. D. (1986). Morphological and immunohistochemical characteristics of T-cell malignant lymphomas in the west of Scotland. *Histopathology*, **10**, 223–34

17. Borowitz, M. J., Reichert, T. A., Brynes, R. K., Cousar, J. B., Whitcomb, C. C., Collins, R. D., Crissman, J. D. and Byrne, G. E. (1986). The phenotypic diversity of peripheral T-cell lymphomas: the Southeastern Cancer Study Group experience. *Hum. Pathol.*, **17**, 567–74

18. Ramsay, A. D., Smith, W. J., Earl, H. M., Souhami, R. L. and Isaacson, P. G. (1987). T-cell lymphomas in adults: a clinicopathological study of eighteen cases. *J. Pathol.*, **152**, 63–76

19. Reitz, M. S., Kalyanaraman, V. S., Robert-Guroff, M., Popovic, M., Sarngadharan, M. G., Sarin, P. S. and Gallo, R. C. (1983). Human T-cell leukemia/lymphoma virus: the retrovirus of adult T-cell leukemia/lymphoma. *J. Inf. Dis.*, **147**, 399–405

20. Stansfeld, A. G. (1985). Peripheral T-cell lymphomas. In *Lymph Node Biopsy Interpretation*. pp. 300–329. (Edinburgh: Churchill Livingstone)

21. Weiss, L. M., Crabtree, G. S., Rouse, R. V. and Warnke, R. A. (1985). Morphologic and immunologic characterization of 50 peripheral T-cell lymphomas. *Am. J. Pathol.*, **118**, 316–24

22. Frizzera, G., Moran, E. M. and Rappaport, H. (1974). Angioimmunoblastic lymphadenopathy with dysproteinaemia. *Lancet*, **1**, 1070–3

23. Lukes, R. J. and Tindle, B. H. (1975). Immunoblastic lymphadenopathy: a hyperimmune entity resembling Hodgkin's disease. *N. Engl. J. Med.*, **292**, 1–8

24. Nathwani, B. N., Rappaport, H. Moran, E. M., Pangalis, G. A. and Kim, H. (1978). Malignant lymphoma arising in angioimmunoblastic lymphadenopathy. *Cancer*, **41**, 578–606

25. Watanabe, S., Sato, Y., Shimoyama, M., Minato, K. and Shimosato, Y. (1986). Immunoblastic lymphadenopathy, angioimmunoblastic lymphadenopathy and IBL-like T-cell lymphoma. A spectrum of T-cell neoplasia. *Cancer*, **58**, 2224–32

26. Weiss, L. M., Strickler, J. G., Dorfman, R. F., Horning, S. J., Warnke, R. A. and Sklar, J. (1986). Clonal T-cell populations in angioimmunoblastic lymphadenopathy and angioimmunoblastic lymphadenopathy-like lymphoma. *Am. J. Pathol.*, **122**, 392–7

27. Lennert, K., in collaboration with Stein, H. (1981). *Histopathology of Non-Hodgkin's Lymphomas (Based on the Kiel Classification)*, pp. 41–44. (Berlin: Springer-Verlag)

28. Lennert, K., in collaboration with Stein, H. (1981). *Histopathology of Non-Hodgkin's Lymphomas (Based on the Kiel Classification)*, pp. 103–111. (Berlin: Springer-Verlag)

29. Horning, S. J., Weiss, L. M., Crabtree, G. S. and Warnke, R. A. (1986). Clinical and phenotypic diversity of T-cell lymphomas. *Blood*, **67**, 1578–82

30. Chan, J. K. C., Ng, C. S., Lau, W. H. and Lo, S. T. H. (1987). Most nasal/nasopharyngeal lymphomas are peripheral T-cell neoplasms. *Am. J. Surg. Pathol.*, **11**, 418–29

31. McMichael, A. J., Pitch, J. R., Galfie, G., Fabre, J. W. and Milstein, C. (1979). A human thymocyte antigen defined by a hybrid myeloma monoclonal antibody. *Eur. J. Immunol.*, **9**, 205–10

32. Howard, F. D., Ledbetter, J. A., Wong, J., Bieber, C. P., Stinson, E. B. and Herzenberg, L. A. (1981). A human lymphocyte differentiation marker defined by monoclonal antibodies that block E-rosette formation. *J. Immunol.*, **126**, 2117–22

33. Beverley, P. C. L. and Callard, R. E. (1981). Distinctive functional characteristics of human T lymphocytes defined by E rosetting or a monoclonal anti-T cell antibody. *Eur. J. Immunol.*, **11**, 329–34

34. Beverley, P. C. L. (1986). Clinical and biological studies with monoclonal antibodies. In Beverley, P. C. L. (ed.) *Methods in Haematology 13. Monoclonal Antibodies*, pp. 247–269.

(Edinburgh: Churchill Livingstone)

35. Haynes, B. F., Eisenbarth, G. S. and Fauci, A. S. (1979). Human lymphocyte antigens: production of a monoclonal antibody that defines functional thymus-derived lymphocyte subsets. *Proc. Natl. Acad. Sci. USA*, **76**, 5829–33

36. Evans, R. L., Wall, D. W., Platsoucas, C. D., Siegal, F. P., Fikrig, S. M., Testa, C. M. and Good, R. A. (1981). Thymus-dependent membrane antigens in man: Inhibition of cell-mediated lympholysis by a monoclonal antibody to the T_{H2} antigen. *Proc. Natl. Acad. Sci. USA*, **78**, 544–8

37. Beverley, P. C. L. (1982). The application of monoclonal antibodies to the typing and isolation of lymphoreticular cells. *Proc. R. Soc. Edin.*, **81**, 212–32

38. Norton, A. J., Ramsay, A. D., Smith, S. H., Beverley, P. C. L. and Isaacson, P. G. (1986). Monoclonal antibody (UCHL1) that recognises normal and neoplastic T-cells in routinely fixed tissues. *J. Clin. Pathol.* **39**, 399–405

39. West, K. P., Warford, A., Fray, K., Allan, M., Campbell, A. C. and Lauder, I. (1986). The demonstration of B-cell, T-cell and myeloid antigens in paraffin sections. *J. Pathol.*, **150**, 89–101

40. Smith, S. H., Brown, M. H., Rowe, D., Callard, R. E. and Beverley, P. C. L. (1986). Functional subsets of human helper–inducer cells defined by a new monoclonal antibody, UCHL1. *Immunology*, **58**, 63–70

41. Poppema, S., Hollema, H., Visser, L. and Vos, H. (1987). Monoclonal antibodies (MT1, MT2, MB1, MB2, MB3) reactive with leukocyte subsets in paraffin-embedded tissue sections. *Am. J. Pathol.*, **127**, 418–29

42. Norton, A. J. and Isaacson, P. G. (1986). Immunocytochemical study of T-cell lymphomas using monoclonal and polyclonal antibodies effective in routinely fixed embedded tissue. *Histopathol.*, **10**, 1243–60

43. Warnke, R. A., Gatter, K. C., Falini, B., Hildreth, P., Woolston, R-E., Pulford, K., Cordell, J. L., Cohen, B., De Woolf-Peeters, C. and Mason, D. Y. (1983). Diagnosis of human lymphomas with monoclonal antileukocyte antibodies. *N. Engl. J. Med.*, **309**, 1275–81

44. Isaacson, P. G., Jones, D. B., Millward-Sadler, G. H., Judd, M. A. and Payne, S. (1981). Alpha-1-antitrypsin in human macrophages. *J. Clin. Pathol.*, **34**, 982–90

45. Hanjan, S. N. S., Kearney, J. F. and Cooper, M. D. (1982). A monoclonal antibody (MMA) that identifies a differentiation antigen on human myelomonocytic cells. *Clin. Immunol. Immunopathol.*, **23**, 172–88

46. Schwarting, R., Gerdes, J. and Stein, H. (1987). BER-H2: a new monoclonal antibody of the Ki-1 family for the detection of Hodgkin's disease in fixed tissue. In McMichael, A. J., Beverley, P. C. L., Crumpton, M., Gotch, F., Horton, M., Hogg, N., Ling, N., MacLennan, I., Mason, D. Y. and Waldmann, H. (eds) *Leucocyte Typing 3*. (Oxford: Oxford University Press)

47. Taylor-Papadimitriou, J., Petersen, J. A., Arklie, J., Burchell, J., Ceriani, R. L. and Bodmer, W. F. (1981). Monoclonal antibodies to epithelium-specific components of the human milk fat globule membrane, production and reaction with cells in culture. *Int. J. Cancer*, **28**, 17–21

48. Epenetos, A. A., Bobrow, L. G., Adams, T. E., Collins, C. M., Isaacson, P. G. and Bodmer, W. F. (1985). A monoclonal antibody that detects HLA-D region antigen in routinely fixed, wax embedded sections of normal and neoplastic lymphoid tissues. *J. Clin. Pathol.*, **38**, 12–17

49. Nasu, K., Said, J., Vonderheid, E., Olerud, J., Sako, D. and Kadin, M. (1985). Immunopathology of cutaneous T-cell lymphomas. *Am. J. Pathol.*, **119**, 436–47

50. Wieczorek, R., Burke, J. S. and Knowles, D. M. II. (1985). Leu-M1 antigen expression in T-cell neoplasia. *Am. J. Pathol.*, **121**, 374–80

51. Kadin, M., Nasu, K., Sako, D., Said, J. and Vonderheid, E. (1985). Lymphomatoid papulosis: a cutaneous proliferation of activated helper T-cells expressing Hodgkin's disease-associated antigens. *Am. J. Pathol.*, **119**, 315–25

52. Weiss, L. M., Bindl, J. M., Picozzi, V. J., Link, M. P. and Warnke, R. A. (1986). Lymphoblastic lymphoma: an immunophenotype study of 26 cases with comparison to T-cell acute lymphoblastic leukemia. *Blood*, **67**, 474–8

53. Stein, H., Lennert, K., Feller, A. C. and Mason, D. Y. (1984). Immunohistological analysis of human lymphoma: correlates of histological and immunological categories. *Adv. Cancer Res.*, **42**, 67–145

54. Bernard, A., Boumsell, L., Reinherz, E. L., Nadler, L. M., Ritz, J., Coppin, H., Richard, Y., Valeusi, F., Dausset, G., Flandrin, G., Lemerle, J. and Schlossman, S. F. (1981). Cell surface characterization of malignant T-cells from lymphoblastic lymphoma using monoclonal antibodies: evidence for phenotypic differences between malignant T-cells from patients with acute lymphoblastic leukemia and lymphoblastic lymphoma. *Blood*, **57**, 1105–10

55. Gallo, R. C., Prem, S. S., Blattner, W. A., Wong-stall, F. and Popovic, M. (1984). T-cell malignancies and human T-cell leukemia virus. *Sem. Oncol.*, **11**, 12–17

56. Southern, E. M. (1975). Detection of specific sequences among DNA fragments separated by gel electrophoresis. *J. Mol. Biol.*, **98**, 503–17

57. Royer, H. D., Acuto, O., Fabbi, M., Tizard, R., Ramachandran, K., Smart, J. E. and Reinherz, E. L. (1984). Genes encoding the Ti ß subunit of the antigen/MHC receptor undergo rearrangement during intrathymic ontogeny prior to surface T3-Ti expression. *Cell*, **39**, 261–6

58. Schwartz, D. C. and Cantor, C. R. (1984). Separation of yeast chromosome-sized DNAs by pulsed field gradient gel electrophoresis. *Cell*, **37**, 67–75

59. Weiss, L. M., Hu, E., Wood, G. S., Moulds, C., Cleary, M. L., Warnke, R. and Sklar, J. (1985). Clonal rearrangements of T-cell receptor genes in mycosis fungoides and dermatopathic lymphadenopathy. *N. Engl. J. Med.*, **313**, 539–44

60. Foon, K. A. and Todd, R. F. (1986). Immunologic classification of leukemia and lymphoma. *Blood*, **68**, 1–31

61. Kadin, M. E., Vonderheid, E. C., Sako, D., Clayton, L. K. and Olbricht, S. (1987). Clonal composition of T cells in lymphomatoid papulosis. *Am. J. Pathol.*, **126**, 13–17

62. Tawa, A., Hozumi, N., Minden, M., Mak, T. W. and Gelfand, E. W. (1985). Rearrangement of the T-cell receptor ß-chain in non-T-cell, non-B-cell acute lymphoblastic leukemia of childhood. *N. Engl. J. Med.*, **313**, 1033–7

63. Foa, R., Pelicci, P-G., Mignone, N., Lauria, F., Pizzolo, G., Flug, F., Knowles, D. M. II and Dalla-Favera, R. (1986). Analysis of T-cell receptor beta chain (Tß) gene rearrangement demonstrates the monoclonal nature of T-cell chronic lymphoproliferative disorders. *Blood*, **67**, 247–50

64. Bertness, V., Kirsch, I., Hollis, G., Johnson, B. and Bunn, P. A. (1985). T-cell receptor gene rearrangements as clinical markers of human T-cell lymphomas. *N. Engl. J. Med.*, **313**, 534–8

65. O'Connor, N. T. J., Feller, A. C., Wainscoat, J. S., Gatter, K. C., Pallesen, G., Stein, H., Lennert, K. and Mason, D. Y. (1986). T-cell origin of Lennert's lymphoma. *Br. J. Haematol.*, **64**, 521–8

66. Isaacson, P. G., O'Connor, N. T. J., Spencer, J., Bevan, D. H., Connolly, C. E., Kirkham, N., Pollock, D. J., Wainscoat, J. S., Stein, H. and Mason, D. Y. (1985). Malignant histiocytosis of the intestine: a T-cell lymphoma. *Lancet*, **2**, 688–91

67. Croce, C. M. (1987). Role of chromosome translocations in human neoplasia. *Cell*, **49**, 155–6

68. Baer, R., Chen, K., Smith, S. D. and Rabbitts, T. H. (1985). Fusion of an immunoglobulin variable gene and a T cell receptor constant gene in the chromosome 14 associated with T cell tumours. *Cell*, **43**, 705–13

11
Tumours of the Macrophage Series

SU-MING HSU

INTRODUCTION

The two major categories of true histiocytic malignancies, which are derived from the mononuclear phagocytic system (MPS) are true histiocytic lymphoma (THL) and malignant histiocytosis (MH). Although the clinicopathologic findings overlap, the two disorders can be distinguished by their unique expression of immunologic markers[1]. The term 'malignant histiocytosis' was first used by Rappaport to describe a systemic malignancy of histiocytes which affects the entire reticuloendothelial system from the beginning[2]. A similar disease entity called 'histiocytic medullary reticulosis' (HMR) was defined by Robb-Smith in 1939[3], but many investigators have regarded the terms MH and HMR as synonymous[4-6]. True histiocytic lymphoma, on the other hand, is a localized malignancy which may or may not progress to disseminated disease[7].

Until recently, true histiocytic malignancies were considered to be rare. Reports from Great Britain, the Netherlands and Taiwan, however, show a relatively high frequency of THL and MH in these countries, suggesting geographic differences in the incidence of this tumour[8-11]. With the aid of newly developed monoclonal antibodies (Mab), we have found that THL or MH may be more common than was previously believed. The diagnosis of THL is hampered by their resemblance to other large-cell lymphomas, i.e. T-and B-immunoblastic lymphomas and centroblastic lymphomas. Although numerous diagnostic criteria (Table 1) for THL and MH have been proposed in the past, none were sufficiently specific or sensitive.

Table 1 Diagnostic criteria for true histiocytic malignancies

1. Phagocytosis (red blood cells, latex particles, etc) by neoplastic histiocytes
2. Presence of lysosomal enzymes (i.e. acid phosphatase non-specific esterase, muramidase, etc)
3. Presence of Fc(r) and/or C3 receptors
4. Presence of lysosomes
5. Lack of surface or cytoplasmic immunoglobulin, and lack of sheep RBC receptors

In this chapter, we will summarize the use of Mabs for the diagnosis of THL and MH. We have established a criterion that is helpful for distinguishing between THL and MH. In addition, the phenotypes of the tumour cells will be described in relation to the clinical and pathologic characteristics of these lymphomas. Furthermore, since a histiocytic origin of Hodgkin's disease (HD) has been emphasized repeatedly, we will compare the immunophenotype of THL with that of HD, and we will propose a hypothetical histogenesis of THL, MH and HD. Before discussing THL and MH, we will briefly summarize the histologic and immunologic characteristics of the cells of the mononuclear phagocytic system.

MONONUCLEAR PHAGOCYTE SYSTEM

Many attempts have been made in the past to classify the phagocytic mononuclear cells and to define the cell system to which they are considered to belong. Among the systems proposed were the macrophage system of Metchnikoff, the reticuloendothelial system of Aschoff, and the reticulohistiocyte system of Volterra and Thomas[12]. In 1972, a new classification, called the mononuclear phagocytic system (MPS), was proposed at a conference in Leiden, Holland[12]. The inclusion of cells in the MPS is based on similarities in the origin, morphology, function and kinetics of phagocytes. The cells of the MPS, which are probably derived from monoblasts in the bone marrow, are monocytes, tissue macrophages (alveolar macrophages in the lung, Kupffer cells in the liver), as well as free and fixed histiocytes in lymphoid tissues.

Cells of the MPS participate in the immune response in different ways: (a) in host defense against microorganisms; (b) as scavengers to remove dying or damaged cells and to sequester inorganic materials that are not metabolized; (c) in bi-directional cellular interactions with lymphocytes; (d) as secretory cells involved in the production of bioactive materials (e.g. interleukin-1) that regulate other cellular functions; and (e) as cells that play an important cytocidal role in the control of neoplasia[13]. The neoplastic transformation of cells in MPS become THL or MH. The tumour cells may preserve some of the functions observed in normal histiocytes (e.g. phagocytosis and production of interleukin-1).

The histiocytes in lymphoid tissue sections can be detected by means of enzyme histochemical reactions (acid phosphatase, non-specific esterase, etc.) and immunofluorescence or peroxidase staining with specific antibodies[14].

MONOCLONAL ANTIBODIES AND OTHER MARKERS

Over the past 5 years, Mab have become available which aid in the identification of members of the MPS[15-18]. Such Mab have proved to be very useful in various ways, such as aiding in the diagnosis of MPS lymphomas. A number of Mab have been produced by immunization of mice with human monocytes or leukaemic cells. Some of these Mab react with the majority of freshly harvested peripheral blood monocytes, whereas others define functional antigens that are shared by monocytes and circulating blood elements such as granulocytes, T-lymphocytes, B-lymphocytes, natural killer cells and platelets[19].

Most of the Mab listed in Table 2 recognize cell membrane antigens associated with monocytes[15-18]. One Mab, anti-Leu M1, however, recognizes lacto-N-fucopentaose III-linked glycoprotein restricted to the Golgi apparatus in histiocytes[20,21]. Recently, we have also produced two Mab by immunizing mice with the histiocytic lymphoma cell line SU-DHL-1. Both of these Mab, 2H9 and 1E9, stain the nuclear membrane of histiocytes[1,22].

Tissue histiocytes (macrophages) may contain unique cytoplasmic proteins that are generally absent from B- and T-cells. These proteins are usually detected by means of heteroantisera, such as anti-lysozyme, anti-α-1-anti-trypsin, or anti-interleukin-1[23-28]. It should be emphasized that none of the markers in current use (Mab or antisera) produce 100% posivity. The marker expression of cells in the MPS may be related to the state of maturation, differentiation, or activation of these cells. It is also important to

Table 2 Summary of monoclonal antibodies used in phenotyping of true histiocytic malignancies

Antibody	Reactivity
OK M1	monocytes, granulocyte natural killer cells, some histiocytes, and some B-cell leukaemia/lymphomas
Mo2	monocytes and some histiocytes
Leu M1	surface – IR cells, Langerhans cells and monocytes Golgi – histiocytes
Leu M3	monocytes, some histiocytes
Leu M5	monocytes, histiocytes, some IR cells, hairy cell (B) leukaemia, some B-cell leukaemia/lymphomas
My 4	monocytes, granulocytes, some histiocytes, B-cells and some B-cell leukaemia/lymphomas
My 7	monocytes, granulocytes, some histiocytes
My 9	monocytes, some histiocytes
HeFi-1 (Ki-1)	rare large cells in normal lymphoid tissues. H-RS cells, true histiocytic lymphoma cells
2H9	nuclear membrane of histiocytes and IR cells. Cell membrane of H-RS cells and tumour cells in true histiocytic lymphoma
1E9	nuclear membrane of IR cells, histiocytes, and tumour cells in THL and MH
1A2	same as HeFi-1
Interleukin-1	histiocytes, some IR cells and Langerhans cells
S-100	neural cells, IR cells and Langerhans cells, and some histiocytes
Tac	interleukin-2 receptors associated with activated T-, B-cells, IR cells and histiocytes
OK T6	cortical thymic T-cells and Langerhans cells, some B-cells

elucidate the phenotype of normal histiocytes before one considers the application of these antibodies for the diagnosis of THL or MH.

PHENOTYPES OF HISTIOCYTES IN LYMPHOID TISSUES

Only the phenotypes of histiocytes in lymphoid tissues will be discussed in this chapter. Like the cells in the T- or B-lymphocyte system, cells in the MPS may be found preferentially in certain favorable locations in the lymph nodes and spleen. There are histiocytes in the germinal centres (tingible-body macrophages) and in the sinus, T-cell zone, or red pulp of the spleen.

Since histiocytes are thought to be derived from monocytes, we have examined the phenotypic expression of histiocytes in lymphoid tissues by using a large panel of Mab directed against monocytes. Details of the results are summarized in Table 3. Most histiocytes in normal lymphoid tissues have been found to be devoid of many of the known markers associated with monocytes, such as OK M1, Mo2, Leu M3, My4, My7 and My9. Monocyte marker-positive (MM+) histiocytes are rare in normal lymphoid tissues, but they may be increased in lymphoid tissues which are involved by tumour (i.e. lymphoma or carcinoma), or by inflammatory or granulomatous changes. These MM+ histiocytes can also be detected in connective tissue such as that of the tonsillar capsule (Figure 1A, B). It may be practical for diagnostic purposes to divide histiocytes into two major groups, MM+ and MM−, regardless of their location. The former group consists of so-called fixed

Table 3 Phenotypes of histiocytes, IR cells and Langerhans cells

	Histiocytes fixed	Histiocytes free	IR cells	Langerhans cells
Leu M1	g+	g+	s+	s+
2H9	nm+	nm+	nm+	−
1E9	nm+	nm+	nm+	−
Leu M5	s+	s+	s+ (some)	−
S-100	+/−	+/−	c+	c+
IL-1	c+ (some)	c+ (some)	c+ (some)	c+ (few)
OK T6	−	−	−	s+
OK M1	−	s+	−	−
anti-lysozyme	c+	c+	−	−

1. Other Mab, Mo2, Leu M3, My4, 7 and 9 show similar reactivities with OK M1
2. HeFi-1, Ki-1 and 1A2 are generally absent from the above cells
3. g, Golgi; nm, nuclear membrane; c, cytoplasmic; s, surface

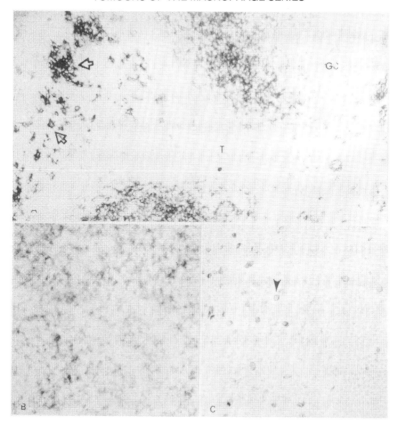

Figure 1 Frozen sections of normal tonsil stained with OK M1 (**A,B**) and 1E9 (**C**). OK M1 stains the histiocytes in the capsule and subcapsular area (arrows). The histiocytes in the germinal centres (GC) and in the T-cell zone (T) are OK M1-negative. The extracellular or dendritic staining in the GC, as illustrated in **B**, should not be mistaken as staining of histiocytes. The nuclear membrane of histiocytes in GC is positively stained by 1E9. **A**, × 70; **B,C**, × 110

histiocytes, and the latter of free histiocytes. The distinction between the two groups is important for an understanding of the nature of true histiocytic malignancies[1]. A hypothetical scheme of histogenesis of phagocytic mononuclear cells and non-phagocytic dendritic cells is summarized in Figure 2.

TRUE HISTIOCYTIC LYMPHOMA

True histiocytic lymphoma is derived from cells in the MPS. Since histiocytes can be identified in numerous locations other than sinuses, a sinusoidal growth pattern is not a necessary criterion for the diagnosis of THL. In lymph nodes, the tumour cells tend to involve the subcapsular region in the early phase of the disease. However, the tumour cells may rapidly invade the parenchyma, such as the T-cell zones, and finally replace the entire node.

169

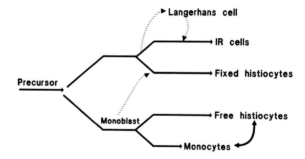

Figure 2 Hypothetical scheme of the histogenesis of mononuclear phagocytic cells and nonphago-cytic accessory cells

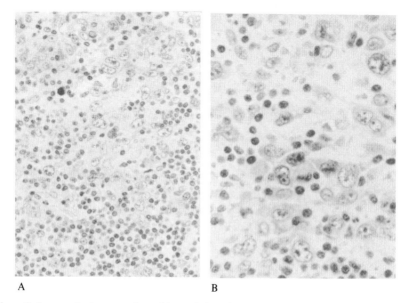

A   B

Figure 3 A non-cohesive type of true histocytic lymphoma. Lymphocytes are prominent in the background. The tumour cells are pleomorphic, and the nuclei are oval, irregular or folded. The chromatin pattern is granular and coarse. The tumour cells usually have 2–5 prominent nucleoli. **A** × 110; **B** × 170

Tumour cells can grow in either a cohesive or a non-cohesive pattern (Figure 3). In the latter, the tumour is characterized by the presence of numerous T-lymphocytes (? reactive) infiltration.

True histiocytic lymphoma may be present in the skin, subcutaneous tissue, gastrointestinal tract, breast, salivary glands or other extranodal sites. The degree of lymphocyte infiltration varies from case to case.

The tumour cells are 30–50 μm in diameter and have a basophilic cyto-plasm. In Giemsa-stained sections, the cytoplasm is greyish blue with a large, distinct paranuclear halo. In methyl pyronine-stained sections, the cytoplasm appears pinkish red. It is sometimes difficult to distinguish between THL cells

Table 4 Phenotypes of true histiocytic lymphomas and Hodgkin's disease

Markers	THL	HD	MH
HeFi-1 (Ki-1)	+	+	–
2H9	s+	s+	–
1E9	nm+	+/–	nm+
1A2	+	+	–
IL-1	+	+	+/–
Lysozyme	+/–	–	+/–
Mo2/OK M1	–	–	+
Leu M1	g+	s+	g+

1. Other Mab Leu M3, My4, My7 and My9 may show similar reactivities with OK M1 and Mo2
2. s, surface; nm, nuclear membrane; g, Golgi
3. +, usually positive; +/–, may be positive; –, usually negative

and immunoblasts of the B-cell type. The nuclei of THL cells are round or oval; they are frequently folded and indented, with a sharply defined nuclear membrane. The chromatin has a fine granular pattern or it may be coarse or slightly clumped. Usually there are 2–5 medium-sized nucleoli of irregular shape. Mitotic figures are frequent. It is often difficult to identify phagocytosis in tissue sections. Occasionally, small numbers of binucleated or multi-nucleated giant cells, resembling Reed–Sternberg (H-RS) cells, are present.

PHENOTYPES OF THL

In the diagnosis of THL, previous diagnostic criteria (Table 1) for THL should be used. In general, THL cells are negative for both B- and T-cell markers. A phorbol ester induction test[29] should be performed, if possible, for examination of the phenotypic expression of TPA-induced THL cells; these tumour cells generally remain negative for T- or B-cell markers.

The cells of THL are generally negative for most monocyte markers even after TPA induction[1] (Table 4). In a series of patients whom we studied, these cells expressed markers similar to those of H-RS cells (Ki-1, HeFi-1, 2H9, 1A2)[30-32] (Figure 4). In H-RS cells, the Leu M1 antigen is localized mainly on the cell membrane and Golgi apparatus, in THL cells, however, it is located only in the Golgi apparatus (Figure 4D)[1,21]. Very few THL cells, especially those containing large nucleoli (Hodgkin's-like cells) may express Leu M1 on their membrane. In addition, THL cells may also express Tac (interleukin-2 receptor), OK T9 (transferrin receptor), Ia, interleukin-1, and 1E9 (Figure 5).

171

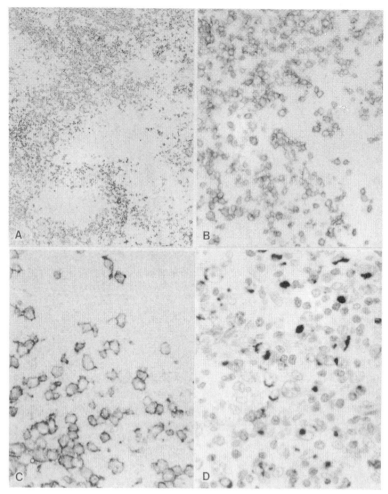

Figure 4 True histiocytic lymphoma cells were stained with HeFi-1 (**A,B**), 2H9 (**C**), and anti-Leu M1 (**D**). Note the Golgi staining pattern in **D**. **A** × 70; **B** × 110, **C,D** × 170

Based on the expression of Leu M1 and 1E9 as well as the lack of other monocyte markers, the neoplastic cells in THL are likely derived from fixed histiocytes, although normal fixed histiocytes do not express Ki-1, HeFi-1 or 1A2[22,30,31]. The marker Leu M5 is normally expressed by fixed histiocytes, but is usually absent from THL cells. However, we have seen few cases of THL in which the tumour cells did not express HeFi-1 or cell membrane 2H9, but expressed Leu M5 and 2H9 on their nuclear membrane. It is likely that some THL are derived from the mature form of fixed histiocytes.

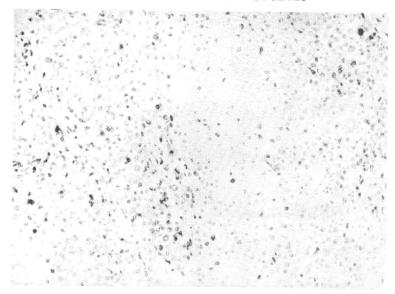

Figure 5 Characteristic nuclear membrane staining of true histiocytic lymphoma cells with Mab 1E9. The small lymphocytes, mostly T-cells, in the background are 1E9 negative. × 110

MALIGNANT HISTIOCYTOSIS

The characteristic feature of MH is a diffuse proliferation of histiocytes and their precursors throughout the reticuloendothelial system[5,6]. Sometimes, the tumour histiocytes may not be distinguishable from normal or reactive histiocytes. In the early stage of the disease, the tumour cells tend to involve the sinuses, and it may be difficult to make the diagnostic distinction from reactive sinus histiocytosis. The tumour cells may rapidly replace the entire lymphoid tissues. The cells are loosely packed (Figure 6).

Malignant histiocytosis may involve almost all visceral organs, including the spleen, liver, lung, kidney, gastrointestinal tract and skin. In the majority of patients, bone marrow and peripheral blood involvement occur during the course of the disease.

The MH cells are frequently indistinguishable from THL cells, however, erythrophagocytosis may be more common in MH (Figure 7). The tumour cells may contain abundant eosinophilic cytoplasm. The nuclei are round, oval or irregular, and are frequently folded or kidney bean-shaped. The chromatin pattern is granular, and the nucleoli are not as prominent as those in THL. Many cells with large, bizzare, multinucleated nuclei may be seen.

PHENOTYPES OF MH

We have studied the phenotypes of eight cases of MH. Most tumour cells are positively stained by Mo2 and 1E9 (Figure 8). Other Mab, such as OK M1,

173

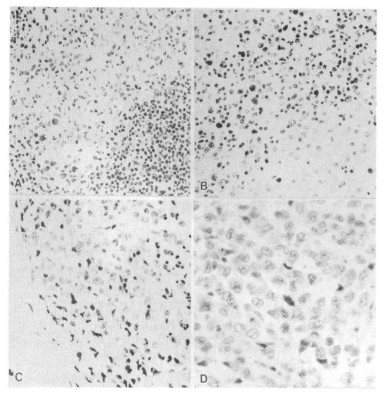

Figure 6 Histopathologic features of malignant histiocytosis in lymph node (**A**), liver (**B**) and skin (**C,D**). Note the high pleomorphism of tumour cells. × 110

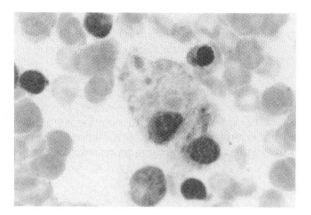

Figure 7 Bone marrow aspirate smear from a patient with malignant histiocytosis shows erythro-phagocytosis by a tumour cell. × 400

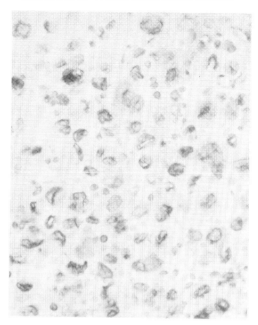

Figure 8 Characteristic nuclear membrane staining with Mab 1E9 in malignant histiocytosis. ×
220

Leu M5, My4, My7, My9 and Leu M1, reacted with varying percentages of
the tumour cells (5-70%). The expression of these markers cannot be pre-
dicted based on the clinical or histopathologic features of the tumour. Among
these markers, 1E9 and 2H9 are located on the nuclear membrane, whereas
Leu M1 is located at the Golgi apparatus (Table 4).

Upon induction with TPA, the tumour cells of MH may show an increase
in the expression of monocyte markers (especially OK M1 and Leu M5). The
MH cells are consistently negative for Tac, HeFi-1, Ki-1, and 1A2; the latter
three markers are known to be associated with H-RS cells[1,32]. The marker of
MH cells is distinctly different from that of THL cells.

Lysozyme is absent from MH cells or present in minimal amounts[25].
Although the use of anti-lysozyme heteroantiserum has been proposed for the
diagnosis of MH[24], we find that this test is of limited use. Unlike THL cells,
MH cells usually contain no interleukin-1 or only very small amounts[33]. The
MH cells usually react positively with acid phosphatase and non-specific
esterase. They tend to show a diffuse reactivity; however, the reaction can also
be punctate or focal.

The marker expression in MH is indistinguishable from that in monocytic
(i.e. acute monoblastic) leukaemia, although there may be heterogeneity in
the phenotypic expression from case to case. As we have stated before, one
cannot expect to find a marker that gives 100% reactivity. Since MH cells are
characterized by the expression of numerous known markers associated with
monocytes and free histiocytes, it is our opinion that MH is derived from free
histiocytes.

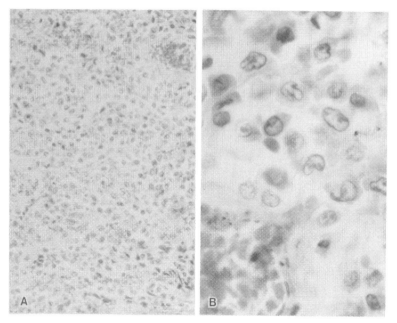

Figure 9 A tissue section of the lung from the U-937 patient. The tumour cells are highly pleomorphic with folded or indented nucleus. **A** × 88; **B** × 280

CELL LINES OF TRUE HISTIOCYTIC MALIGNANCIES

There are certain advantages to the use of cell lines for the study of the biologic behaviour of lymphomas. Numerous B- or T-cell lines are currently available for such studies, however, cell lines of histiocytic origin are rare. The cell lines THP-1 and CTV-2 are derived from patients with acute monoblastic leukaemia (AMoL); these cells may also be used, but they are not exactly like the cells from true histiocytic lymphomas[34,35].

Only two cell lines, U-937 and SU-DHL-1, are probably related to THL or MH[36,37]. U-937 is derived from a 37-year-old patient with a generalized lymphoma. The bone marrow and blood were not involved. The tumour was fast-growing; widespread lymph node enlargement and hepatomegaly were present within 2 months of the initial biopsy. The patient died 3 months after the diagnosis. Autopsy revealed a lymphoma engaging the supraclavicular, axillary, mediastinal and inguinal lymph nodes. Tumour infiltration was also seen in the spleen, liver, pleura, lungs and pericardium (Figure 9). Although erythrophagocytosis was seen, generally this is not a prominent feature. The diagnosis was diffuse histiocytic lymphoma (DHL).

U-937 cells were subsequently found to express features of monoblasts or histiocytes. The cells produce lysozyme and have a strong esterase activity. Marker study of U-937 cells revealed that the cells expressed numerous monocyte markers, especially after induction with TPA[39–40]. The cells are also known to produce IL-1. The phenotypic expression of U-937 indicates that

Figure 10 The lung section from U-937 patient was stained with anti-Leu M1. Note characteristic Golgi staining pattern. × 220

the original tumour was MH rather than DHL[32]. Immunoperoxidase staining with anti-Leu M1 in the original specimen from this patient showed a characteristic Golgi reaction pattern (Figure 10).

The SU-DHL-1 cell line was isolated from the pleural fluid of a 10-year-old caucasian boy with a generalized diffuse histiocytic lymphoma. A lymph node biopsy was previously interpreted as Hodgkin's disease. The spleen, liver and bone marrow showed no evidence of lymphoma. The patient did not respond to treatment and died 6 months after the initial diagnosis.

The nature of SU-DHL-1 cells has only recently become clear. These cells contain non-specific esterase, acid phosphatase and IL-1, but no lysozyme. They are consistently negative for OK T3, Leu 4, OK T4, OK T8, 3A1, Lyt 3 (T-cell markers), and Leu 14, B1, Leu 12, s-Ig and c-Ig (B-cell markers)[32]. SU-DHL-1 cells, however, can be stained by anti-Leu 1 (a T-cell Mab). These cells retain germline Ig heavy and light chain loci, without evidence of gene rearrangement[41]. They are positive for HeFi-1, Ki-1, 2H9 (surface), 1A2, and Tac[32]. The phenotype of SU-DHL-1 cells is very similar to that of H-RS cells. These cells fail to express monocyte markers, such as OK M1, Mo 2, My 4,

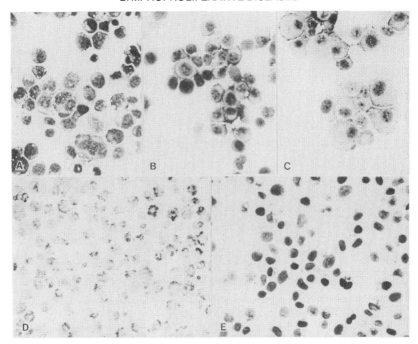

Figure 11 Cytospin smears prepared from SU-DHL-1 (**A**) and SU-DHL-101 cells (**B**). SU-DHL-101 cells were induced to differentiate with phorbol ester, and the cells showed a round, regular nucleus with abundant cytoplasm (**C**). Cells with multiple nuclei were frequently observed. A cytoplasmic granular 1E9 staining pattern is seen in SU-DHL-1 cells (**D**). However, in TPA-induced SU-DHL-101 cells, the staining is restricted to the nuclear membrane (**E**). × 150

My 7, My 9, Leu M1 or Leu M3. SU-DHL-1 cells are only weakly positive for Leu M5, which is known to be associated with monocytes and histiocytes[32]. However, SU-DHL-1 cells contain antigen 1E9 in their cytoplasm. This antigen is normally expressed on the nuclear membrane of histiocytes[22,23].

The study of SU-DHL-1 cells is hampered by their inability to respond to TPA. Recently, we have established a subline from SU-DHL-1 which we termed SU-DHL-101 (Figure 11). The cells express Fc (r) receptors on the cell membrane and contain large amounts of interleukin-1, lysozyme, α-1-chymotrypsin, esterase and acid phosphatase in the cytoplasm. The new cell line responds to TPA quickly, and it is suitable for studies on the nature of THL. SU-DHL-101 cells undergo change into HeFi-1, 2H9 and Ki-1 negative after TPA induction. TPA-induced cells revealed a characteristic 1E9 and Leu M1 antigen distribution on the nuclear membrane and at the Golgi apparatus, respectively. (Table 5). The TPA-induced cells remained negative for all T- (including Leu 1) and B-cell markers. Apparently, the SU-DHL-1 lymphoma is a THL, and these cells are probably derived from fixed histiocytes because they lack expression of monocyte markers.

The expression of Leu 1 in SU-DHL-1, but not in SU-DHL-101, is of interest. It is unlikely that SU-DHL-1 lymphoma is a T-cell lymphoma. The

Table 5 Phenotypes of SU-DHL-1 and SU-DHL-101 cells

	SU-DHL-1	*SU-DHL-101*	*SU-DHL-101 (TPA-induced)*
HeFi-1	+	+	−
Ki-1	+	+	−
2H9	s+	s+	nm+
1E9	c+	c+/nm+	nm+
Tac	+	+/−	−
Lysozyme	−	+/−	++
Chymotrypsin	−	+++	+++
IL-1	+	+	+
Acid phosphatase	+	++	+++
Esterase	+	++	+++
Leu-1	+	−	−
Leu-M1	−	g+/−	g+/−

1. s, surface; c, cytoplasmic; nm, nuclear membrane, g, Golgi
2. +/−, weak positive; +, positive; ++, moderate positive; +++, strong positive

presence of one or few T-cell markers in a lymphoma should not be used as sole evidence for the diagnosis of T-cell lymphoma. An aberrant marker expression in lymphomas and leukaemias is frequently observed. Two monoblastic leukaemic cell lines (CTV-2 and THP-1) were also found to express T-cell markers (i.e. 3A1, or Leu 4).

The similar marker expression between SU-DHL-1 (other THL cells as well) and H-RS cells may suggest a possible histiocytic nature of HD, as previously proposed. However, recent studies favour an interdigitating reticulum (IR) cell origin of H-RS cell[19,42,43].

RELATIONSHIP BETWEEN FIXED HISTIOCYTES AND INTERDIGITATING RETICULUM CELLS

Although interdigitating reticulum cells are called T-zone histiocytes in Japan, these cells are not true phagocytic histiocytes. However, the two-cell types have numerous similarities in their immunologic markers. One could expect that the lymphomas derived from IR cells may possess a diagnostic problem to distinguish them from THL. In this chapter, we will briefly address the immunologic characteristics of IR cells which is important for a precise diagnosis of histiocyte- and IR cell-related lymphomas.

Interdigitating reticulum cells are localized in the T-cell zone, and they function as antigen-presenting cells[44,45]. Like histiocytes, IR cells express markers such as Ki-M1 and interleukin 1[33,46] (Figure 12). It has been

179

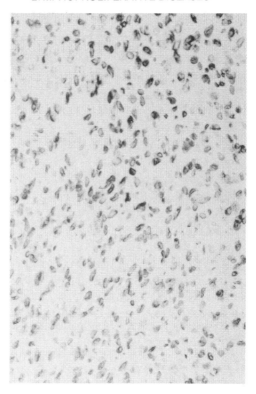

Figure 12 Mab 1E9 staining in interdigitating reticulum cells in a dermatopathic node. The staining reaction is restricted to the nuclear membrane. × 140

suggested that IR cells and fixed histiocytes have the same origin or a similar pathway of differentiation[42,46]. IR cells may be related to the epidermal dendritic cells (Langerhans cells) in the skin because both express markers such as Leu M1 and S-100. However, they differ in other markers, such as 2H9, 1E9, and OK T6 (Table 3). Both IR cells and Langerhans cells are included in the group of non-phagocytic, dendritic accessory cells. A hypothetical scheme of the histogenesis of histiocytes, IR cells and Langerhans cells is summarized in Figure 2.

Like B- and T-cells, IR cells or their related cells in normal or reactive lymphoid tissues may have various morphologic features and markers. Markers such as S-100, Leu M1, and IL-1 are helpful in the identification of these cells (Table 5). We have observed IR cells in three major cytologic categories. All three are characterized by the expression of a surface Leu M1 antigen and various degrees of staining with anti-IL-1. The first type has elongated and twisted nuclei, and these cells are strong S-100 positive. The second type of IR cells are commonly observed in lymph nodes with dermatopathic lymphadenitis. These cells have indented or slightly folded nuclei, and they are also S-100 positive. The third type resembles Hodgkin's mononuclear cells, with a prominent nucleolus, and these cells are usually S-100 negative.

HODGKIN'S DISEASE

The nature of HD has been controversial for decades, but an origin from B-or T-lymphocytes or from histiocytes has been proposed (see Chapter 7). However, the tumour cells, the so called Reed–Sternberg (H-RS) cells, in HD are generally negative for T- and B-cell markers even after TPA induction[32]. These cells are also negative for monocyte markers and have minimal esterase and acid phosphatase activity[47,48]. Although an immunoglobulin gene rearrangement has been discovered in H-RS cells, the rearrangement is not a property specific for B-lymphocytes; it has also been detected in myelomonocytic leukaemias and THL[49].

H-RS cells are characterized by the presence of a surface Leu M1 antigen. This antigen, with a molecular weight of 150 000 Kd, is a lacto-N-fucopentaose III-linked glycoprotein[20]. This antigen is not sialylated, or only minimally, in H-RS cells, whereas it is sialylated in IR cells[43]. The surface Leu M1 antigen is readily detected in IR cells, but not in histiocytes or in other lymphoid cells in normal lymphoid tissues[42]. This suggests that H-RS cells and IR cells are related. In addition, H-RS cells are consistently positive for IL-1 which is a known marker for IR cells[33]. Perhaps, H-RS cells are derived from the Leu M1+, IL-1+, and S-100– subset of IR cells.

H-RS cells express markers such as HeFi-1, Ki-1, s-2H9, and 1A2[1,22,32], all of which can also be detected in THL cells, but are absent from most normal histiocytes and from IR cells (Table 4). This raises the possibility that H-RS cells and THL cells are derived from related cells. We have noted that, in normal lymphoid tissues, IR cells and fixed histiocytes have numerous similarities. It is not surprising that tumours derived from similar types of cells express similar tumour markers.

All of the markers expressed by H-RS cells disappear from the surface of these cells, and of SU-DHL-101 cells, following TPA induction. Antibodies HeFi-1 and Ki-1 stain rare large cells in the T-cell zone of normal lymphoid tissues. There is no evidence indicating that these markers are oncogenic or viral products. Perhaps they are normally associated with an immature or activated form of IR cells or histiocytes.

INTERLEUKIN-1 IN THL, MH AND HD

Interleukin-1 (IL 1) is a low molecular weight peptide produced by monocytes/histiocytes and IR cells. It is not surprising that cytoplasmic IL-1 is detected in tumour cells from THL, MH and HD. (Table 4).

Interleukin-1 has an important role in the initiation and amplification of T-and B-lymphocyte activation[26-28]. In addition, IL-1 may be important in the regulation of body temperature, in fibroblast proliferation and in synovial cell activation[28,50]. IL-1 from various sources has recently been purified to homogeneity, and the gene encoding this protein has been cloned. The human recombinant IL-1 prepared from *Escherichia coli* occurs as two molecular species, termed α and β, with isoelectric points of 5.0 and 7.0, respectively. The α and β forms of IL-1 have approximately the same molecular weight,

17 500, and both are biologically active, proteolytic C-terminal fragments derived from parent molecules of molecular weight 31 000. Rabbit hetero-antiserum against IL-1 also recently have become available. The antibody can be used in B-5 fixed, paraffin embedded tissue sections.

IL-1 is strongly expressed in the non-cohesive type of THL, in which the tumour is characterized by abundant lymphocyte infiltration. It is not known whether these lymphocytes are residual lymphocytes in tissues, or whether they are reactive to the tumour. Interestingly, the non-cohesive type of THL usually has a relatively non-aggressive clinical course as compared to that of cohesive THL. The low expression of IL-1 in cohesive type of THL (MH as well) may attribute, in part, to the poor prognosis of these lymphomas.

Hodgkin's disease is another type of lymphoma with strong expression of IL-1 in the tumour cells. The expression of IL-1 in H-RS cells indicates a possible origin of these cells from IR cells. Several histologic characteristics of HD such as an abundant T-lymphocyte reaction and the presence of fibrosis may partly be explained as being due to the production of IL-1 by H-RS cells.

DIFFERENTIAL DIAGNOSIS

The diagnosis of histiocytic malignancy is probably one of the most difficult tasks even for expert haematopathologists. This can be illustrated by the two cases, U-937 and SU-DHL-1 discussed above. With the aid of immunologic markers, the differential diagnosis of THL and MH from other DHL should become less complicated. It is also important to use multiple Mab for a precise diagnosis because an aberrant marker expression by lymphoma cells may cause a little bit of confusion.

It should be noted that phagocytosis is not absolutely specific for cells in the MPS. Lymphoma or leukaemia cells derived from T- or B-cells infrequently show phagocytosis when growing in culture. In addition, phagocytosis by benign, reactive histiocytes has been reported in malignant lymphomas, especially those of the T-cell type[51,52]. It was postulated that the neoplastic T-cells elaborate a lymphokine that could stimulate the cells of the MPS. This so-called haemophagocytic syndrome (HPS) can also be seen in immunodeficient patients with or without secondary infection. Marker studies may be needed for the differential diagnosis. The histiocytes in HPS should have a phenotype similar or identical to that of normal histiocytes, and the cells are HeFi-1/s-2H9/Ki-1-negative.

Acute monocytic leukaemia (AMoL) is often difficult to distinguish from MH. The differing clinical and pathologic manifestations of these two malignant disorders correlate with the properties of their cell of origins. The malignant cells in AMoL represent the neoplastic equivalent of monocytes/monoblasts, whereas the cells of MH are probably related to free histiocytes. Free (monocyte- marker-positive) histiocytes are closely related to monocytes. It is not surprising, therefore, that AMoL and MH present similar immunologic markers. The differential diagnosis of these two disorders is based on the clinical manifestation of the disease (e.g. bone marrow and peripheral blood involvement in AMoL and visceral organ involvement in MH).

Histiocytosis X (HX) is a proliferative disorder of Langerhans cells. The lesion may involve skin, bone, lung, liver and other reticuloendothelial cell systems. The HX cells have features of differentiated histiocytes[53]. These cells express markers such as OK T6 and S-100, whereas the tumour cells of THL and MH are OK T6 and S-100 negative. In addition, a sialylated Leu M1 antigen is often present on the surface of HX cells. Thus, the demonstration of anti-Leu M1 staining on these cells requires prior digestion of tissue sections with neuraminidase.

CONCLUSIONS

It has become clear that there are two types of histiocytes; one type is monocyte marker-positive, and the other negative, in lymphoid tissues. The monocyte marker-negative histiocytes express no OK M1, Mo2, Leu M3, My 4, My 7, or My 9, but have antigens such as Leu M5 in common with monocytes. The monocyte marker-negative histiocytes are fixed histiocytes in lymphoid tissues. Monocytes and fixed histiocytes share some other markers, such as 2H9 1E9, and Leu M1, however, the subcellular distribution of these antigens may be different. For example, Leu M1 is expressed on the cell surface of monocytes but at the Golgi apparatus in histiocytes. Monocyte marker-positive histiocytes are likely to be free histiocytes. It seems that free histiocytes evolve directly from monocytes.

There are two major types of true histiocytic malignancies. True histiocytic lymphoma is characterized by the absence of monocyte markers, but they express markers such as Ki-1, HeFi-1, 1A2, and s-2H9 which are known to be associated with H-RS cells. Malignant histiocytosis is characterized by the expression of monocyte markers, especially Mo2, OK M1, and Leu M5. It is likely that THL and MH are related to fixed and free histiocytes, respectively.

Hodgkin's disease is likely to be derived from interdigitating reticulum cells (Figure 13). Fixed histiocytes and IR cells have numerous similarities and are

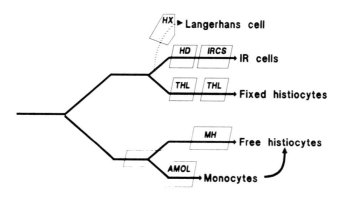

Figure 13 Hypothetical scheme of the histogenesis of lymphomas related to mononuclear phagocytic cells and non-phagocytic accessory dendritic cells. IRCS; interdigitating reticulum cell sarcoma

related. Indeed, lymphomas derived from fixed histiocytes and from IR cells may express similar markers.

ACKNOWLEDGEMENTS

The author wishes to thank Dr Sunström, Department of Pathology, University of Uppsala, Sweden, for providing clinicopathologic information of the U-937 patient, and for providing paraffin slides for study of the Leu M1 distribution in tumour cells. The author also thanks Dr Epstein, University of Southern California, for providing SU-DHL-1 cells.

References

1. Hsu, S.-M., Pescovitz, M. and Hsu, P.-L. (1985). Monoclonal antibodies for histiocyte/inter-digitating reticulum cell-related lymphomas. In Reisfeld, R. A. and Sell, S. (eds) *Monoclonal Antibodies and Cancer Therapy*. ULCA Symposium on Molecular and Cellular Biology, Vol. 27, pp. 53–62. (New York: Alan R. Liss)
2. Rappaport, H. (1966). Tumors of the hematopoietic system. In *Atlas of Tumor Pathology*, pp. 49–63. (Washington, DC; Armed Forces Institute of Pathology)
3. Scott, R. B. and Robb-Smith, A. H. T. (1939). Histiocytic medullary reticulosis. *Lancet*, **2**, 194–8
4. Mann, R. B., Jaffe, E. S. and Berard, C. W. (1979). Malignant lymphomas. A conceptual understanding of morphologic diversity. *Am. J. Pathol.*, **94**, 105–75
5. Warnke, R. A., Kim, H. and Dorfman, R. F. (1975). Malignant histiocytosis (histiocytic medullary reticulosis). 1. Clinicopathologic study of 29 cases. *Cancer*, **35**, 215–30
6. Ho, F. C. S. and Todd, D. (1978). Malignant histiocytosis. Report of five Chinese patients. *Cancer*, **42**, 2450–60
7. Jaffe, E. S. (1985). Malignant histiocytosis and true histiocytic lymphomas. In Jaffe, E. S. (ed.) *Surgical Pathology of the Lymph Nodes and Related Organs*, pp. 381–411. (Philadelphia: Saunders)
8. Isaacson, P., Wright, D. H., Judd, M. A. and Mephan, B. L. (1979). Primary gastrointestinal lymphoma: A classification of 66 cases. *Cancer*, **43**, 1805–19
9. Isaacson, P., Wright, D. H. and Jones, D. B. (1983). Malignant lymphoma of true histiocytic (monocyte/macrophage) origin. *Cancer*, **51**, 80–91
10. Valk, P. van der., Te Velde, J., Jansen, J., Ruiter, D. J., Spaander, P. J., Cornelisse, C. J. and Meijer, C. J. L. M. (1981). Malignant histiocytic lymphoma of true histiocytic origin: histiocytic sarcoma. A morphological, ultrastructural, immunological, cytochemical and clinical study of 10 cases. *Virch. Arch. A. Pathol.*, **391**, 249–65
11. Su, I.-J., Shih, L.-Y., Dunn, P., Kadin, M. E. and Hsu, S.-M. (1985). Pathological and immunological observations of malignant lymphomas in Taiwan: with special reference to the retrovirus-associated adult T cell lymphoma/leukemia. *Am. J. Clin. Pathol.*, **84**, 715–23
12. Van Furth, R., Cohn, Z. A., Hinsch, J. G., Humphrey, J. H., Spector, W. G. and Langevoort, H. L. (1972). The mononuclear phagocyte system: a new classification of macrophages, monocytes, and their precursor cells. *Bull. WHO*, **46**, 845–52
13. Shevach, E. M. (1984). Macrophages and other accessory cells. In Paul, W. E. (ed.) *Fundamental Immunology*, pp. 71–127. (New York: Raven Press)
14. Hsu, S.-M., Raine, L. and Fanger, H. (1981). Use of avidin–biotin–peroxidase complex (ABC) in immunoperoxidase techniques: A comparison between ABC and unlabeled antibody (PAP) procedures. *J. Histochem. Cytochem.*, **29**, 577–80
15. Breard, J., Reinherz, E. L., Kung, P. C., Goldstein, G. and Schlossman, S. F. (1980). A monoclonal antibody reactive with human peripheral blood monocytes. *J. Immunol.*, **124**, 1943–8
16. Todd, R. F., van Agthoven, A., Schlossman, S. F. and Terhurst, C. (1982). Structural analysis of differentiation antigens Mo1 and Mo2 in human monocytes. *Hybridoma*, **1**, 329–35

17. Dimitrium-Bona, A., Burmester, G. R., Waters, S. J. and Winchester, R. J. (1983). Human mononuclear phagocyte differentiation antigens. I. Patterns of antigenic expression on the surface of human monocytes and macrophages defined by monoclonal antibodies. *J. Immunol.*, **130**, 145–52

18. Hanjan, S. N. S., Kearney, J. F. and Cooper, M. D. (1982). A monoclonal antibody (MMA) that identified a differentiation antigen on human myelomonocytic cells. *Clin. Immunol. Immunopathol.*, **23**, 172–9

19. Hsu, S.-M., Zhang, H.-Z. and Jaffe, E. S. (1983). Monoclonal antibodies directed against human lymphoid, monocytic, and granulocytic cells: Reactivities with other tissues. *Hybridoma*, **2**, 403–12

20. Hsu, S.-M., Huang, L. C., Hsu, P.-L., Ge, Z.-H., Ho, Y.-S. and Mulshine, J. (1986). Ultrastructural and biochemical studies on Leu M1 antigens in granulocytes and H-RS cells in Hodgkin's disease. *J. Natl. Cancer Inst.*, **77**, 363–70

21. Hsu, S.-M. and Jaffe, E. S. (1984). Leu M1 and peanut agglutinin stain the neoplastic cells of Hodgkin's disease. *Am. J. Clin. Pathol.*, **82**, 29–32

22. Hsu, S.-M., Pescovitz, M. D. and Hsu, P.-L. (1986). Monoclonal antibodies against SU-DHL-1 cells stain the neoplastic cells of true histocytic lymphoma, malignant histiocytosis and Hodgkin's disease. *Blood*, **68**, 213–19

23. Mendelsohn, G., Eggleston, J. C. and Mann, R. B. (1980). Relationship of lysozyme (muramidase) to histocytic differentiation in malignant histiocytosis. An immunohistochemical study. *Cancer*, **45**, 273–9

24. Tubbs, R. R., Sheibani, K., Sebek, B. A. and Savage, R. A. (1980). Malignant histiocytosis. Ultrastructural and immunocytochemical characterization. *Arch. Pathol. Lab. Med.*, **104**, 26–9

25. Carbone, A., Micheau, C., Caillaud, J.-M. and Carlu, C. (1981). A cytochemical and immunohistochemical approach to malignant histiocytosis. *Cancer*, **47**, 2862–71

26. Mizel, S. B. (1982). Interleukin 1 and T cell activation. *Immunol. Rev.*, **63**, 51–72

27. Howard, M., Mizel, S. B., Lachman, L., Ansel, J., Jonson, B. and Paul, W. E. (1983). Role of interleukin 1 in anti-immunoglobulin-induced B cell proliferation. *J. Exp. Med.*, **157**, 1529–43

28. Murphy, P. A., Simon, P. L. and Willoughby, W. F. (1980). Endogenous pyrogens made by rabbit peritoneal exudate cells are identical with lymphocyte activation factors made by rabbit alveolar macrophages. *J. Immunol.*, **124**, 2498–2501

29. Ho, Y.-S., Chakrabarty, S. and Hsu, S.-M. (1986). Induction of differentiation of Burkitt's lymphoma cell lines by phorbol ester: possible relationship with pre-B cells or immature B cells. *Cancer Invest.*, **5**, 101–7

30. Hecht, T. T., Longo, D. L., Cossman, J., Bolen, J. B., Hsu, S.-M., Israel, M. and Fisher, R. I. (1985). Production and characterization of a monoclonal antibody that binds Reed–Sternberg cells. *J. Immunol.*, **134**, 4231–6

31. Schwab, U., Stein, H., Gerdes, J., Lemke, H., Kirchner, H., Schaadt, M. and Diehl, V. (1982). Production of a monoclonal antibody specific for Hodgkin's and Sternberg–Reed cells of Hodgkin's disease and a subset of normal lymphoid cells. *Nature*, **299**, 65–7

32. Hsu, S.-M. and Hsu, P.-L. (1986). Phenotypes and phorbol ester-induced differentiation of human histocytic lymphoma cell lines (U-937 and SU-DHL-1) and Reed–Sternberg cells. *Am. J. Pathol.*, **122**, 223–30

33. Hsu, S.-M. and Zhao, X. (1986). Expression of interleukin 1 in H-RS cells and neoplastic cells from true histocytic lymphomas. *Am. J. Pathol.*, **125**, 221–6

34. Chen, P.-M., Chiu, C.-F., Chiou, T.-J., Maeda, S., Chiang, H., Tzeng, C.-H., Sugiyama, T. and Chiang, B. N. (1984). Establishment and characterization of a human monocytoid cell line CTV-1. *Jpn. J. Cancer Res. (Gann)*, **75**, 660–4

35. Tsuchiya, S., Yamabe, M., Yamaguchi, Y., Kobayashi, Y., Konno, T. and Tada, K. (1980). Establishment and characterization of a human acute monocytic leukemia cell line (THP-1). *Int. J. Cancer*, **26**, 171–6

36. Epstein, A. L., Levy, R., Kim, H., Henle, W., Henle, G. and Kaplan, H. S. (1978). Biology of human malignant lymphomas: IV. Functional characterization of ten diffuse histocytic lymphoma cell lines. *Cancer*, **42**, 2379–85

37. Sundstrom, C. and Nilsson, J. (1976). Establishment and characterization of a human histocytic lymphoma cell line (U-937). *Int. J. Cancer*, **17**, 565–7

38. Rigby, W. F. C., Shen, L., Ball, E. D., Guyre, P. M. and Fayer, M. W. (1984).

Differentiation of a human monocytic cell line by 1,25-Dihydroxyvitamin D3 (calcitriol): A morphologic, phenotypic, and functional analysis. *Blood,* **64**, 1110–15

39. Hatrari, T., Pack, M., Bougnoux, P., Chang, Z.-L. and Hoffman, T. (1983). Interferon-induced differentiation of U937 cells: comparison with other reagents that promote differentiation of human myeloid or monocytic cell lines. *J. Clin. Invest.,* **72**, 237–44

40. Schmid, A., Hatrari, T. and Hoffman, T. (1984). Differentiation of a human monocyte-like cell line by (2′–5′) oligoisoadenylate. *Exp. Cell Res.,* **150**, 292–7

41. Siminovitch, K. A., Jensen, J. P., Epstein, A. L. and Korsmeyer, S. J. (1986). Immunoglobulin gene rearrangements and expression in diffuse histiocytic lymphomas reveal cellular lineage, molecular defects, and potential sites of chromosomal translocation. *Blood,* **67**, 391–7

42. Hsu, S.-M., Yang, K. and Jaffe, E. S. (1985). Phenotypic expression of Hodgkin's and Reed–Sternberg cells in Hodgkin's disease. *Am. J. Pathol.,* **118**, 209–17

43. Hsu, S.-M., Ho, Y.-S., Li, P.-J., Monheit, J., Ree, H. J., Sheibani, K. and Winberg, C. D. (1986). L & H variants of Reed–Sternberg cells express sialylated Leu M1 antigen. *Am. J. Pathol.,* **122**, 199–204

44. Muller-Hermelink, H. K. and Lennert, K. (1978). The cytologic, histologic and functional bases for a modern classification of lymphomas. In Lennert, K. (ed.) *Malignant Lymphomas* pp. 1–82. (New York: Springer-Verlag)

45. Veerman, A. J. P. (1974). On the interdigitating cells in the thymus-dependent area of the rat spleen: A relation between the mononuclear phagocyte system and T-lymphocytes. *Cell Tissue Res.,* **148**, 247–57

46. Radzun, H. J., Parwaresch, M. R., Feller, A. C. and Hansmann, M. L. (1984). Monocyte/macrophage-specific monoclonal antibody Ki-M1 recognizes interdigitating reticulum cells. *Am. J. Pathol.,* **117**, 441–50

47. Beckstead, J. H., Warnke, R. A. and Bainton, D. F. (1982). Histochemistry of Hodgkin's disease. *Cancer Treat. Rep.,* **66**, 609–13

48. Kadin, M. E. (1982). Possible origin of Reed–Sternberg cells from interdigitating reticulum cells. *Cancer Treat. Rep.,* **66**, 601–8

49. Mirro, J., Zipf, T. F., Pui, C.-H., Kitchingman, G., Williams, D., Melvin, S., Murphy, S. B. and Stass, S. (1985). Acute mixed lineage leukemia: Clinicopathologic correlations and prognostic significance. *Blood,* **66**, 1115–23

50. Schmidt, J. A., Mizel, S. B., Cohen, D. and Green, I. (1982). Interleukin 1, a potential regulator of fibroblast proliferation. *J. Immunol.,* **128**, 2177–82

51. Jaffe, E. S., Costa, J., Fauci, A. S., Cossman, J. and Tsokos, M. (1983). Malignant lymphoma and erythrophagocytosis: Simulating malignant histiocytosis. *Am. J. Med.,* **75**, 741–9

52. Kadin, M. E., Kamoun, M. and Lamberg, J. (1981). Erythrophagocytic Ty lymphoma – A clinicopathologic entity resembling malignant histiocytosis. *N. Engl. J. Med.,* **304**, 648–53

53. Nezelof, C. (1979). Histiocytosis X: A histological and histogenetic study. In Rosenberg, H. S. and Berstein, J. (eds) *Perspectives in Pediatric Pathology,* Vol 3, pp. 153–178. (USA: Masson Publ.)

12
Immunostaining Methods for Frozen and Paraffin Sections

B. L. MEPHAM and K. J. M. BRITTEN

INTRODUCTION

The science of immunocytochemistry has developed from the simple 'direct' immunofluorescence test introduced by Albert Coons and colleagues[1]. The 'direct' method (Figure 1a) in which the antibody is conjugated to a fluoro-chrome or enzyme label has been progressively replaced by the 'indirect' method[2]. This method does not require the primary antibody to be label-led, as a second labelled antibody is used to detect the primary antibody (Figure 1b). Until the introduction of peroxidase labels[3,4] the tech-niques were limited by the fluorescent label to frozen sections. Despite publication of a method applying the immunofluorescence technique to spec-

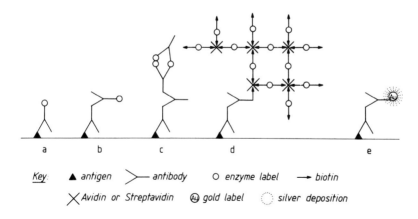

Key: ▲ antigen ⟩— antibody ○ enzyme label → biotin

✕ Avidin or Streptavidin 🅐 gold label ⋯ silver deposition

Figure 1 (a) Direct technique; (b) Indirect technique; (c) unlabelled antibody enzyme technique (this illustration, peroxidase–anti-peroxidase, PAP); (d) avidin or streptavidin/biotin, ABC, SABC; (e) Immunogold–silver technique, IGSS

ially prepared paraffin embedded tissues[5] considerable disadvantages still remain.

Disadvantages of Immunofluorescence Technique

(1) Preparations are not permanent so repeated examination and storage is inconvenient.

(2) Fresh frozen sections are generally used, providing relatively poor histological detail.

(3) Sections are prepared from tissues selected specifically for this technique and, therefore, comparison with others prepared by 'routine' paraffin methods for histological diagnosis is difficult.

(4) A special microscope is necessary, preferably with photographic facility, because immunofluorescence fades rapidly and may need to be recorded.

(5) Interpretation of the results demands experience.

To overcome some of these disadvantages, antibodies labelled with histochemically demonstrable enzymes were developed as an alternative for detection of antigen. Horseradish peroxidase (HRP) and alkaline phosphatase (AP) are mainly used for labelling antibodies, and further work by Sternberger *et al.*[6] resulted in the development of peroxidase–anti-peroxidase complexes (PAP) which retain the properties of antibody and enzyme alike. Antibodies have also been labelled with ferritin for electron microscopy and, more recently with colloidal gold both for electron and light microscopy. One of the major advantages of unlabelled antibody–enzyme methods is that they may be applied to paraffin and frozen sections alike, thus enabling retrospective and prospective studies. The application to paraffin sections was used by Taylor and Burns[7] for studies of lymphoreticular neoplasms, so demonstrating the advantages of immunoenzyme techniques. Initially the method for demonstration of immunoglobulins in formalin-fixed tissues proved unreliable, but after treatment of sections with proteolytic enzymes, immunoreactivity was restored[8,9].

PRINCIPLES OF IMMUNOCYTOCHEMICAL STAINING

Direct technique

This method relies on the combination of antigen present in tissues with an appropriate labelled antibody (Figure 1a). The label may be visualized by fluorescence microscopy or histochemistry. It is seldom used in tissue sections as each different primary antibody has to be labelled. Conjugation is laborious and results in reduction of antibody activity and decreased efficiency of the label.

Indirect technique

As shown in Figure 1b, only one labelled antibody directed against the appropriate animal species is necessary for demonstrating many antigens. The technique is mainly applied to frozen sections or cyto-centrifuged cell preparations (cytopreps) in which immunoreactivity has not been impaired by tissue preparation procedures. In paraffin sections, immunoreactivity may not always be retained by routine fixation, but can often be restored by controlled proteolytic enzyme digestion prior to immunostaining. Alternative fixation procedures may sometimes be necessary, but they can only be employed for prospective studies. Disadvantages of the indirect technique may be that background staining (connective tissue) is often excessive due to the relatively high concentration of antibody required, and it is less sensitive than unlabelled antibody enzyme methods[7,10,11].

Unlabelled antibody enzyme methods

These methods, introduced simultaneously by Sternberger[3] and Mason et al.[4], are sometimes known as 'the immunoglobulin enzyme-bridge method'. The technique involves three antibodies, in which the second stage antibody is directed against the same animal species as the first and third, so forming a 'bridge'. The third antibody is directed against a suitable enzyme, usually horseradish peroxidase or alkaline phosphatase, either of which are subsequently visualized using appropriate histochemical substrates. Purification of antiperoxidase antibody by absorption with peroxidase led to the preparation of soluble complexes of peroxidase–anti-peroxidase (PAP) (Figure 1c)[6]. PAP consists of a ring structure, often pentagonal, comprising two anti-peroxidase units and 2–4 peroxidase molecules[6]. The sensitivity of this technique is increased, in comparison with the indirect method, as judged by a higher working titre of the first stage antibody which can be used[10,12]. In a similar way, alkaline phosphatase can be used to form alkaline phosphatase–anti-alkaline phosphatase complexes (APAAP)[13]. Other enzymes which may be used for immunocytochemistry are glucose oxidase[14], complexed glucose oxidase–anti-glucose oxidase (GAG)[15] and beta-galactosidase[16], none of which are widely used as yet.

Unlabelled antibody enzyme methods have certain advantages over the labelled antibody methods[17].

(1) Multivalency of the immunological reagents leads to amplification of signal.

(2) Conjugates employed in the indirect method are often contaminated with unlabelled or denatured antibody and also free denatured peroxidase, both of which compete with the labelled antibody for antigenic sites.

(3) To produce strong specific staining with minimal background staining labelled antibodies have to be optimally diluted. Unlabelled oligoclonal antibodies can be applied at high dilution resulting in high avidity antibodies being preferentially bound to the antigen.

Enhancement techniques

The sensitivity of the unlabelled antibody enzyme method may be improved by immunological enhancement techniques[13,18]. Prior to the histochemical demonstration of the enzyme label, the second and third stages are repeated, so increasing the bound label. This technique is particularly suitable when monoclonal antibodies are used to detect antigen present in small amounts in tissue.

Enhancement of the peroxidase label has been described, whereby diamino-benzidine (DAB) is treated with silver salts so intensifying its deposition[19]. The colour of the DAB may also be altered by adding imidazole to the final substrate[20] or by post-treatment with salts of cobalt, copper and nickel[21,22].

Avidin–biotin complex method (ABC)

The method, as described by Hsu et al.[23], is now widely employed. Avidin, a glycoprotein present in egg white, has a high affinity for the vitamin, biotin, for which it possesses four binding sites. Biotin can be conjugated both to antibodies and enzymes used in immunocytochemistry. These properties are utilized in the ABC technique; this is a three-stage method whereby the second stage antibody is conjugated not directly to the enzyme but to biotin (Figure 1d). Complexes are formed by the addition of avidin to biotin, previously conjugated via a spacer arm to peroxidase[24] (or other enzymes). Avidin–biotin complexes with at least one free biotin binding site will combine with the biotin present in the conjugated second antibody. If the enzyme in the complex is conjugated to more than one biotin molecule it will combine with two or more avidin molecules. Consequently, a branching network of avidin–biotin and enzyme molecules can be formed providing a large number of enzyme molecules for histochemical demonstration (Figure 1d). The ABC technique is more sensitive than PAP, as judged by the ability to routinely use lower concentrations of primary antibody[23]. One advantage over the PAP method is that the third stage is common to systems employing oligo- or monoclonal primary antibodies. Theoretically, there are a few disadvantages of the ABC technique. Avidin, being a glycoprotein, may react with lectins and other molecules via its carbohydrate moeity. It also has a high isoelectric point, making it highly positively charged at neutral pH and may, therefore, bind to negatively charged molecules. Both of these factors may cause non-specific binding of avidin in tissue sections.

Streptavidin–biotin complex method (SABC)

Streptavidin[25], isolated from the bacterium Streptomyces avidini, has similar binding properties to avidin. However, unlike avidin it is a protein not a glycoprotein, thus eliminating non-specific binding via carbohydrate moeities. It also has an isoelectric point close to neutral pH, possessing only a few strongly charged groups at the slightly alkaline pH used in immunocyto-chemical techniques. In our department we find that the SABC and ABC techniques are technically similar and that they are more sensitive than PAP (Figure 2).

Immunogold silver staining (IGSS)

The immunogold technique was originally described for electron micros-copy[26], but recently it has been developed for light microscopy by the addition

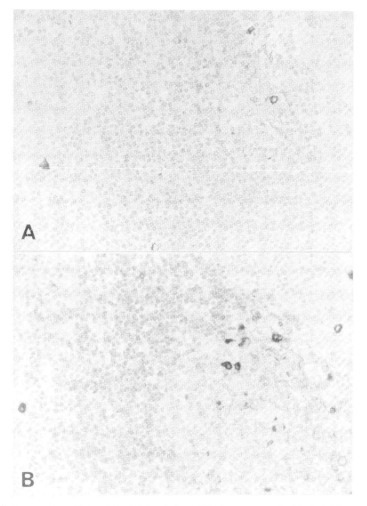

Figure 2 Increased sensitivity of the ABC technique **(B)** when compared with the PAP technique **(A)**. Adjacent sections stained by the different methods using the primary antibody to IgM at the same dilution. × 200

of a silver enhancement step to enhance the deposits of gold colloid at the antigenic site[27,28] (Figure 1e). Second stage antibodies labelled with colloidal gold particles are available in a range of sizes from 1–40 nm. (Janssen Life Sciences Products, Olen, Belgium). The technique is said to be more sensitive than PAP[29]. We find, however, that there are a number of drawbacks:

(1) Although there are only two steps, the overall immunostaining time is not decreased compared to the unlabelled enzyme or ABC methods due to the time-consuming preparation of a number of reagents required for the silver enhancement. Originally, the physical developer was light-sensitive, so the silver deposition procedure had to be carried out in the dark.

191

(2) Weak intracellular and surface staining, both of which are encountered in lymphoid tissues, are difficult to differentiate from background staining.

(3) Background staining cannot be totally eliminated despite many variations of staining technique. Three forms of background staining were identified: (a) silver precipitate, (b) gold 'noise', and (c) 'unwanted' specific staining of collagen.

More recently, Janssen have introduced the 'Intense M' kit containing the main reagents and in which the developer required for silver enhancement is not light-sensitive.

IMMUNOCYTOCHEMICAL STAINING

Immunostaining methods were developed using oligoclonal antibodies which do not necessarily recognize single epitopes; monoclonal antibodies, however, are directed against single epitopes and so we must be aware of their different characteristics if they are to be successfully applied to common techniques.

Oligoclonal antibodies

(1) Immunization may produce a different response to a specific antigen from animal to animal.

(2) Unless purified by absorption, they may not be specific.

(3) In some instances the recognition of a group of epitopes may be advantageous, because if some of the epitopes are destroyed the antigen will still be detected due to recognition of the remaining epitopes by the antibody.

Monoclonal antibodies

(1) Monoclonal antibodies recognize a single epitope and are, therefore, highly specific. This may be a disadvantage if the epitope is rare or if it is common to unrelated cells and structures. Full characterization of the antibody is, therefore, necessary.

(2) Compared to oligoclonal antibodies there is less non-specific binding to unrelated sites, hence precise specific staining with less background is usually achieved.

(3) They are available as tissue culture supernatants, which are low in antibody content, as ascites with a high concentration of antibody, or as a purified protein fraction of ascites, which reduces the non-specific or background staining sometimes seen with the unpurified preparation.

(4) Preservation of clones will ensure that antibodies are replicated without variation.

(5) As some monoclonal antibodies are of the IgM class, it is therefore, essential to have the second stage antibodies directed against IgM

alone, rather than whole serum which often contain comparatively small amounts of IgM.

(6) It may be advantageous to mix several monoclonal antibodies (where specificities have been previously characterized) to make a 'cocktail' of antibodies of a broader spectrum.

(7) A wide range of commercially prepared antibodies, particularly to cell surface antigens, are now available. However, these can have limited diagnostic value due to inaccessibility or destruction of antigen by preparative histological techniques.

Laboratory requirements

In order to maintain reproducible immunostaining, standardization of techniques and an analytical attitude are of paramount importance.

Incubation

When carrying out immunostaining procedures the number of slides handled must not exceed the expertise of the worker. Too many slides will result in drying-out of sections, particularly between washing and the application of antibody. Moist chambers (Figure 3) must be used to prevent evaporation of antibody solution from the sections. These may be quite simple in design and fit into a refrigerator (+4° C) or an incubator (37° C), as it is sometimes necessary to carry out incubation of some primary antibodies under these conditions for up to 24 hours. Incubation for 30 minutes at room temperature (20° C) is convenient and adequate for the majority of antibodies. Longer incubation times may be necessary, particularly for some weakly reacting

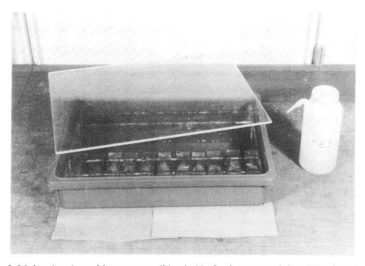

Figure 3 Moist chamber with a perspex lid suitable for immunostaining. The size allows the chamber to be placed in an incubator or refrigerator

primary antibodies. Incubation overnight at +4°C is usually preferable to 2–4 hours at 37°C which may result in similar specific staining but often produces increased background staining. Although particular primary antibodies may require prolonged incubation times, second and third stage antibodies usually only require 30 minutes incubation at room temperature.

Buffers and washes

Many workers use phosphate buffered saline pH 7.4 (PBS) for washing between the immunological stages, but we prefer 0.05 mol/l Tris buffer pH 7.6, diluted 1:10 in saline (TBS)[30]. We have compared these buffers and found the immunostaining results preferable when using TBS rather than PBS (unpublished data). If buffers are not used frequently they should be stored in a concentrated form at 4°C and diluted prior to use.

Most laboratories use deionised or distilled water for the preparation of trypsin solutions, wash and histochemical buffers. However, using single glass-distilled water we have had failure of immunostaining for unidentifiable reasons, but conversion to double glass-distilled water has prevented this. Washing sections between steps may be carried out by placing slides in staining racks on a platform over a magnetic stirrer in a trough containing wash-buffer so providing continuous agitation. To avoid repeated handling of the slides three applications of wash-buffer for 5–10 minutes duration is adequate. It is important that prior to application of each antibody, excess wash-buffer is allowed to drain from the section as insufficient draining will result in dilution of antibody. Sections must never be allowed to dry as this will cause staining artefact.

Endogenous enzymes

Peroxidase

Endogenous peroxidases, present as myeloperoxidase in leukocytes and haemoglobin peroxidase in red blood cells, also react with DAB chromogen. Activity may be inhibited (often referred to as blocked), prior to immunostaining, using one of a number of methods which have previously been described, methanol/hydrochloric acid[31]; sodium borohydride/periodic acid[32] and methanol/hydrogen peroxide[12,33]. On paraffin sections we have used the methanol/hydrogen peroxide method (see methods section of this chapter) for a number of years. Occasionally, inhibition in some sections is difficult, but this may be overcome by extending the time in the reagent from 10 to 30 minutes. On frozen sections, the 'fixative' properties of methanol will often destroy or alter the distribution of antigen, and hydrogen peroxide may cause sections to detach from the slide. An alternative method, in which 0.3% sodium azide is incorporated in the DAB/hydrogen peroxide substrate[34], has been tested with success but not adopted routinely.

Alkaline phosphatase

Endogenous alkaline phosphatase is found in myoepithelial cells, fibroblastic

Figure 4 An example of chessboard titrations designed to establish the optimum dilution of three antibodies which are to be used in conjunction with each other and where the titres are unknown. The second stage antibody is always used in excess to ensure that only high affinity antibody reacts with the primary one and also that it is not lost by subsequent washes. Once all the titres have been established that of a replacement antibody can be determined by a single titration

	Stage	Antibody	Dilutions	Optimum dilution
Titration 1	One	RãHuIgA	1/50–1/3200	1/800
	Two	SwãRIgG	1/50	–
	Three	RPAP	1/50–1/800	1/200
Titration 2	One	RãHuIgA	1/800	–
	Two	SwãRIgG	1/50–1/800	1/200
	Three	RPAP	1/200	–
Titration 3	Verify using optimum dilutions established for all stages			

reticulum cells and endothelial cells of blood vessels, all of which are present in lymph nodes. In paraffin sections its presence does not usually interfere with immunostaining since it is usually destroyed during fixation and processing. In frozen sections its presence may mask or be confused with specific immunocytochemical staining, but inhibition can be achieved by the incorporation of 1 mmol/l levamisole (Sigma L9756) in the substrate[35].

Antibodies

Dilution

Before antibodies are used routinely their optimum dilution must be determined by titration. The titre may differ for frozen and paraffin sections, the latter usually requiring a more concentrated antibody. The optimum titre of an antibody may be defined as the highest dilution which will produce the strongest specific staining with weakest background staining. Sometimes, if a concentrated antibody is used staining may be severely reduced, or even completely negative. This is not due to the absence of antigen, but to an excess of antibody and is similar to the prozone phenomenon encountered in agglutination tests.

Chessboard titrations should be carried out on all antibodies which are required to interact in order to establish their respective optimum dilutions. When three stages are involved, more than one titration is necessary (Figure 4).

Second stage antibodies are not always species specific, so they may need to be absorbed with non-immune serum from the same animal species as the tissue under test.

Storage

Antibodies are often supplied with instructions for storage, but if not the following general rules apply.

Storage depends on the amount of antibody received, its final concentration, its rate of deterioration and frequency of use. It is important to avoid repeated freeze–thawing of an antibody, so once thawed aliquots should be stored at +4°C until totally used. Usually the activity of oligoclonal antibodies deteriorates at a slower rate than monoclonals allowing the majority to be stored at +4°C. If, however, an antibody is used infrequently or at high dilution it is best aliquoted into appropriate amounts and stored at –20°C. Monoclonal antibodies supplied as supernatants are best distributed into aliquots on arrival and stored at –20°C, leaving a small amount stored at +4°C for immediate use. Those received as ascites or a purified protein fraction of ascites are the least stable. However, they are often used at high dilutions so are best stored partially diluted in aliquots at –20°C and then finally diluted when required. Antibodies conjugated to enzymes or antibody–enzyme complexes should be stored at +4°C. If the antibodies are received lyophilized they can be reconstituted with the required amount of sterile water. Often antibodies contain a chemical preservative, sodium azide, which at the usual dilution (10 mmol/l) has no effect on specific staining. Some antibodies remain stable for many months, or several years, but it is prudent to monitor deterioration by periodic checks using a range of dilutions centred around the optimum titre.

Controls

To ensure that the methods produce genuine demonstration of antigen in the sections, various controls should be used. There are several ways to do this and those most commonly used are listed below.

(1) *Positive Control:* The inclusion of a section known to contain the antigen under test.

(2) *Specificity of Primary Antibody:* Absorption of this antibody by addition of specific antigen prior to application to the section. Pure antigens appropriate for blocking are not always available, but a similar test in which competition for the same antigen by antibodies raised in different species may be used. For example, the addition of an excess of *goat* anti-human IgG to *rabbit* anti-human IgG, in a 3-stage unlabelled antibody method using rabbit PAP should result in reduced staining.

(3) *Non-Specific Binding of Second or Third Stages:* Omission of the primary antibody will indicate if staining is due to non-specific binding of the second or third stages of the tissues.

(4) *Intrinsic control:*
  (a) Simultaneous immunostaining of a number of cases in which the staining results are likely to differ.

(b) Simultaneous immunostaining with a variety of antibodies on sections of the same case.

Both of the tests will help to identify spurious staining, confirm that the antibodies are reactive and that the methods have been carried out correctly.

Enzyme histochemistry

Peroxidase – DAB (3,3'-diaminobenzidine tetrahydrochloride)

This method relies upon the reaction of peroxidase with its substrate hydrogen peroxide to form a primary complex which oxidizes the electron donor, DAB, forming a dark brown crystalline product. A number of different formulae have been described, comprising various permutations of buffer pH, amount of DAB and hydrogen peroxide. In our experience, the original method, described by Graham and Karnovsky[36], using 5 mg DAB per 10 ml of 0.2 mol/l Tris/HCl buffer pH 7.6 to which is added 100 μl of 0.1% freshly diluted hydrogen peroxide has proved reliable. The hydrochloride salt (cat. no. D5637 Sigma Chemical Co. Ltd, Poole, UK) is preferable to the free base as it dissolves readily in the buffer. Hydrogen peroxide, particularly when diluted, deteriorates rapidly with a consequent loss of activity. It is preferable to keep aliquots of undiluted hydrogen peroxide at +4°C, and stock solutions should be replaced at regular intervals. The fear surrounding DAB as a dangerous carcinogen has now subsided, but like many other chemicals used in laboratories, it should be regarded as a potential carcinogen and handled accordingly.

Peroxidase – AEC (3-amino-9 ethylcarbazole)[37]

Peroxidase catalyses the oxidation of this chromogen by hydrogen peroxide to produce a bright red colour at sites of peroxidase activity, contrasting well with a blue haematoxylin counterstain. The coloured reaction product is soluble in alcohol and xylene, so sections must be mounted in aqueous media resulting in difficulty in the storage of slides and some loss of resolution with microscopy. Counterstaining should be carried out using a progressive haematoxylin stain such as Mayer's haemalum to avoid the need for differentiation in acid alcohol.

Peroxidase – PPD-PC (phenylenediamine-pyrocatechol)[38]

This technique is based on the principle that in the presence of phenols there is oxidative coupling of aromatic amines forming a dark brown coloured product which is not soluble in alcohol or xylene, however, fading may occur over a period of time. The reagent consisting of 1 part para-phenylenediamine dihydrochloride + 2 parts pyrocatechol, is available ready blended (Cat. no. H7507, Sigma Chemical Co. Ltd, Poole, UK) and is used as a substitute for DAB. It has been reported that this reagent is specific for plant peroxidase, so the endogenous animal peroxidase should not react.

Alkaline phosphatase

A number of techniques are available for the demonstration of alkaline phosphatase in tissue sections[39], but the two most commonly used in immuno-cytochemistry are the azo dye methods, either using simple organic phosphate or phosphates with substituted naphthol groupings. The latter methods are preferable because the reagents are more stable and there is better localization of the final reaction product. The method works by hydrolysis of the substituted naphthols to give an insoluble naphthol derivative which then couples to a suitable diazonium salt to produce a coloured reaction product. Different coloured reaction products may be achieved by altering the diazonium salts. Fast red TR and new fuchsin (actually a hexazonium salt) produce a red reaction product giving good contrasts with a haematoxylin counterstain[13,35]. We prefer the technique of Ponder and Wilkinson[35] as the combination of veronal acetate buffer and Fast Red TR produces clean preparations with precise localization of alkaline phosphatase label. In double labelling techniques Fast Blue BB is a good second chromogen[13,40]. The coloured reaction products of all these methods are soluble in alcohol and, therefore, require mounting in an aqueous media such as glycerin jelly or Apathy's medium. If stained paraffin sections are allowed to dry in air, prior to placing in xylene, resin mounting media such as DPX are suitable, although this technique does not seem to be suitable on frozen sections.

Paraffin sections

Fixation

The most commonly used fixative in the United Kingdom is 10% neutral buffered formalin (NBF), but treatment of paraffin sections with proteolytic enzymes prior to immunostaining is necessary for the demonstration of many antigens useful in the study of lymphoreticular disease[41]. Most surface antigens are best demonstrated in frozen sections (p. 204), but with ideal fixation conditions and a sensitive immunostaining technique some surface antigens can also be demonstraed in paraffin sections. The term '10% formalin' is frequently used for many formalin fixative solutions, irrespective of their actual composition. Neutral buffered formalin pH 7 is preferred in surgical pathology because pigment formed in acidic solutions, although microscopically insignificant, is prevented. There are a number of ways in which formalin solutions are buffered. The most common incorporate phosphates[42] but simpler methods, such as the addition of 2% calcium acetate[42] or simply keeping solutions over calcium or magnesium carbonate are also used[43]. Tissues from the autopsy room may not be fixed in solutions of the same formula as surgical specimens; often a crude fixative, consisting of 10% formalin in tap water is used. It is likely that tissues from different laboratories will have been fixed in formalin solutions of various compositions, differing pH and, most importantly, for different lengths of time. All of these factors will affect immunoreactivity. Demonstration of intracellular immunoglobulins in formalin-fixed sections was initially unreliable, as illustrated by reports in which new fixatives were introduced or existing ones modified[44,45]. By routinely treating fixed sections with proteolytic enzyme intracellular immunoglobulins can be demonstrated[8,9], demonstrating that fixatives may not always destroy immunoreactivity but merely mask it

(Figure 5). A simple formalin fixative, suitable for routine use and not requiring sections to be treated with proteolytic enzymes, consisting of 10% formalin and 2.5% acetic acid, has been described by Curran and Gregory[46]. Other fixatives, eg. formol–mercury, Bouins' and Carnoy's facilitate demonstration of immunoglobulins, but Zenker–acetic or B5 are unsuitable as specific staining is often indistinguishable from the background[47]. Not all antigens remain immunoreactive after fixation, for example alpha-1-antitrypsin in mercuric chloride containing fixatives or, similarly, in formalin–acetic acid fixative. However, a monoclonal antibody designated TAL-IB5 will detect HLA-D antigen in tissues which have been fixed in formalin–acetic acid, Bouins' and sometimes unbuffered formol–saline but not NBF[48]. Leukocyte Common Antigen, CD45, available from Dako, is similar in that it gives good results in tissues fixed in neutral buffered formalin, but often only weak staining is seen in sections from neutral buffered formol–saline fixed tissues. A recently described method[49] using 'methacarn' which is a modification of Carnoy's fixative[50] may, in the future, prove to be useful for some antigens in lymphoid tissue.

The composition and hence the properties of a fixative solution determine its pH and osmolarity and to some extent its rate of penetration. However, penetration is also affected by the temperature and length of time in fixative, and by the cellular composition and size of the tissue blocks. Unbisected lymph nodes, greater than 1–1.5 cm in diameter, will exhibit poor fixation in the centre when fixed for periods of time that, due to the necessity of diagnosis, are less than 24 hours. Although the sections may be acceptable for diagnostic purposes with routine Haematoxylin and Eosin (H&E) staining (Figures 6B and 6C) they are unsuitable for immunocytochemistry as, after treatment with proteolytic enzyme, the poorly fixed centre of the node may be over-digested (Figures 6D and 6E). Conversely, over-fixation will occur in tissues remaining in fixative solutions for long periods of time or when the temperature at which fixation occurs is increased, resulting in a corresponding loss of immunoreactivity. Although not ideal, NBF may be regarded as a suitable compromise fixative in that underfixed tissues may be corrected by immersing slides in trypsin for shorter times and over-fixed ones for longer times. It is advisable to establish a fixation and processing protocol which will enable the immunocytochemical techniques to be standardized. We prefer specimens to be dispatched straight from the operating theatre to the laboratory in dry, sterile containers. Lymph nodes are then bisected and imprint smears are made and stained by Rapidiff II Romanowsky stain (Infrakem Ltd, Standish, UK). A provisional diagnosis then determines the procedure to adopt. Part of the lymph node is always fixed in NBF and processed to paraffin wax, another portion may be quenched in liquid nitrogen (−196°C) and stored in a liquid nitrogen refrigerator in anticipation of frozen section staining.

Tissue processing

The majority of laboratories use some form of automatic tissue processing in which dehydration in alcohol is followed by 'clearing' in an ante-medium, of

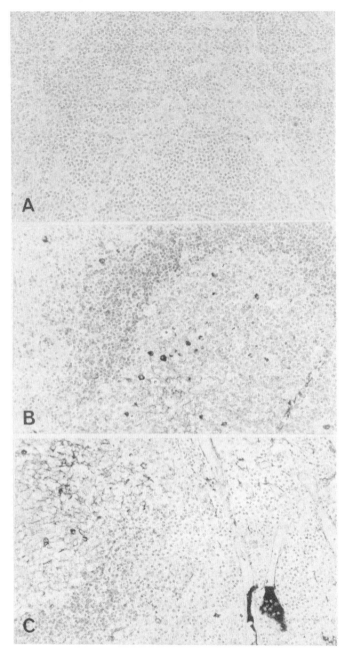

Figure 5 Paraffin sections of tonsil fixed in NBF showing the effect of enzyme digestion prior to immunostaining for IgM. **(A)** Sections not treated with trypsin – no staining; **(B)** Section treated with 0.1% trypsin for 15 minutes – positive staining of cells and some follicular and mantle staining; **(C)** 30 minutes trypsin produces over-digestion which is exhibited by loss of cellular material, particularly cytoplasm, and some reticulin staining. × 150

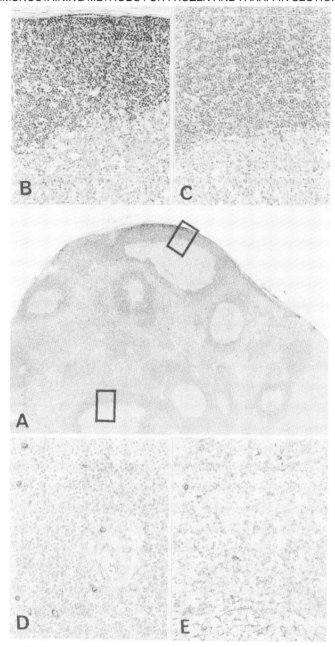

Figure 6 Paraffin sections of NBF-fixed lymph node **(A)** stained by H&E showing sites of the following photomicrographs (magnification × 15). Higher powers H&E (× 120) taken at the edge of the section **(B)** and the centre **(C)** showing cellular details in which there is little difference. The lower photomicrographs stained for kappa light chains by the ABC technique after treatment with trypsin. In **(D)** (edge of section) there is no evidence of digestion, but in the centre **(E)** there is digestion as the result of inadequate fixation which is either due to poor fixative penetration or insufficient time in the fixative

201

which there are a number to choose from. Traditionally, toluene and chloroform are still used, but some laboratories are now using less toxic ones such as CNP30 and Histosol (Shandon Southern Products Ltd, Runcorn, UK).

If the initial fixation process is incomplete, alcohol used for dehydration will also fix the tissues with a coagulant denaturing effect of proteins[51] which, in our experience, impairs immunoreactivity. The time taken to process tissues from fixation to paraffin embedding will vary from laboratory to laboratory. It may be either a short process, combining heat and vacuum, taking approximately 4 hours, or a commonly used process taking 16–20 hours at 18°C and, in some laboratories, infiltration of wax under vacuum. Over the last 12 years we have carried out immunocytochemistry on paraffin sections from many laboratories. Poor immunostaining results have generally been attributable to faults in fixation and never to the different processing schedules.

Wax and infiltration

Paraffin wax for histology is available pure or with microcrystalline waxes or polymers added, supposedly to improve section cutting properties. None of these waxes have apparently affected immunoreactivity. However, all traces of wax must be removed prior to staining. Infiltration of tissues is usually carried out at a temperature between 60–65°C. Excessive temperature and time in molten wax should be avoided in order to prevent tissue damage and also to prevent reduced immunoreactivity.

Microtomy

Section cutting and floating on water does not seem to affect immunocytochemical staining, but thin sections (3–4 microns) of lymph node are preferable for microscopy. Disposable microtome blades now make these easy to achieve.

Section adhesives

The traditional adhesive for tissue sections is glycerine–albumin which, containing protein, is best avoided. Sections cut from properly fixed and processed tissues should not generally require adhesives. If sections do become detached this may be prevented by treating the slides with a small amount of 0.01% poly-L-lysine[52], prior to section mounting.

Section drying

Sections of lymphoreticular tissues are best dried at 37°C overnight. Drying on a hot plate at temperatures in excess of 50°C will cause 'cracking' of the section, but more importantly may also be detrimental to immunoreactivity.

Storage of sections

It is preferable to carry out the immunostaining technique as soon as possible after the sections have been prepared. Some antigens seem to lose their immunoreactivity if they are stored for any length of time, but we have no evidence that those currently useful in the diagnosis of lymphoreticular disease are affected in this way. It is likely that fixation affords some protection from the deleterious effects of tissue processing, wax infiltration and mechanical disruption caused by section cutting and drying.

Unmasking immunoreactivity with proteolytic enzymes

The demonstration of the majority of antigens useful for the diagnosis of lymphoreticular disease in tissues fixed in NBF requires treatment of sections with proteolytic enzymes prior to immunostaining. A number of suitable enzymes are available: trypsin[9], protease[8] and pepsin[53]. We have found trypsin to be the most suitable because it is cheap and its activity is easily controlled[54]. The exact mechanism by which it works is unknown, but it probably cleaves peptide bonds of protein chains between arginine and lysine, so causing the chains to partially separate and allow antibody access to antigenic sites masked by fixation. The degree of proteolysis (often referred to as 'digestion') must be related to the extent to which the protein has been fixed, a process which can only be estimated by trial and error. Over-exposure will result in obvious 'digestion' of tissue which can be recognized by the absence of cellular components and increased background staining in the sections (Figure 5c). Under-exposure will produce negative, or weak, immunostaining (Figure 5A). If demonstration of antigens in sections is to be reproducible the proteolytic techniques must be reliable and standardized so that the only variable is the degree of fixation. It is, therefore, essential to precisely control the trypsin treatment with particular regard to preparation, pH, temperature and the time of exposure. Faults in this part of the technique often occur and note should be taken of the following points:

(1) Activity of trypsin from different suppliers will vary, as will different batches. Trypsin from porcine pancreas (product number T8128, Sigma Chemical Co Ltd, Poole, UK) has generally been consistent and of proven reliability.

(2) It is essential that 0.1% calcium chloride is included in the trypsin solution to supply calcium ions necessary for activation of the enzyme.

(3) Preparation in de-ionised or distilled water is generally suitable, but double glass-distilled water will ensure *consistent* purity.

(4) A solution of trypsin and calcium chloride will be approximately pH 4.5–5.0. 0.1 mol/l sodium hydroxide must be added to adjust the pH to 7.8 which is optimal for trypsin activity.

(5) The temperature of the prepared trypsin solution should be stabilized at 37°C by placing the container in a waterbath. Another container of distilled water should also be placed in the waterbath for temperature

equilibration of the slides prior to placing in the prepared enzyme solution.

(6) Once prepared, the activity of the trypsin decreases significantly[54]. It is essential to follow the same sequence of events so that the elapsed time from beginning the preparation of trypsin to immersion of sections is always the same.

Frozen sections

There are several models of cryostat available, but we prefer the 'open top' type because the temperature inside does not noticeably increase when a large number of sections are required from each case.

Tissue 'quenched' and stored in a liquid nitrogen refrigerator is unsuitable for immunocytochemistry after a period of time which, in the case of some antigens, may be as short as one year. Long-term storage at the higher temperature of $-70°C$ has also proven unsatisfactory as the tissues dehydrate producing changes in their morphology and immunoreactivity.

Freezing tissues

Small slices, 2 mm or less in thickness and approximately 5×10 mm in area, wrapped in aluminium foil are snap-frozen by immersion in liquid nitrogen to ensure that the tissue is frozen throughout. The foil packets are then placed in polypropylene screw-cap tubes (Sterilin Ltd, Feltham, UK) which are then transferred to a nitrogen refrigerator and stored in the nitrogen vapour ($-130°C$ to $-196°C$).

Storage of sections

Several methods for the preparation and storage of frozen sections, prior to immunostaining have been described. Some involve freeze-drying the sections before storing at $-20°C$[55]. We use a development of this method in which the sections are 'freeze dessicated'. Sections are put into a metal staining rack standing on a layer of silica gel (BDH Ltd, Poole, UK) which is then placed in an airtight polythene sandwich box and then put into a freezer at $-20°C$. Sections may be stored in this way for up to 3 weeks before immunoreactivity is impaired. Alternatively, if the sections are to be stained within 18 hours they may be left overnight at room temperature.

Fixation of cryostat sections

When removed from the $-20°C$ freezer sections should be left at room temperature, 18–20°C, for several minutes to allow the condensation to dry-off, prior to fixing in acetone for 15 minutes. Contrary to the technique described by Warford[56] in which water is added to the acetone, we prefer dried acetone stored over a type 4A molecular sieve (BDH Ltd, Poole, UK) to absorb any water present. Once sections have been brought to room temperature they should not be re-frozen. Frozen sections from some tissues, notably skin, are prone to detach from the slides during staining, but this can be prevented by using poly-L-lysine (p. 203).

METHODS

Introduction

Descriptions of many immunocytochemical methods have now been published. The following ones are used in our laboratories and are the result of continual development.

Peroxidase–anti-peroxidase (PAP) technique using oligoclonal antibodies

Suitable for paraffin-embedded tissues.

(1) Deparaffinize sections in xylene (twice, 10 minutes each) and take to 70% alcohol.
(2) Inhibit endogenous peroxidase by treating with freshly prepared 0.5% hydrogen peroxide in methanol; 10 minutes.
(3) Wash well in tap water.

If sections are *not* to be trypsinized omit step 4–6.

(4) Prewarm in distilled water at 37°C; 5 minutes.
(5) Treat with 0.1% trypsin (Sigma T8128) in 0.1% calcium chloride (adjust to pH 7.8 with 0.1 M NaOH) at 37°C. 15–30 minutes**.
(6) Rinse in cold running water with agitation, 2–3 minutes.
(7) Wash in Tris buffered saline (TBS); twice, 5 minutes each.
(8) Apply rabbit anti-human antibody*; 30 minutes.
(9) Wash in TBS; three times, 5 minutes each.
(10) Apply swine anti-rabbit IgG*; 30 minutes.
(11) Wash in TBS; three times, 5 minutes each.
(12) Apply rabbit peroxidase–anti-peroxidase*; 30 minutes.
(13) Wash in TBS; three times, 5 minutes each.
(14) Apply DAB/H_2O_2 substrate; 10 minutes.
(15) Rinse in TBS followed by a wash in running tap water; 5 minutes.
(16) Counterstain with haematoxylin, and blue in running tap water.
(17) Dehydrate, clear and mount.

**Time may vary with batch of trypsin, fixative and/or length of fixation
*At current dilution in TBS as determined by titration

Avidin–biotin complex (ABC) technique using oligoclonal antibodies

The ABC using monoclonal antibodies is now routinely used.

Suitable for fixed paraffin-embedded tissues.

(1) Deparaffinize sections in xylene (twice, 10 minutes each) and take to 70% alcohol.

(2) Inhibit endogenous peroxidase by treating with freshly prepared 0.5% hydrogen peroxide in methanol; 10 minutes.

(3) Wash well in tap water.

If sections do *not* require trypsinization omit steps 4–6

(4) Prewarm in distilled water at 37°C; 5 minutes.

(5) Treat with 0.1% trypsin (from porcine pancreas, Sigma T8128) in 0.1% calcium chloride (adjust to pH 7.8 with 0.1 M NaOH) at 37°C; 15–30 minutes**.

(6) Rinse in cold running water with agitation; 2–3 minutes.

(7) Wash in Tris buffered saline (TBS); twice, 5 minutes each.

(8) Apply mouse monoclonal antibody*; overnight at +4°C.

(9) Wash in TBS; three times, 5 minutes each.

(10) Apply biotinylated rabbit anti-mouse Ig*; 30 minutes.

(11) Wash in TBS; three times, 5 minutes each.

(12) Apply avidin–biotin complex (peroxidase)*; 30 minutes.

Prepare complexes at least 30 minutes before use

(13) Wash in TBS; three times, 5 minutes each

(14) Apply DAB/H_2O_2 substrate; 10 minutes.

(15) Rinse in TBS followed by a wash in running tap water; 5 minutes.

(16) Counterstain with haematoxylin, and blue in running tap water.

(17) Dehydrate, clear and mount.

**Time may vary with batch of trypsin, fixative and/or length of fixation
*At current dilution in TBS as determined by titration

Indirect immunoperoxidase technique using monoclonal antibodies

Suitable for use with frozen sections, cytocentrifuge preparations and smears.

(1) Cut cryostat sections (6 μm).

(2) Air dry at room temperature; 30 minutes.

(3) Store slides at −20°C wrapped in foil or in a rack over silica gel in an airtight box for a maximum of 14 days.

(4) Unwrap slides or remove from box and rack and lay on bench until the condensation has evaporated, 10 minutes.

(5) Replace slides in racks and fix in water-free acetone at room temperature; 15 minutes.

(6) Lay slides in immuno-trays and allow acetone to evaporate; 10 minutes.

(7) Wash in TBS; twice, 5 minutes each.

(8) Apply mouse monoclonal antibody*; 30 minutes.

(9) Wash in TBS; three times, 5 minutes each.

(10) Apply rabbit anti-mouse Ig peroxidase conjugate*; 30 minutes.

(11) Wash in TBS; three times, 5 minutes each.

(12) Apply DAB/H_2O_2 substrate; 10 minutes.

(13) Rinse in TBS followed by a wash in running tap water; 5 minutes.

(14) Counterstain in haematoxylin, and blue in running tap water.

(15) Dehydrate, clear and mount.

*At current dilution in TBS as determined by titration

Alkaline phosphatase–anti-alkaline phosphatase (APAAP) technique using monoclonal antibodies

Suitable for use with frozen sections, cytocentrifuge preparations and smears.

(1) Cut cryostat sections (6 μm).

(2) Air dry at room temperature for 30 minutes.

(3) Store at –20° C wrapped in foil or in a rack over silica gel in an airtight box for a maximum of 14 days.

(4) Unwrap slides or remove from box and rack and lay on bench until condensation has evaporated; 10 minutes.

(5) Fix in water-free acetone at room temperature; 15 minutes.

(6) Lay slides in immuno-trays and allow acetone to evaporate; 10 minutes.

(7) Wash in TBS; twice, 5 minutes each.

(8) Apply mouse monoclonal antibody*; 30 minutes.

(9) Wash in TBS; three times, 5 minutes each.

(10) Apply goat anti-mouse Ig*; 30 minutes.

(11) Wash in TBS; three times, 5 minutes each.

(12) Apply mouse alkaline phosphatase–anti-alkaline phosphatase complexes*; 30 minutes.

   Prepare complexes at least 5 hours before use

(13) Wash in TBS; three times, 5 minutes each.

(14) Apply goat anti-mouse Ig*; 10 minutes

(15) Wash in TBS; three times, 5 minutes each } optional

(16) Apply mouse AAPAP complexes*; 10 minutes. } enhancement

(17) Wash in TBS; three times, 5 minutes each.

(18) Apply Fast red TR/naphthol AS-BI phosphate substrate.

(19) Rinse in TBS followed by a wash in running tap water; 5 minutes.

(21) Counterstain in Mayer's haematoxylin, and blue in running tap water; 10 minutes.

(23) Mount in an *aqueous* mountant.

   *At current dilution in TBS as determined by titration

Substrates and reagents

Tris buffered saline, pH 7.6 (TBS)

Sodium chloride	80 g
Tris (hydroxymethyl) aminomethane	6.05 g
1 N hydrochloric acid	38 ml (approx.)
Distilled water to	10 litre

Check pH and adjust to pH 7.6, if necessary.

Inhibitor for endogenous peroxidase

Hydrogen peroxide – AnalaR 30% w/v (100 volumes) (BDH Prod: 10128)	0.2 ml
Methanol – general purpose reagent (BDH Prod: 29192)	11.8 ml

Trypsin

Trypsin from porcine pancreas (Sigma Type T8128)	0.5 g
Calcium chloride 12–24 mesh (BDH Prod: 27588)	0.5 g
Double glass-distilled water	500 ml

Use 0.1 mol/l sodium hydroxide to adjust pH to 7.8 at 37°C

DAB/H_2O_2 substrate

Prepare all reagents just before use.

(1) 3,3′ Diaminobenzidine tetrahydrochloride (DAB)
(Sigma D5637)   5 mg
(2) Tris/HCl buffer pH 7.6*   10 ml
(3) 1% H_2O_2 (freshly prepared by adding
0.1 ml 30%w/v H_2O_2 to 2.9 ml distilled water)   0.1 ml

Dissolve 1 in 2 and immediately before use add 3. Incubate for 10 minutes

Tris–HCl buffer

0.2 mol/l Tris (Sigma T1503)	12 ml
0.1 N hydrochloric acid	19 ml
Distilled water	19 ml

Fast red TR/naphthol AS-BI phosphate substrate

Prepare all reagents just before use.

(1) Veronal acetate buffer pH 9.2*   10 ml
(2) Fast red TR (Sigma F1500)   5 mg
(3) Levamisole (Sigma L9756)   2.5 mg
(4) Naphthol AS BI phosphate (Sigma N2250)   5 mg
(5) Dimethylformamide (BDH Prod: 10322)   0.1 ml

Dissolve 2 and 3 in 1, dissolve 4 in 5. Mix the two solutions. Filter and incubate for 10–60 minutes.

Veronal acetate buffer pH 9.2

Sodium barbitone	1.472 g
Sodium acetate trihydrate	0.972 g
0.1 mol/l hydrochloric acid	2.5 ml
Distilled water to	250 ml

ACKNOWLEDGEMENTS

We should like to thank Julie Foster for typing the manuscript and being extremely patient.

References

1. Coons, A. H., Creech, H. J., Jones, R. N. and Berliner, E. (1942). The demonstration of pneumococcal antigen of tissues by the use of fluorescent antibody. *J. Immunol.*, **45**, 159–70

2. Weller, T. H. and Coons, A. H. (1954). Fluorescent antibody studies with agents of Varicella and Herpes Zoster propagated *in vitro*. *Proceedings of the Society for Experimental Biology and Medicine*, **86**, 789–94

3. Sternberger, L. A. (1969). Some new developments in immunocytochemistry. *Mikroskopie*, **25**, 346–61

4. Mason, T. E., Phifer, R. F., Spicer, S. S., Swallow, R. A. and Dreskin, R. B. (1969). An immunoglobulin–enzyme bridge method for localising tissue antigens. *J. Histochem. Cytochem.*, **17**, 563–9

5. Sainte-Marie, G. (1962). A paraffin embedding technique for studies employing immunofluorescence. *J. Histochem. Cytochem.*, **10**, 250–6

6. Sternberger, L. A., Hardy, P. H. Jr., Cuculis, J. J. and Meyer, H. G. (1970). The unlabelled antibody enzyme method of immunohistochemistry. *J. Histochem. Cytochem.*, **18**, 315–33

7. Taylor, C. R. and Burns, J. (1974). The demonstration of plasma cells and other immunoglobulin-containing cells in formalin fixed, paraffin embedded tissues using peroxidase-labelled antibody. *J. Clin. Pathol.*, **27**, 14–20

8. Denk, H., Radaszkiewicz, T. and Weirich, E. (1977). Pronase pre-treatment of tissue sections enhances sensitivity of the unlabelled antibody–enzyme (PAP) technique. *J. Immunol. Meth.*, **15**, 163–7

9. Curran, R. C. and Gregory, J. (1977). The unmasking of antigens in paraffin sections of tissue by trypsin. *Experimentia*, **33**, 1400–1

10. Petrali, J. P., Hinton, D. M., Moriarty, G. C. and Sternberger, L. A. (1974). The unlabelled antibody enzyme method of immunocytochemistry. Quantitative comparison of sensitivities with and without peroxidase–antiperoxidase complex.(PAP). *J. Histochem. Cytochem.*, **22**, 782–801

11. Burns, J., Hambridge, M. and Taylor, C. R. (1974). Intracellular immunoglobulins: A comparative study on three standard tissue processing methods using horseradish peroxidase and fluorochrome conjugates. *J. Clin. Pathol.*, **27**, 548–57

12. Burns, J. (1975). Background staining and sensitivity of the unlabelled antibody (PAP) method. Comparison with the peroxidase labelled antibody sandwich method using formalin fixed, paraffin embedded material. *Histochemistry*, **43**, 291–4

13. Cordell, J. L., Falini, B., Erber, W. N., Ghosh, A. K., Abdulaziz, Z., MacDonald, S., Pulford, K. A. F., Stein, H. and Mason, D. Y. (1984). Immunoenzymatic labelling of monoclonal antibodies using immune complexes of alkaline phosphatase and monoclonal alkaline phosphatase (APAAP complexes). *J. Histochem. Cytochem.*, **32**, 219–29

14. Suffin, S. C., Muck, K. B., Young, J. C., Lewin, K. and Parten, D. D. (1979). Improvement of the glucose oxidase immunoenzyme technique. *Am. J. Clin. Pathol.*, **71**, 492–6

15. Clark, C. A., Downs, E. C., Primus, F. J. (1982). An unlabelled antibody method using glucose oxidase–antiglucose oxidase complexes (GAG): A sensitive alternative to immunoperoxidase for the detection of tissue antigens. *J. Histochem. Cytochem.*, **30**, 27–34

16. Bondi, I., Chieregatti, G., Eusibi, V., Fulcheri, E. and Bussolati, G. (1982). The use of beta-galactosidase as a tracer in immunocytochemistry. *Histochemistry*, **76**, 153–8

17. Sternberger, L. A. (1986). *Immunocytochemistry*. 3rd Edn. (New York: John Wiley & Sons)

18. Ordronneau, P., Lindstrom, P. B-M. and Petrusz, P. (1981). Four unlabelled antibody bridge techniques: A comparison. *J. Histochem. Cytochem.*, **29**, 1397–404

19. Gallyas, F., Gorcs, T. and Merchenthaler, I. (1982). High grade intensification of the end-product of the diaminobenzidine reaction for peroxidase histochemistry. *J. Histochem. Cytochem.*, **30**, 183–4

20. Borowitz, M. J., Croker, B. P. and Burchette, J. (1982). Immunocytochemical detection of lymphocyte surface antigens in fixed tissue sections. *J. Histochem. Cytochem.*, **30**, 171–4

21. Hsu, S. M. and Soban, E. (1982). Color modification of diaminobenzidine (DAB) precipitation metallic ions and its application for double immunohistochemistry. *J. Histochem. Cytochem.*, **30**, 1079–82

22. Adams, J. C. (1981). Heavy metal intensification of DAB-based HRP reaction product. *J. Histochem. Cytochem.*, **29**, 775

23. Hsu, S. M., Raine, L. and Fanger, H. (1981). Use of avidin–biotin–peroxidase complex (ABC) in immunoperoxidase techniques: A comparison between ABC and unlabelled antibody (PAP) procedures. *J. Histochem. Cytochem.*, **29**, 577–80

24. Hoffman, K., Titus, G., Montibeller, J. A. and Finn, F. M. (1982). Avidin binding of carboxyl-substituted biotin and analogues. *Biochemistry*, **21**, 978–84

25. Bonnard, C., Papermaster, D. S. and Kraehenbuhl, J. P. (1984). The streptavidin–biotin bridge technique: Application in light and electron microscope immunocytochemistry. In Polak, J. M. and Varndell, I. M. (eds), *Immunolabelling for Electron Microscopy*, pp. 95–111. (Amsterdam: Elsevier Scientific)

26. Faulk, W. P. and Taylor, G. M. (1971). An immunocolloid method for the electron microscope. *Immunochemistry*, **8**, 1081–3

27. Danscher, G. (1981). Localisation of gold in biological tissue. A photochemical method for light and electron microscopy. *Histochemistry*, **71**, 81–8

28. Holgate, C. S., Jackson, P., Cowen, P. N. and Bird, C. C. (1983). Immunogold–silver staining: A new method of immunostaining with enhanced sensitivity. *J. Histochem. Cytochem.*, **31**, 938–44

29. Springall, D. R., Hacker, G. W., Grimelius, L. and Polak, J. (1984). The potential of the immunogold–silver staining method for paraffin sections. *Histochemistry*, **81**, 603–8

30. Burns, J. (1975). An appraisal of immunocytochemical methods in routine histology. *Proc. R. Microsc. Soc.* **10**, 97

31. Straus, W. (1976). Use of peroxidase inhibitors for immunoperoxidase procedures. In Felman, (ed.) *International Symposium on Immunoenzymatic Techniques*. INSERM Symposium No. 2, pp. 117–124

32. Heyderman, E. (1979). Immunopathology technique in histopathology: Applications, methods and controls. *J. Clin. Pathol.*, **2**, 971–8

33. Streefkerk, J. G. (1972). Inhibition of erythrocyte pseudoperoxidase activity by treatment with hydrogen peroxide following methanol. *J. Histochem. Cytochem.*, **20**, 829–31

34. Brooks, D. A., Zola, H., McNamara, P. J., Bradley, J., Bradstock, K. F., Hancock, W. W. and Atkins, R. C. (1983). Membrane antigens of human cells of the monocyte/macrophage lineage studied with monoclonal antibodies. *Pathology*, **15**, 45–52

35. Ponder, B. A. and Wilkinson, M. M. (1981). Inhibition of endogenous tissue alkaline phosphatase with use of alkaline phosphatase conjugates in immunocytochemistry. *J. Histochem. Cytochem.*, **29**, 981–4

36. Graham, R. C. Jr. and Karnovsky, M. J. (1966). The early stages of absorption of injected horseradish peroxidase in the proximal tubules of mouse kidney: Ultrastructural cytochemistry by a new technique. *J. Histochem. Cytochem.*, **14**, 291–302

37. Graham, R. C. Jr., Ludholm, U. and Karnovsky, M. J. (1965). Cytochemical demonstration of peroxidase activity with 3-amino-9-ethylcarbozole. *J. Histochem. Cytochem.*, **13**, 150–2

38. Hanker, J. S., Yates, P. E., Metz, C. B. and Rustioni, A. (1977). A new specific, sensitive and non-carcinogenic reagent for the demonstration of horseradish peroxidase. *Histochem. J.*, **9**, 789–92

39. Bancroft, J. D. and Stevens, A. (1982). *Theory and Practice of Histological Techniques*. 2nd Edn, pp. 381–384. (London: Churchill Livingstone)

40. Mason, D. Y., Sammons, R. E. (1978). Alkaline phosphatase and peroxidase for double immunoenzymatic labelling of cellular constituents. *J. Clin. Pathol.*, **31**, 454–62

41. Isaacson, P. G. and Wright, D. H. (1986). In Polak, J. M. and van Noorden, S. (eds) *Immunocytochemistry Modern Methods and Applications*. 2nd Edn. (Bristol: Wright)

42. Lillie, R. D. (1965). *Histopathologic Technique and Practical Histochemistry*. (London: MacGraw-Hill)

43. Bancroft, J. D. (1967). *An Introduction to Histochemical Technique*. Chapter 5, pp. 54–59. (London: Butterworths)

44. Garvin, A. J., Spicer, S. S., Parmley, R. T. and Munster, A. M. (1974). Immunohistochemical demonstration of IgG in Reed–Sternbert and other cells in Hodgkin's disease. *J. Exp. Med.*, **139**, 1077–83

45. Nakane, P. K. (1975). Recent progress in the peroxidase labelled antibody method. *Ann. NY Acad. Sci.*, **254**, 203–11

46. Curran, R. C. and Gregory, J. (1980). Effects of fixation and processing on immunohistochemical demonstration of immunoglobulin in paraffin sections of tonsil and bone marrow. *J. Clin. Pathol.*, **33**, 1047–57

47. Mepham, B. L. (1982). Influence of fixatives on the immunoreactivity of paraffin sections. *Histochem. J.*, **14**, 731–7

48. Epenetos, A. A., Bobrow, L. G., Adams, T. E., Collins, C. M., Isaacson, P. G. and Bodmer, W. F. (1985). A monoclonal antibody that detects HLA-D region antigen in routinely fixed,

wax embedded sections of normal and neoplastic lymphoid tissues. *J. Clin. Pathol.*, **38**, 12–17

49. Mitchell, D., Salih Ibrahim and Gusterson, B. A. (1985). Improved immunohistochemical localization of tissue antigens using modified methacarn fixation. *J. Histochem. Cytochem.*, **33**, 491–5

50. Puchtler, H., Sweat Waldrop, F., Meloan, S. N., Terry, M. S. and Conner, H. M. (1970). Methacarn (Methanol-Carnoy) fixation. Practical and theoretical considerations. *Histochemie*, **21**, 97–116

51. Baker, J. R. (1963). In *Principles of Biological Microtechnique*. (London: Methuen)

52. van Noorden, S. (1986). Tissue preparation and immunostaining techniques for light microscopy. In Polak, J. M. and van Noorden, S. (eds) *Immunohistochemistry: Modern Methods and Applications*. 2nd Edn. (Bristol: Wright)

53. Reading, M. (1977). A digestion technique for reduction of background staining in the immunoperoxidase method. *J. Clin. Pathol.*, **30**, 88–90

54. Mepham, B. L., Frater, W. and Mitchell, B. S. (1979). The use of proteolytic enzymes to improve immunoglobulin staining by the PAP technique. *Histochem. J.* **11**, 345–57

55. Stein, H., Bonk, A., Tolksdorf, G., Lennert, K., Rodt, H. and Gerdes, J. (1980). Immunohistologic analysis of the organisation of normal lymphoid tissue and non-Hodgkin's lymphomas. *J. Histochem. Cytochem.*, **28**, 746–60

56. Warford, A. and Ketchin, G. S. (1986). The effect of fixation upon monoclonal cryostat immunohistochemistry. *Med. Lab. Sci.*, **43**, 128–34

Index